MATERNAL MEASURES:
FIGURING CAREGIVING IN THE EARLY MODERN PERIOD

To those dear "others" who helped us to become "mothers":
Hugh Miller and Ray Shattenkirk; and to our children,
who teach us what it means to be mothers every day:
Fiona, Isaiah, Damaris and Elias Miller,
and Shoshana, Raphael, Isabella and Lily Shattenkirk.

Maternal Measures

Figuring caregiving in the early modern period

Edited by

Naomi J. Miller and Naomi Yavneh

Ashgate

Aldershot • Burlington USA • Singapore • Sydney

Published by
Ashgate Publishing Limited
Gower House
Croft Road
Aldershot
Hants GU11 3HR
England

Ashgate Publishing Company
131 Main Street
Burlington
Vermont 05401-5600
USA

Ashgate website: http://www.ashgate.com

British Library Cataloguing-in-Publication data

Maternal measures: figuring caregiving in the early modern period. – (Women and gender in the early modern world)
    1. Motherhood in literature   2. Caregivers in literature   3. Literature and society – History   4. Literature, Modern – 15th and 16th centuries – History and criticism
    I. Miller, Naomi   II. Yavneh, Naomi
    809.9'3353'0903

Library of Congress Cataloging-in-Publication data

Maternal measures: figuring caregiving in the early modern period / edited by Naomi J. Miller and Naomi Yavneh.
        p.   cm. (Women and gender in the early modern world)
    Includes index.
    1. Motherhood – History.   2. Mothers – History.   3. Caregivers – History.
    I. Miller, Naomi.   II. Yavneh, Naomi.   III. Series
    HQ759 M3733 2000
    306.874'3'09—dc21   99-055005
                                                                                                                    CIP

ISBN 0 7546 0031 9

Printed on acid-free paper and bound in Great Britain by
MPG Books Ltd, Bodmin, Cornwall

Contents

PART V   MORTALITY

Acknowledgements

Our collaboration as editors has been a true gestation of spirit, mind, and heart, resulting in this collection of essays that speaks to the issues of "mothers and others" in the early modern world as well as our own. We ourselves met when we were looking at the same book at an MLA book exhibit in Chicago in December 1990, and realized that we shared the same first name, and the same interests, and even the same alma mater of Princeton from undergraduate days. We also shared our experience as young mothers, leading to our first collaboration, the following December 1991, in an MLA session entitled 'This Self Which Is Not One: Childbearing, Childrearing, and the Profession'.

Further MLA sessions followed, as well as professional collaboration in Renaissance Society of America conferences and the marvelous Attending to Early Modern Women conferences every three years at the University of Maryland, College Park, where we first sketched out our hopes and ideas for this collection of essays on mothers and others, that has come to be titled "Maternal Measures", and has found a home with the Ashgate Publishing series on Women and Gender in the Early Modern World. In the meantime, children followed as well, so that our collaboration as co-editors [known to our contributors as 'the Naomis'] has also been marked by our shared experience of each giving birth to four children before receiving tenure. Thus, the dedication to this volume …

We should like to thank many individuals who have contributed to the labor and delivery of this special volume of essays, not the least our outstanding contributors, who have seen the volume through many stages, and whose essays speak for themselves. We should like to give particular thanks and gratitude to Betty Travitsky and Patrick Cullen, whose instructive comments and patient encouragement and advice have brought the volume to full term. Thank you, Betty and Patrick, for your caregiving in the truest sense.

We should also like to thank Erika Gaffney, Ashgate Publishing, for being editor, friend, and colleague all in one. The fact that our work on this volume brought us into contact with Erika has been one of many unexpected blessings for which we give thanks. We are grateful, too, for the help and guidance of Ellen Keeling, senior editor, Ashgate Publishing, and look forward to meeting her some day. And we should like to express our appreciation to Rachel Lynch, the original commissioning editor at Ashgate who welcomed our volume.

We appreciate the comments and encouragements of many fellow scholars along the way, including Elaine Beilin, Heather Dubrow, Valeria Finucci, Margaret Hannay, Barbara Lewalski, Margaret Rosenthal and Walter Stephens.

We learned a great deal from the readers' comments on the volume as well, and have been fortunate to have the opportunity to revise and reshape the volume in accord with the many suggestions we received.

We leave the volume, now, to the care of our current series editors, Allyson Poska and Abby Zanger, with whom we are happy to be working.

Naomi Miller wishes to thank, first, her own mother Dr. Nobuko Ishii, who has so often lit the way ahead, as teacher and scholar as well as mother. Next, she wishes to thank her unflappable friends and fellow scholars in early modern studies, whose humor and wisdom have assisted her not only in her work on this volume, but in many other endeavors: Emily Bartels, Carol Ann Johnston, Laura Lunger Knoppers, and, particularly, Mary Thomas Crane, with whom she first shared the experience of motherhood, then, and now, and always. Throughout the experience of working on this volume, Naomi Miller has been supremely grateful for the presence of Naomi Yavneh: friend, confidante, co-editor, and other mother for all seasons.

From the University of Arizona, a Small Grants Award and a Humanities Research Initiative Grant supported the necessary archival research that has provided the basis for Naomi Miller's work on this volume, as well as on other research projects on maternity in early modern England.

Finally, Naomi Miller thanks her husband, Hugh, and her children, Fiona, Isaiah, Damaris, and Elias, for bringing joy, challenge, and wonder in contrapuntal harmony to each day of her life.

Naomi Yavneh would like to thank Deborah Steinberger, Susan Overton, Giovanna Benadusi, Fraser Ottanelli, Silvio Gaggi, Daniel Belgrad, Ruth Banes, Priscilla Brewer, Jim D'Emilio, Paula Lee. She also appreciates the help of Nancy Baisden, Aline Wilson and Hopeanne Pendelton, and of her students, especially Dorothy Brockman, Claudia Conti and Aristoula Mandelos.

A Dean's Development Grant from the College of Arts and Sciences at the University of South Florida supported the research for Naomi Yavneh's portion of the volume.

Finally, she would like to thank the matriarchs of her family: Anne Marcus and Anna Yavneh, Kuni Yavneh, Tenli Yavneh, Nina Steinberg and Lee Shattenkirk; her dear friend Naomi Miller (the Other Naomi and the first to b4); her husband, Ray Shattenkirk; and, most of all, her children – Shoshana, Raphael, Isabella Hannalee and Lily Ariana – who fill her life with joy, music and excitement.

List of Figures

Notes on Contributors

Linda Phyllis Austern is Associate Professor of Music History at Northwestern University. She has published widely on early modern music, gender and culture, particularly in sixteenth- and seventeenth-century England.

Emilie L. Bergmann is Professor of Spanish at the University of California, Berkeley. She is a co-author of *Women, Culture and Politics in Latin America* (California, 1990) and co-editor of *"Entiendes": Queer Readings, Hispanic Writings* (Duke University Press, 1995), and has published on sixteenth- and seventeenth-century Spanish literature, representations of the maternal in early modern Spanish and colonial Latin American culture, the poetry of Sor Juana Inés de la Cruz, and twentieth-century Spanish women writers.

Caroline Bicks is Assistant Professor of English at The Ohio State University. She has published essays on the Anglican churching ritual, Diana at Ephesus, and childbirth communities. She is currently working on a book-length study of the early modern midwife as original narrator of England's genealogical and gynecological tales.

Mary Thomas Crane is Associate Professor of English at Boston College. She is the author of *Framing Authority: Sayings, Self, and Society in Sixteenth-Century England* (Princeton University Press, 1993) and of *Shakespeare's Brain: Reading with Cognitive Theory* (forthcoming from Princeton in 2000).

Frances E. Dolan is Professor of English, and an Affiliate of the History Department and the Women's Studies Program, at Miami University in Ohio. She is the author of *Dangerous Familiars: Representations of Domestic Crime in England, 1550–1700* (Cornell University Press, 1994) and *Whores of Babylon: Catholicism, Gender, and Seventeenth-Century Print Culture* (Cornell University Press, 1999), from which her contribution to this volume has been reprinted.

Heather Dubrow, Tighe-Evans Professor and John Bascom Professor at the University of Wisconsin-Madison, is the author of five books, most recently *Shakespeare and Domestic Loss* (Cambridge, 1999). Her other publications include a co-edited collection, numerous articles on teaching and early modern literature, and two chapbooks of poetry.

Glenn Ehrstine is Assistant Professor of German at the University of Iowa. His study "Theater, Culture, and Community in Reformation Bern, 1523–1555" is forthcoming from E.J. Brill in 2001.

Claire Fontijn is Assistant Professor of Music at Wellesley College, where she teaches Music History and directs the Collegium Musicum. Her previous publications on Baroque music include articles on flute-playing techniques as well as on women musicians. She is currently completing her first book, for Oxford University Press, entitled *Desperate Measures: The Life and Music of Antonia Padoani Bembo (c. 1640–c. 1720)*.

Susan Frye is Associate Professor of English and Women's Studies at the University of Wyoming. The author of *Elizabeth I: The Competition for Representation* (Oxford University Press, 1993; 1997) and co-editor with Karen Robertson of *Maids and Mistresses, Cousins and Queens: Women's Alliances in Early Modern England* (OUP 1999), she has published on Spenser, Shakespeare, and early modern women.

Nancy Hayes teaches English at St. Ambrose University in Davenport, Iowa, her hometown. She has degrees in English from Smith College and the University of Connecticut, an MFA in Literary Translation (medieval German love songs) and a Ph.D. in Comparative Literature from the University of Iowa.

Kari Boyd McBride teaches in the Women's Studies Department at the University of Arizona. Articles forthcoming in 2000 include "Gender and Judaism in Meditations on the Passion: Middleton, Southwell, Lanyer, and Fletcher" in *Discovering and Recovering the Seventeenth-Century Religious Lyric*, ed. Eugene Cunnar and Jeffrey Johnson (from Duquesne). She maintains an online bibliography on Aemilia Lanyer and is writing on country house discourse in early modern England.

Naomi J. Miller is Associate Professor of English Literature and Women's Studies at the University of Arizona. Her publications on early modern women writers and gender include a book-length study of Lady Mary Wroth, entitled *Changing the Subject: Mary Wroth and Figurations of Gender in Early Modern England* (University Press of Kentucky, 1996), a collection of essays on Wroth, co-edited with Gary Waller, entitled *Reading Mary Wroth: Representing Alternatives in Early Modern England* (University of Tennessee Press, 1990), and various essays on Shakespeare, Elizabeth Cary, and Aemilia Lanyer, as well as renaissance mothers' advice books and polemical pamphlets. She is currently working on a book-length study of early modern constructions of maternity.

Patricia Phillippy is Associate Professor of English and Coordinator of Comparative Literature at Texas A&M University. She is the author of *Love's

Remedies: Recantation and Renaissance Lyric Poetry (1995), and numerous articles on early modern women writers. Her chapter in this volume is part of a book in progress, *The Sisters of Magdalene: Women, Death and Mourning in Post-Reformation England*, which examines material and representational aspects of women's works of mourning in the period.

Judith Rose is Assistant Professor of English and Women's Studies at Allegheny College in Pennsylvania. A poet and fiction writer as well as an academic, she has published in *The Iowa Review, Prairie Schooner, The Virginia Quarterly*, and other journals. The chapter included here will also appear in a book-in-progress, *"The First Fruits of a Woman's Wit": Reappropriation of the Metaphor of Conception by Early Modern Women*

Kathryn Schwarz is Assistant Professor of English at Vanderbilt University. She has published several essays on representations of female martiality in the early modern period, and is the author of a book, *Tough Love: Amazon Encounters in the English Renaissance*, forthcoming from Duke University Press.

Edith Snook is a doctoral candidate at the University of Western Ontario in London, Ontario. She is completing her dissertation on representations of reading and metaphors of vision in early modern women's writing.

Susan C. Staub is a Professor of English at Appalachian State University. She has published articles on various aspects of Renaissance prose and poetry and has recently completed a book-length manuscript entitled *Nature's Cruel Step-Dames: Representations of Early Modern Women and Domestic Violence in the Street Literature of Seventeenth-Century England*. Her current research focuses on motherhood in early modern England.

Deborah Steinberger is Assistant Professor of French and Comparative Literature at the University of Delaware. Her research areas include seventeenth-century theater and writing by women of the early modern period. She has published articles on the theater of Molière, Donneau de Visé, Destouches and Nivelle de la Chaussée, and on the works of Françoise Pascal. Her critical edition of Françoise Pascal's epistolary collection *Le Commerce du Parnasse (1669)* is forthcoming.

Rachel Trubowitz is Associate Professor of English at the University of New Hampshire, Durham. She has published essays on a variety of topics in early modern English literature, most recently "'Nourish Milke': Breast-Feeding and the Crisis of Englishness, 1600-60" in *Journal of English and Germanic Philology*, 99.1 (2000), 29–49. Her book-in-progress is on nursing and nation-building in seventeenth-century England.

Naomi Yavneh is Associate Professor of Renaissance Culture in the department of Humanities and American Studies at the University of South Florida. The author of numerous articles on reproduction and breastfeeding in the early modern period, as well as on Italian literature, gender and spirituality, she is currently completing a book, *The Body of the Virgin*.

Mothering Others:
Caregiving as Spectrum and Spectacle in the Early Modern Period

Naomi J. Miller

During the early modern period, maternity was constantly evaluated, conceptualized and redefined, from a range of social and artistic perspectives, even as maternal practices shaped standards of care. The spectrum of early modern maternal roles and responsibilities extended well beyond actual mothers to the many female caregivers who participated and assisted in childbirth and lactation, nurtured and instructed their own and others' offspring with advice, managed the domestic production of their own and others' households, wrote polemics, ruled courts, and administered the final stages of care in illness and death. The participation of female caregivers in all areas of early modern life offered not only a spectrum of care from birth to death, but also a spectacle of caregiving powers, potentially life-threatening as well as life-giving, that were scrutinized, idealized, criticized, and represented in a range of social and literary texts as well as visual works of art and musical compositions.

The spectrum, and spectacle, of maternity in particular and of female caregivers at large in the early modern period, is the subject of the essays in this volume. Exploring such figures as mothers and stepmothers, midwives and wet nurses, wise women and witches, saints and amazons, murderers and nurturers, the contributors to the present volume examine a striking range of positive and negative constructions of female caregiving in the sixteenth and seventeenth centuries (with individual examples dated as early as 1340 and as late as 1812), in countries that include England, Italy, Spain, France, Germany, Latin America, Mexico, and the New World. Linking the disciplines of literature, social history, music history, and art history, and attending to differences of gender, class, and race, this volume highlights a spectacular spectrum of early modern women caregivers, from prototypes to antitypes.

Recent multidisciplinary volumes of essays in the field of early modern gender studies have posed important questions regarding the variations among different disciplinary approaches. James Grantham Turner, for example, introduces his collection of essays on sexuality and gender in early modern Europe by drawing connections among historians of society, literature, and art, and by calling attention to the concomitant challenge and advantage of establishing moments of common ground among literary characters, visual images, and "real" individuals, as well as among the different national cultures of Europe.[1] In her essay collection on Renaissance culture and the everyday, Patricia Fumerton identifies a "new social historicism of the everyday," which juxtaposes material details and conceptualizations of everyday life, attending not only to factual historical data, but also to collective meanings, values, representations, and practices.[2] Similarly, Susan Frye and Karen Robertson's recent collection of essays on women's alliances in early modern England brings together a variety of literary and historic texts, examining material culture and social practice.[3]

In the present volume on early modern caregivers, the methods and materials of several disciplines appear not simply in alternating essays, but at times in the same essay, resulting in a conjunction of different disciplines and cultures that serves to revise and deepen our understanding of maternal measures both within and beyond traditional cultural and disciplinary boundaries. It is important to point out that the focus of this multidisciplinary volume on representations of maternity and female caregiving in the early modern period at once arises from and builds upon the extraordinary work of social historians over the past two decades, whose detailed archival investigations and transformative visions of the nature of history itself have reshaped our understanding of gender and culture in early modern society. As Merry Wiesner observes in her landmark study of women and gender in early modern Europe, scholars working in women's history have had to search for new sources to reveal the experiences of women and have used traditional sources in innovative ways, drawing upon sociology, anthropology, art history and literary studies for theories and methodology.[4] Sara Mendelson and Patricia Crawford note in their extensive survey of women in early modern England that "women are everywhere and nowhere in the archives," impelling historians to reconstruct evidence of women's lives from a wide range of indirect source material, including literary and visual representations, and necessitating techniques of "reading against the grain, of asking where women are absent as well as present in the documents."[5] The roster of social historians of gender in early modern Europe who offer an array of historical data accompanied by analyses of their own methodologies and usage of sources, and whose work contains detailed discussions of women's experiences as mothers, includes Olwen Hufton, Anthony Fletcher, Susan Dwyer Amussen, and Christiane

Klapisch-Zuber, to note only a few.[6] Standing out as a particularly important predecessor to the present volume, among a number of valuable essay collections on topics related to women and gender in the early modern period, is Valerie Fildes's *Women as Mothers in Pre-Industrial England*, which gathered together an illuminating group of essays on social constructions of maternity that provided a starting point for further interpretive analyses of maternity in a variety of disciplines.[7]

Mendelson and Crawford, Wiesner, and many of the other historians cited above discuss how research by social historians has expanded to include the use of sources such as literary texts and visual images. So, too, the literary, musical, and art historians included in the present volume draw upon historical data and social texts to inform their analyses of early modern conceptualizations and practices of caregiving and maternity. At the same time, while historical studies of maternity have tended to present women's experiences primarily in terms of the female life-cycle denoted by the familial roles of maid, wife and widow, the multidisciplinary essays in the present volume explore a wider variety of female caregiving roles, extending from birth to death within overlapping arenas of health, education, labor, religion, and politics, as well as the family.

What gave early modern women caregivers some measure of power to shape the very societies that worked to delimit and define their roles, both within and outside the home? One answer lies in the often strikingly malleable boundaries of those social roles for women: not only as mothers and daughters, wives and widows, but also as educators and advice-givers, role models and friends.[8] The wide range of writings by and about early modern women that address social issues and experiences offers contemporary scholars the opportunity to identify interconnected realms of social existence, and to consider the flexible operation in practice of theoretical social boundaries. On the one hand, representations of women by men, whether in texts or images, at once reflected and dominated many of the gendered assumptions of the society at large. On the other hand, across a spectrum of differences in class and culture and medium, women's voices extended from intimate musings in letters and diaries to assertive and even polemical engagements, not only with skeptical male onlookers, but also with a mixed audience of other women. Whether confronting social and political customs at large, or charting a passage through life-cycles at home, from birth, childrearing, education, and household management to death, early modern women worked to define roles for themselves that tested the assumptions and sometimes reformed the practices of the societies in which they lived.

Not surprisingly, early modern women were often identified and represented, both by themselves and by men, in terms of their caregiving functions. Within the family, the roles of mothers, grandmothers, stepmothers, and mothers-in-law, as well as daughters, wives, and widows, provided women with opportunities for authority as well as service, and for instruction as well as training. At the same time, an increasing range of caregiving roles *outside* the family placed women in positions of nurture, instruction, and even power in a variety of social settings. Women who served as midwives, wetnurses and family nurses were respected in many cases, and yet denigrated in others, when their influence and knowledge came to be perceived as a threat to existing structures of authority.[9] In instances where women served as tutors or educators in upper class families, or even as teachers through the venue of middle class mothers' advice books, both the range of their influence and the perceived challenge to more traditional sources of authority was heightened.[10] The very issue of education for women was marked by vehement debates, with variations across class lines, in which advocates of early modern women's learning, particularly women, faced opposition and hostility, and yet managed to both attain and transmit literacy in a striking range of circumstances.[11] In the case of wise women or witches, notions of sustenance and destruction were linked in ways that made explicit the implicit links between forces of nurture and rejection already associated with women in general.[12]

When scrutinizing measures of maternity, it is useful to juxtapose representations of actual and mythic mothers in different mediums of representation and different countries, in order to attend to some of the cultural undercurrents, encompassing both norms and aberrations, that shaped the spectacle as well as the spectrum of early modern women caregivers. Maternity itself was both a physical and social construct in the early modern period. The physicality of the woman's body was measured quite frequently in terms of maternal functions and responsibilities that received varying emphases across classes and cultures, raising questions as to when and how the breast and the womb serve as signs signifying "woman."[13]

A female organ associated at once with sexuality and maternity, the breast often functioned as a site for the sexual definition of women. Mythic representations of the breast as a symbol of femininity in the early modern period ranged from Greek legends of Amazons, described as female warriors who burned off their right breasts in order to enhance their ability to draw their bows and who destroyed or sent away their male children, to the figure of the Virgin Mary, whose breast milk served as an image of infinitely divisible grace. Representations of women's breasts in literature and the visual arts frequently alluded to metonymic images, such as lilies, ivory, and snow, which eroticized the breast as an object of masculine desire while divorcing it from connotations of unstable flow and change.[14]

In social texts, women's breasts were constructed in both maternal and erotic terms, sometimes conflating their significance as symbols of caregiving nurturance with their function as sexual spectacle. In early modern Europe, breast milk was believed to be a purified form of menstrual blood, which changed color as it passed back and forth between the breast and the womb, bearing witness to the fluid materiality of women's bodies and their reproductive function.[15] In the same period, the breast was subject to newly eroticized interest and signification, accompanied by increased exposure and decoration of women's breasts in clothing fashions.[16] Attesting to a different set of issues, treatises on breastfeeding which proliferated in a number of early modern countries conveyed class tensions associated with the use of the breast. Although the hiring of lower class women as wet nurses for infants from upper class families had a long and established history, it gradually became an increasingly controversial practice, due to perceived associations between the quality of breast milk and maternal social status.[17]

The uterus was another female organ that came to be associated both with powers of femininity in physical reproduction, and with apparently female weaknesses such as fluidity and instability, through its link with the physical flows of blood in menstruation and childbirth and through historical associations connecting disorders such as hysteria with a "wandering womb." In the Hippocratic writings that influenced medical practices in the early modern period, certain behavioral disorders were given the name "hysteria," from *hystera*, the Greek word for womb, and treatments were prescribed in order to induce the uterus to move downward to its proper position.[18] Plato and Aristotle described the womb as an animal within an animal, with its own consciousness, capable of moving around within the lower part of the body and upsetting the bodily economy with its disturbed state.[19] Such conceptions supported stereotypes of feminine error and changeability. In midwifery manuals of sixteenth-century England, the womb was represented as so greedy for male seed that it could descend to snatch and suck semen, indicating the unsettling power of female sexual desire.[20]

In the early modern period, both breast and uterus represented life-giving nurturance and reproduction as well as the potential disruption of patriarchal order. Beyond the purview of masculine control or regulation, the female reproductive organs could serve simultaneously to validate women's caregiving roles and to undermine male social authority. When mothers and other female caregivers claimed positions for themselves as generators of their own words and images, issues of authority and authorship collided.[21]

Among many examples of male-authored treatises on maternity, Jacques Guillemeau's influential treatises on childbirth and nursing in seventeenth-century France, later translated and widely circulated in England, focus on women's functions as caregivers.[22] Guillemeau includes explicit descriptions, in some cases illustrated by woodcuts, of women's sexual organs, while addressing the issue of female sexuality seemingly only in terms of medical concerns regarding pregnancy, labor, and delivery. Although Guillemeau's nursing text opens with a straightforward recommendation that mothers nurse their own children, substantial space is devoted to discussion of the size, shape and color of suitable breasts for nursing when wet-nurses must be selected. By contrast, in seventeenth-century England, Elizabeth Clinton offers an explicitly maternal perspective on the same issue in a treatise addressed to her daughter-in-law, in which she urges mothers to nurse their own children for reasons of spiritual as well as physical nourishment – without concomitant attention to breast size and nipple shape.[23] Female caregiving in Elizabeth Clinton's text, whether through breast milk or words of wisdom, is valued for its powerful shaping force rather than purely for the physicality of the originary female body.

"Therefore let no man blame a mother, though she something exceed in writing to her children," declares Dorothy Leigh in England in 1616, "since every man knows that the love of a mother to her children is hardly contained within the bounds of reason." Explaining the significance of her task, Leigh adds: "my mind will continue long after me in writing."[24] Expressing maternity, for Dorothy Leigh, signifies writing to excess, beyond the bounds of reason and concomitantly "hardly contained" within the boundaries of generic constraints. In fact, early modern women's varying expressions of maternity not only could not be contained within traditional generic boundaries, but also served to extend the boundaries of their caregiving roles in other capacities.

Dorothy Leigh focuses specifically upon the authority of maternal expression in writing, explaining in her dedicatory preface to her children that she could conceive of no better way of directing them than "to write them the right way."[25] While acknowledging that writing is considered "a thing so unusual" among women, Leigh locates the origins of her authorship in her "motherly affection," and asserts the authority of her words over her sons. Moreover, Leigh's claim that her mind will "continue long after me in writing" maintains the lasting power of her maternal expression. At several moments, expanding the generic boundaries of her maternal advice text, Leigh even links the authority of her written words with the text of the Bible, which her sons may learn to read "in their own mother tongue," under the direction of her "many words," so that they may gather food for the soul "out of the word as the children of Israel gathered manna in the wilderness."[26] While Leigh takes care never to substitute the authority of her text for that of the Bible, the conflation of her maternal words with the "mother tongue" of the Bible suggests her power as a mother to provide verbal and spiritual nourishment for her children.

In a variety of early modern texts and images associated with female caregivers, mothers and others offer the potential for both nurture and rejection, sustenance and destruction. Maternity was associated with a doubleness of identity that only partially coincides with the doubleness commonly associated with feminity at the time. Whereas women in general might be directed to be chaste, silent, and obedient in order to counteract the perceived power of their sexuality, mothers in particular emerged as figures who combined the sexuality required for procreation and reproduction with considerable authority over their offspring, male as well as female. In the popular genre of mothers' advice books, authored by figures such as Dorothy Leigh, early modern women emphasized the dignity and strength that they brought to their roles as caregivers, allowing them to direct their children in particular, and their households in general, with confidence.

Authority inextricably linked with female sexuality: a powerful combination in a period that exhibited marked anxieties over the positions of women. Mothers and other female caregivers appear as both objects and agents of sacrifice in early modern texts and images, sometimes represented as madonna and monster at once. Early modern pamphlets that eulogized or condemned individual women construct maternity in particular with heightened metaphors, repeatedly locating a starting point for description in excess. In the case of Margaret Vincent, a woman who murdered two of her children in the belief that she could save their souls, since she was being forced by her husband to raise them as Protestants despite her own conversion to Catholicism, a condemnatory pamphlet entitled *A pitiless Mother* (1616) attacks her as "Tigerous" and "wolfish" for her "unnaturall" violation of the dictates of maternity.[27]

In Vincent's case, early modern codes of maternity provide the standard of measure for condemning a woman "who by nature should have cherished [her children] with her own body, as the Pelican that pecks her own breast to feed her young ones with her blood," and instead behaves more monstrously than "the Viper, the envenomed Serpent, the Snake, or any Beast whatsoever," in taking her children's blood, "nay, her own dear blood bred in her own body, cherished in her own womb."[28] Embedded in the narration of the pamphlet on Vincent is the implication that this tragedy resulted from a woman's misguided attempt to oppose an incipient and subversive maternal authority to her husband's rule. The unsettling spectacle of Margaret Vincent bears witness to the fact that maternal care, at once contested and contestatory, potentially monstrous and self-sacrificial, was an issue not simply of physical reproduction, but of domestic power as well.

While Dorothy Leigh and Margaret Vincent serve to mark opposite ends of the spectrum of maternal caregiving in early seventeenth-century England, the historical circumstances of mothers and other caregivers differed considerably, not only in different countries and centuries within the early modern time period, but also across class lines, with the voices of poorer or working mothers less directly represented in many written sources.[29] Moreover, patterns of child care in particular encompassed a range of practices and behaviors beyond the explicitly instructive framework offered by many mothers' advice books, as has been well-documented by social historians of childhood.[30] Nevertheless, caregivers were often represented and judged, celebrated or condemned, in terms of maternal measures, precisely because the spectacle of maternity offered a spectrum of female practices against which to measure the acceptable or disturbing extent of early modern women's caregiving powers.

* * *

The essays in the present volume span the disciplines of literature, music, and art history and explore a spectrum of caregiving roles and practices in Europe and the New World. The essays are grouped topically into five sections that reflect the variety of circumstances of caregiving as well as measures of maternity in the early modern period: conception and lactation, nurture and instruction, domestic production, social authority, and mortality. Each group of essays sheds light upon some of the opportunities and restrictions that marked early modern women's caregiving roles, and draws individual disciplinary and geographical views into complementary juxtaposition. Addressing both verbal and visual spectacles, social and musical "measures," and often covering overlapping topics and issues, the essays offer an interconnected series of perspectives on early modern caregivers, caretakers, and care itself.

Conception, Childbirth and Lactation

The labor of women attends the very beginnings of life, from childbirth to the nursing of newborns. The processes of conception and birth, as well as the caregiving associated with labor, delivery, and lactation, were very much the province of women in the early modern period. Indeed, while most of the published writings concerning childbirth were authored by men, women's practical influence in the birthing room remained significant throughout much of the fifteenth, sixteenth and seventeenth centuries.[31] The immense significance of childbirth and nursing in figurative as well as literal terms surfaces repeatedly in a wide variety of countries and mediums throughout the early modern period, revealing some striking preoccupations with the powers of mothers and others that intertwine issues of class and race as well as gender.

Focusing on the very concept of conception, Judith Rose explores the ways in which early modern women artists manipulated "conceptual paradigms" in both verbal and visual mediums, in order to realign the relationship between maternity and artistic procreativity. In "Mirrors of Language, Mirrors of Self: The Conceptualization of Artistic Identity in Gaspara Stampa and Sofonisba Anguissola," Rose investigates the relationship between Aristotelian paradigms of conception and the sixteenth-century genesis of Stampa's *nove stile* and Anguissola's self-portraits. Rose finds that both women located in the maternity of the Virgin Mary a conceptual point of origin for their own positions as female artists. Demonstrating how Stampa differentiates her position from that of Petrarch by representing herself as the terrestrial reflection of the Virgin, while Anguissola constructs a gallery of mirrors that link her self-portraits with her paintings of the Madonna and child, Rose locates in the spectacle of holy maternity an enabling conception of procreativity for early modern women.

Moving from conception to birth, Caroline Bicks focuses her attention upon early modern preoccupations with the caregiving authority of midwives. In "Midwiving Virility in Early Modern England," Bicks argues that the material connections among the tongue, the genitals, the umbilical cord and the hand of the midwife were inflected by larger cultural concerns about female power over the virility of the early modern male subject. Examining treatises such as *The Byrth of Mankynde* (1540), Jacques Guillemeau's *Childe-birth, or the Happy Deliverie of Women* (1612), Nicholas Culpeper's *A Directory for Midwives* (1651), and William Sermon's *The Ladies Companion, or the English Midwife* (1671), Bicks demonstrates how these texts construct female speech so as to negotiate the authors' unease with both the birthing community and the power of the midwives over the bodies of newborn males. By contrast, in the first English, female-authored midwifery handbook for women in England, *The Midwives Book* (1671), Jane Sharp reminds midwives of the need for caution, while recognizing their potential to enslave and effeminize England's virile members.

Naomi Yavneh's essay shifts the focus of the section from conception and childbirth to lactation. In "To Bare or Not Too Bare: Sofonisba Anguissola's Nursing Madonna and the Womanly Art of Breastfeeding," Yavneh compares Anguissola's realistically depicted *Madonna che alatta il bambino* (1588) with Ambrogio Lorenzetti's *Madonna del latte* (1340) in particular, and with early Renaissance *Madonna lactans* in general, questioning why this almost uniquely naturalistic representation of a breastfeeding Virgin painted by a major woman artist appears at a time when the *Madonna lactans* had largely fallen out of favor as a subject. Examining post-Tridentine treatises on both images and Mary, treatises on beauty and the nature of women, and medical tractates on breastfeeding, Yavneh concludes that Anguissola's painting not only evokes the ideas of religious reformers such as Cardinal Paleotti and Filippo Neri, but draws a parallel as well between the shaping qualities of mother's milk and the power of the female artist.

Rachel Trubowitz's essay "'But Blood Whitened': Nursing Mothers and Others in Early Modern Britain," closes the section with an interrogation of the celebration of maternal breastfeeding by such domestic guidebook writers as Jacques Guillemeau (*The Nursing of Children*, 1612), Robert Cleaver and John Dod (*A godly Form of Household Government*, 1614), and William Gouge (*Of Domesticall Duties*, 1621). Her essay further charts images of nursing motherhood and wet-nursing in early modern travel narratives which, like the domestic guidebooks, reveal a singular preoccupation with breast-milk, blood, and the racialized construction of English national identity. Trubowitz focuses upon texts that both assess and help to shape and stabilize the maternal body, the foreign body, and the body politic, in conditions of rapid social change and cultural chaos and fragmentation. Trubowitz demonstrates that the idealized images of nursing maternity enshrined by the domestic guidebooks, which construct fraught relations between lactating mothers and "others," both reflect and disseminate seemingly disparate cultural anxieties about race, Jews, wet-nurses, and the (in)coherence of English national identity – anxieties that are similarly conjoined in the works of travel writers such as Samuel Purchas (*Purchas His Pilgrimage*, 1626).

Nurture and Instruction

Early modern women themselves claimed the labor of childbirth and nursing as a justification for their continuing authority over their offspring in the form of maternal nurture and instruction. Mothers and others often chose to offer not only their bodies, but concomitantly their words, to provide their own and others' offspring with the nourishment of affection and instruction, from childhood to adulthood. Revealingly, mothers were often the figures most empowered, and even expected, to conjoin passion with instruction in the early modern period. By contrast to some masculine models of learning, in which instruction was divorced from the liabilities associated with maternal caregiving, other models, particularly those associated with maternal figures and voices, linked instruction with nurture.[32]

Emilie L. Bergmann draws attention to sixteenth-century Spanish and Latin American colonial didactic, fictional, and historical texts that construct the reproductive role of the feminine in an ideological context. In "Language and 'Mother's Milk': Maternal Roles and the Nurturing Body in Early Modern Spanish Texts," Bergmann analyses the disjunction between the proverbial commonplace ("language we drank in at our mothers' breasts") and humanistic representations of the maternal role. Bergmann finds that these texts implicitly separate the pregnant maternal body from the physical processes of nurturing through lactation, and cultural initiation through language acquisition. The essay contextualizes key texts by sixteenth-century didactic writers, including Juan Luis Vives and Fray Antonio de Guevara, as well as less well-known medical, theological and linguistic treatises, in light of the cultural discourses of empire represented by such works as Juan de Valdes' *Dialogo de la lengua* (c. 1535), the Inca Garcilaso's *Comentarios reales* (1609), and Cervantes's *El coloquio de los perros* (1613). Bergmann demonstrates the extent to which both

Valdes's and Garcilaso's use of the naturalizing metaphor of culture and language as "mother's milk" challenges the conceptual separation between maternal culture and patriarchal language.

Glenn Ehrstine's "Motherhood and Protestant Polemics: Stillbirth in Hans von Rüte's *Abgötterei* (1531)" addresses contrasting spectacles of femininity during the German Reformation, when idealized images of maternity served as one standard against which disorderly women were measured and found wanting. Hans von Rüte's carnival play, *Abgötterei*, transforms generic boundaries by bringing matters of maternity into a carnival context, juxtaposing licentious elements of pre-Lenten celebration with the plight of two childless women praying to Mary for luck in longed-for childbirth. Ehrstine demonstrates how Rüte coopts the socially sanctioned concerns of maternity in order to criticize the cult of saints in early modern Germany, while representing mothers themselves as both caregivers and unruly women in a carnivalesque display. Contextualizing his argument with reference to contemporary representations of maternity, Ehrstine suggests that the very appearance of two would-be mothers among the victims of ecclesiastical impiety in Rüte's play acknowledges the interests of female audience members, who were active in religious instruction as well as nurture.

In "The Virgin's Voice: Representations of Mary in Seventeenth-Century Song," Claire Fontijn attends to a striking and uncollected repertory of pieces depicting the occasions of Christ's birth and crucifixion that feature the Blessed Virgin Mary, who sings in a direct, first-person voice infused with character. The strong traditions of Marian devotion in southern Europe, particularly in seventeeth-century Italy, prompted songs in which Mary dramatizes her situation, such as lullabies around Christmastime sung by the young nursing mother, and laments for Holy Week and Easter sung by the weeping mother mourning the death of her son on the cross. The essay examines eight representative works, ranging from Tarquinio Merula's "Hor ch'e tempo di dormire" (*Curtio precipitato et altri Capricij*, 1638) and Antonia Bembo's "Per il Natale" (*Produzioni armoniche*, 1697–1701) to Claudio Monteverdi's "Pianto della Madona" (*Selva morale e spirituale*, 1641) and Francesco Capello's "Dic mihi, sacratissima virgo" (*Motetti a voce sola*, 1610), in which a soprano portraying the Virgin Mary interprets her maternal role through dramatic performance. Fontijn's analysis reveals the extent to which, in many of these cases, maternal nurture and instruction are magnified through the figure of the mother of the Lord.

Edith Snook's "'His open side our book': Meditation and Education in Elizabeth Grymeston's *Miscelanea Meditations Memoratives*" explores the strategies utilized by Grymeston in her posthumously published mothers' advice book (1604) that enabled her to present herself as both mother and educator. Elaborating upon the relevance of Grymeston's feminized educational approach to our understanding of the position of women in the history of education and of women's spirituality, the essay demonstrates how Grymeston uses her authority as a mother to instruct her son in a way that transforms both the mode and matter of his education, and thus provides a potentially disruptive moment in gendered social divisions, in religious hierarchies, and as a consequence, in disciplined ideas about gender. By establishing a connection between education and the meditative tradition, Grymeston instills the potential for the dissolution of rigid spiritual hierarchies, offering the meditative world of women as a model for men as well. Snook demonstrates that Grymeston creates a version of masculinity for her son that is not dependent upon her absence or the expurgation of femininity, even as she writes a positive intellectual, spiritual, and social identity for herself as author, mother, and woman.

Domestic Production

In a very real sense, the "working mothers" of the early modern period were responsible for a multitude of domestic duties associated with household caregiving. Women's authority within the family as a social system often originated with their maternity, while their responsibilities sometimes extended beyond their roles as mothers to other issues of domestic governance and material production.[33] In the cases of women whose class standing allowed them to use the household as a locus of social action, caregiving responsibilities enabled a certain measure of authority and definition within the domestic sphere.[34] Overall, moreover, as the data amassed by such historians as Sara Mendelson, Patricia Crawford and Merry Wiesner indicates, although upper class and laboring women performed different tasks, women's work almost always included both household responsibilities and child care.[35] At the same time, increased domestic power was not without attendant risks arising from anxieties or misinterpretations regarding the nature of women's work and the scope of their influence, as the present essays under the heading of "Domestic Production" suggest.

Nancy Hayes' "Negativizing Nurture and Demonizing Domesticity: The Witch Construct in Early Modern Germany," for example, examines the domesticity of witch figures in German tract and sermon illustrations from the late fifteenth to the late sixteenth centuries. In these illustrations, the conventional nature of such female "domestic" duties as milking or cooking has been subverted by the apparently anti-maternal intentions of their doers. When the work is represented not at the traditional hearth or in the barn, but rather outside domestic structures, its transfer to unenclosed spaces seemingly unleashes destructive forces against established social order. Depicted in the act of milking axe handles to steal milk from a neighbor's cow, or preparing noxious concoctions over an open fire to seed hail storms, the women in these illustrations are engaged in withdrawing means of nurturance from their fellow villagers. The essay identifes a further paradox in the discrepancies between the written texts and the woodcuts that purportedly illustrate them, when the texts argue that the actual maleficia is executed by demons, with the witches merely providing signals, while the illustrations typically portray the women as acting without demonic assistance, and thus literally embodying the evil in themselves. Hayes analyses how the German witch figures negativize maternal nurture, representing the Other to the Mother.

Deborah Steinberger's "The Difficult Birth of the Good Mother: Donneau de Visé's *L'Embarras de Godard, ou l'Accouchée*" focuses upon the significance of the central theme of domestic maternity, hitherto unprecedented on the French stage, in the 1667 production by Molière's troupe of Jean Donneau de Visé's one-act comedy, *L'Embarras de Godard, ou l'Accouchée* (*Godard's Predicament, or the New Mother*). Diverging from the long comic tradition of portraying older female characters as blocking figures who obstruct the happiness of others, Donneau de Visé's Mme Godard prefigures the compassionate *mère confidentes* (mother-confidantes) of eighteenth-century sentimental comedy. Steinberger suggests that Donneau de Visé's domestic realism and his introduction of the figure of the good mother represent a larger movement that she terms the "domestication" of French comedy, which reflects changes in patterns of social space in early modern France, as well as the elaboration of the concepts of private life and family intimacy. Moving from the public space of the city square to the private space of the domestic interior, French comic stage settings begin to link measures of maternity with domestic production, although mother figures ultimately fail to maintain their presence on the stage.

Domestic reputation as well as production is the subject of Mary Thomas Crane's essay, "Conflicting Identities of Early Modern English Housewives," which explores the tensions marking the sexual and social identities of English "huswives" in the late sixteenth and early seventeenth centuries. The term "huswife" itself was particularly problematic and contested in the early modern period, when it could mean simultaneously *both* "a woman (usually married) who manages her household with skill and thrift," *and* "a light, worthless, or pert woman or girl, or hussy." At a time when women's domestic roles were changing at all levels of society, the conflicting uses of this term provide a kind of paradigm of issues at stake as women became increasingly confined to and associated with domestic matters. Descriptions of "the huswife," then, can illuminate some of the roles manufactured for women as they were increasingly dissociated from the actual manufacture of goods. Crane examines an array of uses of the term in order to trace patterns of anxiety, first, over working class women's wage-earning potential within the home (with fears of concomitant sexual independence) and, later, over upper class women's increasing idleness (with fears of concomitant sexual freedom) as they were confined to a domestic sphere where servants did most of the work.

In "Maternal Textualities," Susan C. Frye takes issue with the common critical assumption that in the early modern period the world of letters and writing was almost wholly a masculinist world. Frye examines some of the ways in which written texts – and in particular, alphabets, initials, and calligraphy – permeated women's domestic lives and helped to make those domestic lives fertile ground for later published writing by women. She argues that women's literary production, while of necessity in conversation with and in competition with that of males, may also be seen as stemming from the domestic production involved in endowing the home with textile markers of class, in cooking, food preserving, midwifery, and healing tasks. For girls and women literate enough to form letters, if only as needlework patterns, female textuality was an everyday occurrence which grew out of the forms of women's culture that simultaneously conformed to and challenged the masculinist, outsider view of their domestic roles. The essay illustrates how texts that were important in everyday women's lives were preserved in a spectrum of media, including needlework, architecture, calligraphy, and diaries, all of which provide evidence that women's domesticization of the text coincided with their entrance into the textual marketplace.

Social Authority

The social authority of early modern women often originated in extensions of their caregiving powers from within the home to society at large. Combining the sexuality of generative wombs with the authority of generative words and roles, mothers and other female caregivers shared a potential for social influence that extended far beyond the boundaries of their immediate families, in association with emblematic power as well as actual political and cultural authority. Although the spectacle of such authority inevitably engendered attacks on the part of writers concerned with upholding masculinist social order, many men as well as women laid claim to the enabling spectrum of powers associated with maternity in the early modern period, whether to illuminate their own creative processes, to question the conventional parameters of domestic roles, or to authorize narratives of religious faith or historical conquest.

Linda Phyllis Austern's essay, "'My Mother Musicke': Early Modern Music and Fantasies of Embodiment," scrutinizes an array of ways in which music was allegorized as a woman in music theoretical treatises and related accounts from the sixteenth and seventeenth centuries, particularly in northern Protestant Europe. Sometimes likened to the mother who gave birth to strong sons who would spring to her defense against rapists and abusers, Music alternatively became the beauteous virgin, allowing male composers to claim their progeny by such a bride in a linguistic attempt to usurp the feminine creative processes of gestation and birth, or the sexual temptress seducing unwary hearers. Moreover male composers and theorists attributed to abstract, audible music the powers and capacities most often ascribed to female caregivers. Austern analyses the strongly gendered and highly sexualized language of creative embodiment in treatises on music theory, demonstrating the ways in which male composers, theorists, performers and listeners thought of their relationship to their art in the same way in which they related to women as mother, bride, and temptress. Crossing disciplinary lines, the essay explores the ways in which the same ideas were translated into visual allegories of music, and used in portraits and images of historical, mythological, and holy figures.

Completing the internal link among essays in the volume that consider the significance of the powerful maternal model of the Virgin Mary in the early modern cultures of Italy, Spain, and Latin America, Frances E. Dolan focuses upon the practices and consequences of Marian devotion in England. Dolan examines how the yoked fear of and fascination with maternal power in the early modern period prompted efforts to grasp as well as resist such power, in a spectrum of venues that included medical treatises about reproduction, prescriptive writings on breastfeeding and other maternal conduct, legal constructions of infanticide, or autobiographical writings, witchcraft discourses and prosecutions, and national iconography. In "Marian Devotion and Maternal Authority in Seventeenth-Century England," Dolan demonstrates how the fierce debates over the extent and value of maternal authority that marked early modern England can be seen to have shaped attitudes toward such problematic issues as the apparently exceptional power of the Virgin Mary. Dolan explores the social attitudes and preoccupations that structured both attacks on and defenses of the Virgin Mary, most of which focused on three crucial, and controversial, stages in a mother's relationship to her child: pregnancy, lactation, and adulthood. Dolan points out that however misogynist their dismissals of women in general, Catholic writers' zealous reverence for the figure of the Virgin countered the sweeping misogyny of Protestant writers, creating the possibility of positive evaluations of women's caregiving contributions to society.

Even exotic spectacles of female authority in the early modern period could not be divorced from domestic associations. Kathryn Schwarz's "Mother Love: Clichés and Amazons in Early Modern England" points out that although Amazons may not seem conventionally domestic, early modern texts refuse to leave Amazonian domesticity at the edge of the world. Instead, from exploration narratives to domestic guidebooks to the frame narrative of *A Midsummer Night's Dream*, Amazons are imagined at home, in familiar spaces where they most emphatically should not belong. Amazons appear not only as political analogues, exotic spectacles, or the wives of heroes, but also as examples in the rhetoric of courtship and conduct, where they do not oppose conventional domesticity, but rather are taken up to idealize it or explain the ways in which it might go wrong. Schwarz argues that, through the tension between the roles they play in myth and the function they serve as exempla, Amazons suggest the ways in which socialized heterosexuality functions as a system of roles. Imagined in intimate as well as disruptive relationship to domestic structures, Amazons as mothers both are and are not the other, presenting at once strange and familiar versions of masculinity that play out male anxieties about female powers.

Mediating between myth and history in "Native Mothers, Native Others: La Malinche, Pocahontas, and Sacajawea," Kari McBride calls attention to three historico-mythical indigenous female figures who have been canonized as central to Euro-American founding narratives: Dona Marina or La Malinche, Matoaka or Pocahontas, and Sacajawea. All three women were mothers during the period of their lives spotlighted by these originary tales, and their maternity can be seen to inflect these histories in significant ways. McBride suggests that the experiences of La Malinche with Cortez in early sixteenth-century Mexico, Pocahontas with John Smith in seventeenth-century colonial America, and Sacajawea with the Lewis and Clark expedition at the turn of the following century, can be viewed as situations where the maternal body makes possible particular narratives of conquest by its ability to delineate cultural boundaries. McBride shows how these three maternal figures come to serve as "natural" go-betweens, translating native culture to European conquerors and vice versa. All three women functioned as commodities for the traffic in women, exchangeable chattel, and yet all three were ultimately mythologized, for good or for ill, as mothers of a new people, a new dispensation, a new world. The essay considers both early modern and contemporary texts about these native mothers, in order to show how maternity functions to authorize their limited and liminal participation in dominant historical narratives.

Mortality

While the final stage of the life cycle, death, exerted destructive force over the many mothers who suffered the deaths of their children, it could paradoxically prove enabling for other early modern women, whose voices at times achieved their greatest power at the close of their own and others' lives. Even as with birth, early modern women were the primary attendants on bodies in death, to such an extent that Mendelson and Crawford conclude that deathbed scenes were "dominated by women," offering a "feminized locale" that fostered "opportunities to construct feminine spheres of social dominance."[36] Some women, moreover, took care to ensure that their experiences lived beyond them in their words. It was the occasion of potentially impending death, after all, that allowed women who authored mothers' advice books such as Dorothy Leigh to justify the excess of their speech, given that "the love of a mother to her children is hardly contained within the bounds of reason."[37] Moving from instructional to financial legacies, an examination of wills for both women and men in early modern England indicates that women favored daughters over sons in no uncertain terms, working even on their deathbeds to offer lasting testaments to women's voices and positions in society.[38] Interestingly, male authors also used the potentially excessive passions associated with maternity to measure their own approaches to mortality, as indicated in the first essay in this section.

In "London's Mourning Garment: Maternity, Mourning and Royal Succession," Patricia Phillippy argues that maternity was constructed in the early modern period as a unique site of affective and emotional license, whose suspension of orthodox responses to loss was particularly useful to male authors in scripting difficult or ambivalent social performances. Phillippy examines the numerous elegies, lamentations, and memorials produced by London publishers in the wake of Queen Elizabeth's death in March 1603, as well as William Muggins' *London's Mourning Garment, or Funerall Teares*, published in the same year, mourning the loss to the plague of nearly 38,000 citizens between July and November 1603. Muggins' elegy shares with the elegies for Elizabeth a preoccupation with the figure of the mother as the central image through which death, its pathos, and its implications are negotiated, represented, and measured. In these examples, male writers construct maternity as a site at which customary forms of mourning are suspended and subsumed within figures of profound, inconsolable grief. By contrast, Phillippy demonstrates that representations of maternal mourning in early modern women's works focus less on transcendence than on the physical fact of death, and employ the mother's lament to empower and authorize textual performances by rooting them within the resistant body of the maternal mourner herself.

Maternal excess provided the locus for recurrent examinations of mortality in monstrous as well as enobling spectacles, as in the figure of Margaret Vincent, discussed above. Early modern preoccupations with infanticide emphasized the horrors of murderous mothers to a much greater degree than murderous fathers, revealing the extent to which maternity provided a measure of life-threatening as well as life-giving powers.[39] In "Early Modern Medea: Representations of Child Murder in the Street Literature of Seventeenth-Century England," Susan Carol Staub focuses upon early modern street literature that documented instances where motherhood went awry, most particularly in examples of murderous mothers. Newsbooks and cheap pamphlets issued after a crime or execution sought both to capitalize on the public's appetite for the sensational and, ostensibly, to spread official ideas about crime and punishment. Staub calls attention to the notable focus of this street literature on spectacles of female criminality, particularly domestic violence, with two kinds of violent crime receiving the most attention: husband murder and infanticide or child murder. While domestic texts and conduct books sought to valorize motherhood, the popular press displayed an almost obsessive concern with mothers who murdered their children. Despite the prevalence of "spinsters" in seventeenth-century court cases involving infant or child murder, the popular press chose to focus instead on married mothers who murdered their children, emphasizing the threatening aspects of female disruption of marital authority associated with these crimes. Staub demonstrates how these texts negotiate notions of sexuality and womanhood in order to maintain their conceptions of a stable, ordered society, criminalizing maternal authority in order to expose its potential danger and limit its scope.

Finally, when mothers themselves are dead, other caregivers must fill the vacuum left by their absence. Heather Dubrow explores some of the anxieties about surrogate parents that shape – and misshape – not only conceptions of caregivers in early modern England, but also many other cultural attitudes. In "'I fear there will a worse come in his place': Surrogate Parents and Shakespeare's *Richard III*," Dubrow points out that the major mortality crisis experienced by England from 1557 to 1559 produced an unusually high percentage of writers and their audience who either had stepparents, or witnessed their presence close at hand. The presence of many types of surrogate parents in the society, including wet nurses, guardians in the wardship system, and so on, indicates some measure of the complex, if vexed, relationship between caregiving, mortality, and authority in the early modern period. In particular, Dubrow observes that because surrogate parents both are and are not the parents they represent, they draw attention to the vulnerability of the individual family members they replace, while at the same time testifying to the longevity of family roles. Focusing on the widespread concern with surrogacy in *Richard III*, Dubrow analyses Shakespeare's treatment of the paradoxes and problems informing the concept of protection, as well as the interplay between loss and recovery. In *Richard III*, as in other early modern texts, the situation of a child surrounded by dubious surrogate caregivers after the loss of a parent serves as a synecdoche for the situation of families as a whole and for the family that is the state.

* * *

As the essays in this volume so amply attest, the pervasive powers of influence associated with maternity in early modern society extended not simply to actual mothers, but to other female caregivers as well, whose standing was variably and yet inextricably linked with the strengths as well as the shortcomings of maternal authority. Midwives and wet nurses, wise women and witches, polemicists and queens: many female positions of authority fostered definitions and comparisons that used maternity as a touchpoint or measure of validation or denigration. For each woman who claimed maternal measures as a strategy of power, one can find another woman who endeavored to stake out a position that extended beyond the purview of reproduction. Often, however, it was in caregiving roles and responsibilities, whether as mothers or others, that many early modern women found the knowledge and power to connect with one another, and variably resist or even reform some of the practices and expectations that determined their standing in society. Mothering others, for better or for worse, female caregivers in the early modern period participated in a spectrum of spectacles whose collective record, explored in part by the essays in this volume, offers an opportunity to measure our current understandings of women's voices and positions as mothers and others, both in the early modern period and in our own.

Notes

1. James Grantham Turner, ed., *Sexuality and Gender in Early Modern Europe: Institutions, Texts, Images* (Cambridge: Cambridge University Press, 1993, xvi; see also Turner's introduction to the volume, "A history of sexuality?", esp. 2–4, 7–8.
2. Patricia Fumerton, "Introduction: A New New Historicism," in *Renaissance Culture and the Everyday*, ed. Fumerton and Simon Hunt (Philadelphia: University of Pennsylvania Press, 1999), esp. 4–7.
3. Susan Frye and Karen Robertson, eds., *Maids and Mistresses, Cousins and Queens* (Oxford: Oxford University Press, 1999), vii; see also their introduction, esp. 3–8, 13.
4. Merry Wiesner, *Women and Gender in Early Modern Europe* (Cambridge: Cambridge University Press, 1993), 1, 3–4. Wiesner devotes an entire chapter to "Women and the creation of culture," 146–75, where she examines women's artistic creations, musical compositions, and literary works, and examines varied restrictions on women's ability to participate in the creation of culture across time and from one geographic area to another.
5. Sara Heller Mendelson and Patricia Crawford, *Women in Early Modern England, 1550–1720* (Oxford: Clarendon Press, 1998), 9. In their section on "Maternity," 148–64, Mendelson and Crawford emphasize that "far from being a 'natural' experience, motherhood was socially and historically constructed," while maternal experiences and responsibilities "differed according to marital status, social level, and a range of personal factors" (148).
6. While not attempting to duplicate the range of references to be found in more detail in some of the essays in this volume and in the extensive bibliographies of the studies cited here, the following list offers a starting point for further investigation:

Olwen Hufton, *The Prospect Before Her: A History of Women in Western Europe* (New York: Alfred A. Knopf, 1996); Anthony Fletcher, *Gender, Sex and Subordination in England 1500–1800* (New Haven: Yale University Press, 1995); Susan Dwyer Amussen, *An Ordered Society: Gender and Class in Early Modern England* (Oxford: Basil Blackwell, 1988); and Christiane Klapisch-Zuber, *Women, Family, and Ritual in Renaissance Italy*, transl. Lydia Cochrane (Chicago: University of Chicago Press, 1985). Given the overlapping boundaries of the medieval and early modern periods, it seems important to note as well the related work of influential medieval historians, including Barbara Hanawalt, *'Of Good and Ill Repute': Gender and Social Control in Medieval England* (Oxford: Oxford University Press, 1998), and David Herlihy, *Women, Family and Society in Medieval Europe: Historical Essays, 1978–1991* (Oxford: Berghahn Books, 1995), and *Opera Muliebria: Women and Work in Medieval Europe* (Philadelphia: Temple University Press, 1990). Relevant collections of essays include Marilyn Migiel and Juliana Schiesari, eds., *Refiguring Woman: Perspectives on Gender and the Italian Renaissance* (Ithaca: Cornell University Press, 1991); Margaret MacCurtain and Mary O'Dowd, eds., *Women in Early Modern Ireland* (Edinburgh: Edinburgh University Press, 1991); Jean R. Brink, Allison P. Coudert, and Maryanne C. Horowitz, eds., *The Politics of Gender in Early Modern Europe* (Kirksville, Miss.: Sixteenth Century Journal Publishers, 1989); Renate Bridenthal, Claudia Koonz, and Susan Stuard, eds., *Becoming Visible: Women in European History*, 2nd edn (Boston: Houghton Mifflin, 1987); Barbara Hanawalt, ed., *Women and Work in Pre-Industrial Europe* (Bloomington: Indiana University Press, 1986); Margaret Ferguson, Maureen Quilligan, and Nancy Vickers, eds., *Rewriting the Renaissance: The Discourses of Sexual Difference* (Chicago: University of Chicago Press, 1986); Mary Beth Rose, ed., *Women in the Middle Ages and the Renaissance: Literary and Historical Perspectives* (Syracuse: Syracuse University Press, 1986); Mary Beth Prior, ed., *Women in English Society, 1500–1800* (London: Methuen, 1985); and Lindsey Charles and Lorna Duffin, eds, *Women and Work in Pre-Industrial England* (London: Croom Helm, 1985). For informative discussions of gender in art history, see Geraldine A. Johnson, *Picturing Women in Renaissance and Baroque Italy* (Cambridge: Cambridge University Press, 1998), and Christa Grossinger, *Picturing Women in Late Medieval and Renaissance Art* (New York: St. Martin's Press, 1997).

7. Valerie Fildes, ed., *Women as Mothers in Pre-Industrial England* (London: Routledge, 1990).

8. Mendelson and Crawford, *Women in Early Modern England*, 231–51, provide an illuminating analysis of a variety of records concerning early modern women's friendships, ranging from social alliances to passionate love.

9. For more detailed historical analysis of midwives, see Hilary Marland, ed., *The Art of Midwifery: Early Modern Midwives in Europe* (London: Routledge, 1993), and Jean Donnison, *Midwives and Medical Men* (New York: Schocken Books, 1977), as well as the more specialized references to midwifery practices in David Gentilcore, *Healers and Healing in Early Modern Italy* (Manchester: Manchester University Press, 1998), and in David Cressy, *Birth, Marriage and Death: Ritual, Religion and the Life-Cycle in Tudor and Stuart England* (Oxford: Oxford University Press, 1997). For historical analysis of wet nurses, see Valerie Fildes, *Wet Nursing: A History from Antiquity to the Present* (Oxford: Basil Blackwell, 1988), and *Breasts, Bottles, and Babies: A History of Infant Feeding* (Edinburgh: Edinburgh University Press, 1986), as well as George Sussman, *Selling Mother's Milk: The Wet-Nursing Business in France, 1715–1914* (Urabana: University

of Illinois Press, 1982). For more comprehensive discussion of childbirth itself, see Jacques Gelis, *History of Childbirth: Fertility, Pregnancy and Birth in Early Modern Europe* (Cambridge: Polity, 1991). See also Wiesner, "The female life-cycle," in *Women and Gender in Early Modern Europe*, 41–81, and Mendelson and Crawford, "Maternity," in *Women in Early Modern England*, 148–64.

10. General studies of mothers' advice books include Valerie Wayne, "Advice for women from mothers and patriarchs," in *Women and Literature in Britain 1500–1700*, ed. Helen Wilcox (Cambridge: Cambridge University Press, 1996), 56–79; Betty S. Travitsky, "The New Mother of the English Renaissance: Her Writings on Motherhood," in *The Lost Tradition: Mothers and Daughters in Literature*, ed. Cathy N. Davidson and E. M. Broner (New York: Ungar, 1980), 33–43, and Elaine Beilin, *Redeeming Eve: Women Writers of the English Renaissance* (Princeton: Princeton University Press, 1987), 266–71.

11. Of particular value for an understanding of gendered learning is Merry Wiesner's in-depth consideration of the obstacles and opportunities for women's education, "Literacy and learning," in *Women and Gender in Early Modern Europe*, 117–45. See also: Fletcher, "Educating Girls," in *Gender, Sex, and Subordination*, 364–75; Hilda L. Smith, "Humanist education and the Renaissance concept of woman," 9–29, and Jacqueline Pearson, "Women reading, reading women," 80–99, in *Women and Literature in Britain*, ed. Wilcox. More general studies of early modern educational offerings and practices include Barbara Hanawalt, "Child-rearing, Training, and Education," in *Growing Up in Medieval London: The Experience of Childhood in History* (Oxford: Oxford University Press, 1993), 69–89; Paul F. Grendler, *Schooling in Renaissance Italy: Literacy and Learning 1300–1600* (Baltimore: Johns Hopkins University Press, 1989); R. A. Houston, *Literacy in Early Modern England: Culture and Education 1500–1800* (London: Longman, 1988); Anthony Grafton and Lisa Jardine, *From Humanism to the Humanities: Education and the Liberal Arts in Fifteenth- and Sixteenth-Century Europe* (Cambridge, Mass.: Harvard University Press, 1986); and Warren Wooden, *Children's Literature of the English Renaissance* (Lexington: University Press of Kentucky, 1986).

12. Recent studies of witches include Jonathan Barry, Marianne Hester, and Gareth Roberts, eds., *Witchcraft in Early Modern Europe* (Cambridge: Cambridge University Press, 1996); Diane Purkiss, *The Witch in History: Early Modern and Twentieth-Century Representations* (London: Routledge, 1996); Anne Llewellyn Barstow, *Witchcraze: A New History of the European Witch Hunts* (London: HarperCollins, 1995); Deborah Willis, *Malevolent Nurture: Witch-Hunting and Maternal Power in Early Modern England* (Ithaca: Cornell University Press, 1995); and Bengt Ankarloo and Gustav Henningsen, eds., *Early Modern European Witchcraft: Centers and Peripheries* (Oxford: Oxford University Press, 1989). Earlier studies that linked witches with female healers and midwives, including Barbara Ehrenreich and Deirdre English, *Witches, Midwives and Nurses: A History of Women Healers* (New York: Feminist Press, 1973), and Thomas Rogers Forbes, *The Midwife and the Witch* (New Haven: Yale University Press, 1966), have been challenged by more recent historical studies, from Merry Wiesner, *Women and Gender in Early Modern Europe*, 230–35, to David Harley, "Historians as demonologists: the myth of the midwife-witch," *Social History of Medicine*, 3 (1990), 1–26. Nevertheless, Wiesner does point out that "though midwives were not more likely to be accused than other women, the older women who hired themselves out temporarily as lying-in maids were" (230).

13. For a brief introduction to these issues, see Naomi J. Miller, "Breast" and "Uterus,"

in *Feminist Literary Theory: A Dictionary*, ed. Elizabeth Kowaleski-Wallace (New York: Garland, 1997). For more detailed analysis, see Jane Silverman Van Buren, *The Modernist Madonna: Semiotics of the Maternal Metaphor* (Bloomington: Indiana University Press, 1989); Thomas Laqueur, *Making Sex: Body and Gender from the Greeks to Freud* (Cambridge: Harvard University Press, 1990); Marcia Ian, *Remembering the Phallic Mother: Psychoanalysis, Modernism, and the Fetish* (Ithaca: Cornell University Press, 1993); Luce Irigaray, *je, tu, nous: Toward a Culture of Difference*, trans. Alison Martin (New York: Routledge, 1993); Elizabeth Grosz, *Volatile Bodies: Toward a Corporeal Feminism* (Bloomington: Indiana University Press, 1994); and Alice Adams, *Reproducing the Womb: Images of Childbirth in Science, Feminist Theory, and Literature* (Ithaca: Cornell University Press, 1994). Studies that focus on the early modern period include Gail Kern Paster, *The Body Embarrassed: Drama and the Disciplines of Shame in Early Modern England* (Ithaca: Cornell University Press, 1993), esp. Chapters 4 and 5, and David Hillman and Carla Mazzio, eds., *The Body in Parts: Fantasies of Corporeality in Early Modern Europe* (New York: Routledge, 1997).

14. Wide-ranging studies of the breast include Marilyn Yalom, *A History of the Breast* (New York: Alfred A. Knopf, 1997), and Fildes, *Breasts, Bottles, and Babies* (1986).

15. See Wiesner, "The female life-cycle," in *Women and Gender in Early Modern Europe*, esp. 44–6; Crawford and Mendelson, "Menstruation," "Parturition," and "Lactation," in *Women in Early Modern England*, 21–9; and Audrey Eccles, *Obstetrics and Gynaecology in Tudor and Stuart England* (Kent, Ohio: Kent State University Press, 1982), 52.

16. Anne Hollander, *Seeing Through Clothes* (Harmondsworth: Penguin, 1988), 194–9.

17. For analyses of these tensions, see Valerie Fildes, *Breasts, Bottles, and Babies* and *Wet Nursing*, as well as Christiane Klapisch-Zuber, "Blood Parents and Milk Parents: Wet Nursing in Florence, 1300–1530," in *Women, Family, and Ritual in Renaissance Italy*, 132–64.

18. For more detailed analysis, see Mendelson and Crawford, "Menstruation," in *Women in Early Modern England*, 21–6, and Ilza Veith, *Hysteria: The History of a Disease* (Chicago: University of Chicago Press, 1965), 10, 13.

19. For a useful summary of Platonic and Aristotelian conceptions, see Robert A. Erickson, *Mother Midnight: Birth, Sex, and Fate in Eighteenth-Century Fiction* (New York: AMS Press, 1986), 15–16.

20. *The Complete Midwife's Practice Enlarg'd* (London, 1569), cited in Eccles, *Obstetrics and Gynaecology*, 29. See also Renate Blumenfeld-Kosinski, *Not of Woman Born: Representation of Caesarean Birth in Medieval and Renaissance Culture* (Ithaca: Cornell University Press, 1990), and Fildes, ed., *Women as Mothers in Pre-Industrial England*, esp. Patricia Crawford, "The construction and experience of maternity in seventeenth-century England," 3–38, Linda A. Pollock, "The experience of pregnancy in early modern society," 39–67, and Adrian Wilson, "The ceremony of childbirth and its interpretation," 68–107.

21. Structures and practices of early modern families within different classes and cultures are covered by Herlihy, *Women, Family and Society in Medieval Europe* (1995); Alan Macfarlane, *Marriage and Love in England: Modes of Reproduction 1300–1840* (London: Blackwell, 1986); Klapisch-Zuber, *Women, Family, and Ritual in Renaissance Italy* (1985); Ralph A. Houlbrooke, *The English Family, 1450–1700* (London: Longman, 1984); and Herlihy and Klapisch-Zuber, *Tuscans*

and Their Families: A Study of the Florentine Catasto of 1427 (New Haven: Yale University Press, 1983). Several anthologies of early modern writings in England provide a wealth of references to this topic, including Joan Larsen Klein, ed., *Daughters, Wives, and Widows: Writings by Men about Women and Marriage in England, 1500–1640* (Urbana: University of Illinois Press, 1992); Houlbrooke, ed., *English Family Life, 1576–1716: An Anthology from the Diaries* (London: Blackwell, 1988); and Suzanne W. Hull, ed., *Women According to Men: The World of Tudor-Stuart Women* (Walnut Creek, CA.: Altamira Press, 1996) and *Chaste, Silent and Obedient: English Books for Women, 1475–1640* (San Marino, CA.: Huntington Library, 1982).

22. Jacques Guillemeau, *Childe-birth, or, The Happy Deliverie of Women* and *The Nursing of Children* (London, 1612).

23. Elizabeth Clinton, *The Countess of Lincolnes Nurserie* (Oxford, 1622).

24. Dorothy Leigh, *The Mother's Blessing* (London, 1616); excerpted *Daughters, Wives, and Widows: Writings by Men about Women and Marriage in England, 1500–1640*, ed. Joan Larsen Klein (Urbana: University of Illinois Press, 1992), 293–4.

25. Leigh, *Mother's Blessing*: this selection alone excerpted in Linda Pollock, *A Lasting Relationship: Parents and Children over Three Centuries* (London: Fourth Estate, 1987), 174.

26. Leigh, *Mother's Blessing*, in Klein, 292, 295.

27. *A pitiless Mother* (London, 1616); excerpted in *Half-Humankind: Contexts and Texts of the Controversy about Women in England, 1540–1640*, ed. Katherine Usher Henderson and Barbara F. McManus (Urbana: University of Illinois Press, 1985), 363.

28. *A pitiless Mother*, in Henderson and McManus, 364.

29. The situation of working women has received considerable attention in recent years, beginning with the influential work of Alice Clark in *Working Life of Women in the Seventeenth Century* (London: Routledge & Kegan Paul, 1919, rpt. 1982), and continuing with a range of more recent studies, including: P. J. Goldberg, *Women, Work, and Life Cycle in a Medieval Economy* (Oxford: Clarendon Press, 1992); David Herlihy, *Opera Muliebria: Women and Work in Medieval Europe* (1990); Merry Wiesner, *Working Women in Renaissance Germany* (New Brunswick: Rutgers University Press, 1986), as well as her more recent chapter on "Women's economic role," in *Women and Gender in Early Modern Europe*, 82–114; Martha Howell, *Women, Production and Patriarchy in Late Medieval Cities* (Chicago: University of Chicago Press, 1986); and Barbara Hanawalt, *The Ties That Bound: Peasant Families in Medieval England* (Oxford: Oxford University Press, 1986). Valuable collections of essays on this topic include: Daryl M. Hafter, ed., *European Women and Preindustrial Craft* (Bloomington: Indiana University Press, 1995); Barbara Hanawalt, ed., *Women and Work in Preindustrial Europe* (1986); and Lindsey Charles and Lorna Duffin, eds., *Women and Work in Pre-Industrial England* (1985). A widespread study of early modern women and class issues is offered by Susan Dwyer Amussen, *An Ordered Society: Gender and Class in Early Modern England* (1988), while more focused attention to the upper classes can be found in Joel T. Rosenthal, *Patriarchy and Families of Privilege in Fifteenth-Century England* (Philadelphia: University of Pennsylvania Press, 1991).

30. See, for example, Louis Haas, *The Renaissance Man and His Children: Childbirth and Early Childhood in Florence, 1300–1600* (New York: St. Martins Press, 1998); Barbara Hanawalt, *Growing Up in Medieval London: The Experience of*

Childhood in History (1993); Shulamith Shahar, *Childhood in the Middle Ages* (London: Routledge, 1990); John Boswell, *The Kindness of Strangers: The Abandonment of Children in Western Europe from Late Antiquity to the Renaissance* (New York: Pantheon Books, 1988); Linda Pollock, *A Lasting Relationship: Parents and Children Over Three Centuries* (1987) and *Forgotten Children: Parent–Child Relations from 1500–1900* (Cambridge: Cambridge University Press, 1983). Useful discussions of patterns of child care appear as well in Mendelson and Crawford, *Women in Early Modern England* (1998); Herlihy, *Women, Family and Society in Medieval Europe* (1995); Klapisch-Zuber, *Women, Family, and Ritual in Renaissance Italy* (1985); Houlbrooke, *The English Family, 1450–1700* (1984); and Herlihy and Klapisch-Zuber, *Tuscans and Their Families: A Study of the Florentine Catasto of 1427* (1983).

31. Mendelson and Crawford, "Maternity," in *Women in Early Modern England*, 148–64; Hufton, "Motherhood," in *The Prospect Before Her*, 177–220; Wiesner, "Pregnancy, childbirth, and motherhood," in *Women and Gender in Early Modern Europe*, 63–73; Wilson, "The ceremony of childbirth," in Fildes, *Women as Mothers*, 96–97.

32. See Note 11 for studies of women and education in the early modern period. For more detailed discussion of the implications of passion in the mothers' advice books, see Naomi J. Miller, "Playing 'the mother's part': Shakespeare's Sonnets and Early Modern Codes of Maternity," in *Shakespeare's Sonnets: Critical Essays*, ed. James Schiffer (New York: Garland Shakespeare Criticism Series, 1998), 403–27, and "'Hens should be served first': Prioritizing Production in Early Modern Pamphlets and Mothers' Advice Books," in *Debating Gender in Early Modern England*, ed. Cristina Malcolmson and Mihoko Suzuki (*forthcoming*).

33. Mendelson and Crawford, *Women in Early Modern England*, offer a wealth of observations regarding women's roles in domestic production, from the fact that "labouring women had a say in their own matrimonial decisions because of their critical position in the family economy" (122), to the explanation that "in the female world of material goods, the official market economy was only the visible tip of a large iceberg of diverse kins of transactions, many of them structured by informal bonds of female friendship and neighborhood" (221). Wiesner, "Women's economic role," in *Women and Gender in Early Modern Europe*, 82–114, observes that men and women had very different relationships to work and work identities in the early modern economy, so that "female work rhythms were … determined by age and class, but even more so by individual biological and social events such as marriage, motherhood, and widowhood" (83); she also notes, in "Women and the creation of culture," 146–75, that crafts such as embroidery lost their professional status during the early modern period and became "increasingly identified as feminine" (148).

34. Felicity Heal, *Hospitality in Early Modern England* (Oxford: Clarendon Press, 1990), 179, 182–3.

35. See, for example, Mendelson and Crawford, "Occupational Identities and Social Roles," in *Women in Early Modern England*, 301–44. Additional sources of historical data regarding female domestic production include: Lena Cowen Orlin, "Three Ways to be Invisible in the Renaissance: Sex, Reputation, and Stitchery," in *Renaissance Culture and the Everyday*, ed. Fumerton and Hunt, 183–203, as well as her collection of excerpts from early modern sources in *Elizabethan Households: An Anthology* (Washington, D.C.: Folger Shakespeare Library, 1995); and Fletcher, "Men's Work, Women's Work," in *Gender, Sex, and Subordination*, 223–55.

36. Mendelson and Crawford, *Women in Early Modern England*, 156, 195, 210.
37. Leigh, *The Mother's Blessing*, in Klein, 293.
38. Amussen, *An Ordered Society*, 34, 38, 91–4.
39. For more detailed discussion of the spectacle of maternal infanticide, see Peter Hoffer and N. E. Hull, *Murdering Mothers: Infanticide in England and New England, 1558–1803* (New York: New York University Press, 1981).

PART I

CONCEPTION AND LACTATION

Mirrors of Language, Mirrors of Self: The Conceptualization of Artistic Identity in Gaspara Stampa and Sofonisba Anguissola

Judith Rose

> *... io provo ben che per mia gran ventura*
> *mi sento il cor di novo stile impresso.*
>
> (But yet I feel, because of my great fortune,
> My heart imprinted with a strong new style.)
>
> (Gaspara Stampa, *Selected Poems*, 14–15)

In sixteenth-century Italy, two women of extraordinary ability, the poet, Gaspara Stampa, and the painter, Sofonisba Anguissola, subtly realigned the relationship between motherhood and artistic "procreativity." Closely investigating the genesis of Gaspara Stampa's *novo stile* and Sofonisba Anguissola's unusual self-portraits, this chapter examines the way in which each of these women manipulated 'conceptual' paradigms in her work. As they redefined Aristotelian paradigms of conception common in the Renaissance, in which the male 'spirit' informs female 'matter,' Stampa and Anguissola redefined their own artistic capability. Concurrently, each invoked and explored her culture's vision of the Virgin Mary in order to provide a new definition of the female artist. In Gaspara Stampa's poetry, an alternative vision of Petrarch's Latinate universe appears; in Sofonisba Anguissola's paintings, the singular female artist mirrors and manipulates linguistic and iconic symbols.

Petrarchan Moments Revised

Any reader of Renaissance poetry (now or then) is familiar with the moment when Petrarch first glimpses the quasi-divine, and perhaps metaphorical,

Laura. It occurs, of course, upon April 6, 1327, a Good Friday. The parallels
with suffering, resurrection, and rebirth are unquestionably deliberate:

> *Era il giorno ch' al sol si scoloraro*
> *per la pietà del suo fattore i rai*
> *quando I' fui preso, et non me ne guardai*
> *che I be' vostr' occhi, Donna, mi legaro.*

> (It was the day when the sun's rays turned pale
> with grief for his Maker when I was taken,
> and I did not defend myself against it,
> for your lovely eyes, Lady, bound me)[1]

On this "day when the sun's rays turned pale with grief for his Maker," the
exposed and penitent Petrarch fails to guard himself against "colpi d'Amor,"
(Love's blows), and finds himself "tutto disarmato" (altogether disarmed) by
the onslaught of love. On a day of communal mourning, Petrarch's own
amorous misfortunes begin, "nel commune dolor" (in the midst of universal
woe). As Patricia Phillippy remarks, the choice of April 6th "exploits the
liturgical associations of the sixth day with the day of creation [of man himself],
and of that date with both the Crucifixion and the Fall."[2] Thus Petrarch can
privilege his poetic creation with echoes of God's creation of man on the sixth
day, as well as with the emblematic moments of loss within the Judaeo-
Christian tradition.

When Gaspara Stampa reworks the trope two centuries later, she echoes
Petrarch's opening line, but relocates the vision of the lover in the ecclesiastical
year. Stampa's moment of apprehension occurs just before Christmas:

> *Era vicino il di che 'l Creatore,*
> *che ne l'altezza sua potea restarsi,*
> *in forma umana venne a dimostrarsi,*
> *dal ventre virginal uscendo fore*

> (It was near the day when the Creator,
> Who might have remained on high,
> Came to show himself in human form,
> Emerging from the Virgin's womb)[3]

Rather than positioning her glimpse of the Count in a time ostensibly associated
with death and mourning, as well as with creation *ex nihilo*, Stampa
deliberately places her inaugural vision at the single moment when the church
unreservedly honors human birth and fecundity. In contrast to Petrarch's more
coded and obscure allusion to creation – a specifically male creation, God's
spirit "moving over the waters" – Stampa's moment of artistic creation occurs
at a moment of festive celebration of the incarnation of the spirit in bodily form,
the soul given access to the world through the female body. Petrarch's allusion
also recalls the Aristotelian moment of 'male' conception, when the male spirit
animates female matter, while the creative moment in Stampa's poem seems to

evoke an alternate 'conceptual' model. Choosing the celebratory moment of Christ's birth also allows the poet to place the Virgin Mary at the emotional center of the poem – it is from her womb that the Creator emerges as a human being. In the following quatrain, Stampa deftly substitutes her poetic persona for the fertile and compassionate Virgin, and her heartless Count for Christ:

> *quando degno l'illustre mio signore,*
> *per cui ho tanti poi lamenti sparsi,*
> *potendo in luogo più alto annidarsi,*
> *farsi nido e ricetto del mio core.*

> (When my illustrious Lord, for whom
> I have written so many scattered laments,
> Who might have nestled in a higher place,
> Made for himself a nest and refuge in my heart.)

Emphasizing the Count's role in evoking her *lamenti sparsi*, the poet telescopes past and present to create an almost static moment of introjection. As she associates her nascent genius with the *ventre virginal* (the Virgin's womb), relocating and reappropriating *concetto* (conception) as an activity of the female poet, Stampa employs a deliberate strategy to lay claim to the "fruits" of her love – her poetry. Moreover, this poetry arises not from "a higher place," but from the body itself; like the vernacular, it is part of lived experience.

When she audaciously positions herself as the Virgin's double in the second poem of her sequence, Stampa not only revises her predecessor's trope on several levels, but also deliberately usurps the role of the most revered female figure in Western civilization. "Negotiating" her guise as an artist in relation to the accepted female role of the Virgin, Stampa creates a multi-faceted, vigorous poetic persona, which contrasts with the passive vision of Mary accepted by the Church. In a single poem she invokes canonical poetry and canonical religion, only to displace, revise, and rewrite them both.

Before closely examining the ways in which Stampa employs the figure of the Virgin, however, I want briefly to look at the some of the ways that Petrarch writes and re-writes *his* vision of the mother of Christ. The *Vergine bella* appears only at the end of Petrarch's *Rime Sparse*; throughout the sequence it is the figure of Laura around whom the narrative – or perhaps the anti-narrative – revolves. As many critics have observed, Laura simply is a pretext for Petrarch's fashioning of his poetic identity. A product of the artistic imagination, she seems to have no independent existence (even within the poems that supposedly celebrate her). In contrast, the Virgin who appears in Petrarch's final poem, after Laura has died and become a quasi-spiritual mentor, is the "anti-type of [the] beloved."[4] In poem 366, the culmination of the *Rime*, the penitent poet addresses the "beautiful Virgin":

Vergine bella, che di sol vestita,
coronata di stelle, al sommo Sole
piacesti si che 'n te sua luce acose:
amor mi sping a dir di te parole,
ma non so 'ncomincia senza tu' aita
et di colui ch' amando in te si pose.

(Beautiful Virgin who, clothed with the sun and crowned with stars, so pleased
the highest Sun that in you He hid His light: love drives me to speak words of you,
but I do not know how to begin without your help and His who loving placed
Himself in you).

(Petrarch, *Rime*, 574–75)

Unlike the earthly Laura, who, as Nancy Vickers has eloquently explained, is
"repeatedly, although reverently, scatter[ed] throughout his scattered rhymes,"
the Virgin who appears at the end of these *rime sparse* is *d'ogni parte
intera*, "whole in every part."[5] This is in fascinating contrast to the state of
Christ in this last poem – here the Virgin's *belli occhi*, "beautiful eyes" see
the *tristi la spietata stampa,* "the pitiless wounds" on the "sweet limbs" of
her dear son. Christ, as *verace omo et verace Dio*, "true man and true God,"
paradoxically seems a less integrated figure than his mother, who is *stabile in
eterno*, "stable for eternity." One might almost interpret this poem as a reversal
of Petrarch's earlier aesthetic position as well as a paradoxical "ethical
recantation" of his former desire, as Phillippy argues (79–88). The poet, as
Christ, assumes the place of the fragmented Laura in relation to the *intera* and
stabile Virgin, who is seen as *nostra Dea*, "our goddess," in some sense, the
"author" of Christ himself. She is *del tuo parto gentil figliuola et madre*,
the "noble daughter and mother of [her] offspring," as well as the *sacrato et
vivo tempio*, the "consecrated living temple" which nourishes Christ (lines 28
and 57).

When Stampa envisions herself as the Virgin in whose heart the *illustre
Conte* may "nest," she appropriates the position that Petrarch himself granted to
the *Vergine bella* of author, privileging her own fecundity and creativity. From
this metaphorical position, the poet can undertake the difficult task of the
female writer, overcoming the multitudinous injunctions of the period against
women's public speech; moreover, she can identify herself with a divine
language, even though she is writing in the vernacular.

The count, whose cruelty so torments her, has caused her to bear "fruits of
love."[6] This *frutto,* her poetic creativity, is the spiritually logical offspring of the
enclosed garden, the *hortus conclusus* which medieval iconography equated
with the Virgin's womb. Stampa employs this ancient image paradoxically,
playing upon its allusions to perfect purity, and, as I will explore below,
punning upon some less exalted associations. The forms Stampa draws for
herself and her lover also imply a new relationship between the poet –
specifically female – and her strangely introjected muse.

In the preface to her poems, "Allo Illustre Mio Signore" (To My Illustrious Lord), Stampa characterizes the *Conte* as:

O obietto nobile, o obietto chiaro, o obietto divino, poi che tormentando ancora giovi e fai frutto.

(O noble object, O bright object, O object divine, since even in tormenting me, you still delight and produce fruit.) [7]

This "divine object" does not, like the Holy Ghost, spiritually impregnate the pliant Virgin; rather the almost perverse "delight" that arises in the poet seems to depend upon *her own* creative response to "torment." Sonnet Four, *Quando fu prima il mio signor concetto* ("When my beloved lord was first conceived") focuses upon a metaphorical moment of conception, where the embryonic lover is blessed (and damned) by a host of surrounding deities. The writer becomes the "conceiving" entity, bestowing upon the *Conte* an array of *le grazie* ("graces") and *doti* ("gifts"); the poet *authors* her lover, aligning herself with Venus, Mars and Mercury, as well as with *la luna*, the Moon, who "freezes" his heart. The poet creates her heartless lover with a certain deliberation, noting that the stars have *m'infiammo de la chiara fiamma mia* ("inflamed me with my own clear fire"). More than a Petrarchan poetic foil, the *Conte* focuses the act of creation itself; in imagining him, Stampa imagines herself as poet.

Thus the Count acts almost as a traditional muse; yet his power rests in his cruelty rather than in his beauty (though Stampa does catalogue his attractions in various poems, among them Poems 4, 7 and 68, the *perfetti* which she notes in his person always contrast with his heartlessness). Stampa takes the "proud disdain" of the Petrarchan love object one step further, portraying the *Conte* as deliberately *empio in amore* (faithless in love).

That callousness provides the catalyst for her writing becomes even more evident in the often noted conflation of *pena* (pain) and *penna* (pen) in Stampa's poetry. As she asks in Poem 8,

S'Amor con novo, insolito focile,
ov'io non potea gir, m'alzo a tal loco,
perche non può non con usato gioco
far la pena e la penna in me simile?

(If Love with a new, uncommon flint
lifts me to such a place where I could never climb,
why am I not able, in an unusual gamble,
to make pain and pen equal in myself?)

Burned by the flame that love has kindled, the poet aspires to write out her pain, making the pen a metaphor for her sorrow. As Juliana Schiesari observes, the poet also invokes a chorus of female voices (in Poem 151) to bewail her situation, but

> instead of being asked simply to partake in a general chorus of woe ... the women
> are also asked, significantly enough, to *write* – as if the scriptural extension of
> mourning were a feminist response to a male melancholia appropriative of the
> symbolics of women's loss.[8]

Writing becomes the essential, appropriate response to the pain of abandonment, as well as to the loss of voice, both for the individual and for the sex. The feather quill – *penna* – becomes, as Stortoni and Lillie suggest, the *penne d'aquila o colomba* (the wings of an eagle or a dove), with which she flies *da l'Indo al Mauro* (from India to Mauretania).[9] The poet's persona, *qua* writer, can transcend physical and psychic boundaries, as well as the encumbrances of gender. Thus the initial image in Sonnet Two, which conflates the connotations of the Virgin – as author, as fertile spring, as the *hortus conclusus* which bears the fruit of poetry – with the poet herself, provides a complex mix of enabling metaphors for creativity.[10] As the sonnet continues, Stampa further complicates its network of allusions.

In the second stanza of Sonnet Two, the poet develops a conceit that curiously recalls the small devotional statues of the Virgin known as *Vierge Ouvrante*, not uncommon in the late middle ages. When the *Conte* "makes for himself a nest and refuge in [her] heart," the poet's body seems literally to enclose her lover. The small *Vierge Ouvrante* figure similarly encloses the Savior; it opens to reveal a still smaller Christ, sometimes on the cross, sometimes seated in calm meditation, surrounded by illustrations of his death and passion.[11] The enclosure of the Christ figure within the body of his mother seems to imply a greater role for the Virgin in the creation story than the Gospels, or the Church, would countenance. Rather than a peripheral figure, she becomes the source both of Christ and his story. Stampa's simultaneous enclosure of the *Creatore* and of her *signore* within a maternal body would seem to privilege the site of female creativity in a similar fashion. Such a construction of poetic creativity suggests a relocation of *concetto* (in all its senses) as a female activity; the woman is no longer mere "matter," the passive recipient, but the wellspring of creation. Still, the strangeness of the image itself – the lover "nested" within the body of the poet – gives the reader pause. This image works on several levels which incorporate the various aspects of the *Conte* as muse and catalyst.

Stampa clearly is aware of an ancient tradition of Christian iconography in which Christ and the Virgin are represented as man and wife;[12] in Poem 366 Petrarch himself, without great elaboration, notes that *sposa* is one of the three *dolci et cari nomi* (sweet and dear names) of the Virgin, and that she is *donna del Re* (the lady of the King). In the basilica of Santa Maria Maggiore in Rome one may find a particularly beautiful mosaic which depicts the Savior and his mother seated side by side in the traditional pose of bride and groom, surrounded by a host of saints and by scenes from her life. In this stunning mosaic, the seated Christ offers the Virgin a bridal crown. A Florentine diptych, another of many similar depictions, shows the two of them with hands clasped in the traditional pose of nuptial union. The tradition also exists in a number of written texts, the most luminous probably that of Bernard of Clairvaux:

> Happy indeed were the kisses he pressed on her lips when she was nursing ... But ... happier those kisses which ... she receives today from the mouth of him who sits on the right hand of the Father, when she ascends to the throne of glory, singing a nuptial hymn and saying: "Let him kiss me with the kisses of his mouth."[13]

The language from the biblical Song of Songs in this passage further underscores the spiritualized sexuality that underlies this imagery, a sexuality which Stampa, unlike her predecessor, deliberately exploits in her revisionary portrait of the Virgin. The poet's specific choice of the word *nido* (nest) implies an encoded sexual pun, since the word for bird, *uccello,* is also a euphemism for the phallus.[14] The bird is also, of course, an ancient symbol of the spirit (graphically illustrated in the miracle of plays of medieval Europe, where, as Marina Warner notes, a bird tethered to a string was pulled toward the heavens when a player 'died' (*Alone of All Her* Sex, 38)). When the *signore* "nests" in the heart of the poet/Virgin, therefore, an implied sexual, as well as "conceptual" union takes place. Stampa imagines a Virgin with an almost palpable body, who unites with her Lord in an embrace that combines sensuality and spirituality, combining her *tre dolci et cari nomi* in a way Petrarch might have shuddered to imagine. In contrast to his vision of a purely integrated, purely spiritual *Vergine santa*, Stampa's Virgin contains the paradoxical elements of human woman, sexuality and desire included. Whereas Petrarch splits off the elements of the female persona he finds disturbing – Laura's mortality becoming *terra* (dust), and her sexuality assuming the form of the Medusa – his female successor chooses to integrate these aspects into her poetic persona – and into her language.

Thus the poet portrays herself as the complex combination of the two disparate poles of feminine identity in the Renaissance: virgin and whore. The continuation of Sonnet Two further develops this image:

> Ond'io si rara e si alta ventura
> accolsi lieta; e duolmi sol che tardi
> mi fe'degna di lei l'eterna cura.
>   Da indi in qua pensieri e speme e sguardi
> volsi a lui tutti, fuor d'ogni misura
> chiaro e gentil, quanto 'l sol giri e guardi.

> (So with joy I took upon myself this rare and lofty fate
> only regretting that it had been given to me so late
> to be made worthy of the Eternal Care.
> Since that moment in my thoughts and hopes and glances
> I am turned wholly to him, luminescent and noble,
> beyond all measure of those the sun circles and beholds.)

In her role as Virgin, the speaker accepts the annunciatory moment, only regretting that *eterna cura* (God himself) has waited so long to find her worthy. Echoing Mary's *Magnificat* in Luke I:46–55, the poet rejoices in her *alta ventura*, which will provide earthly, rather than spiritual fame (reflecting the Virgin's realization that "all generations shall call me blessed").

Just as she has mythologized her own role, Stampa imagines a *chiaro e gentile* Count, whose virtues exceed all measure (in direct proportion to his cruelty). The *Conte* thus becomes the idealized, if heartless, Platonic lover linked to the paradoxically passionate Virgin. Using the imagery of Pico della Mirandola developed from the philosophy of Marsilio Ficino, Stampa experiments with the possibilities of neo-Platonic thought. Pico's meditation culminates in a moment wherein the soul (which is specifically – and traditionally – gendered female) invites the "King of Glory":

> [L]et us wish [peace] for our own soul, that through it she herself shall be made the house of God, and to the end that as soon as she has cast out her uncleanness through moral philosophy and dialectic ... the King of Glory may descend and ... make his stay with her ... [S]he shall ... in golden raiment like a wedding gown, and surrounded by a varied throng of sciences, receive her guest ... as a spouse from whom she will never be parted.[15]

Pico's "female" soul, in an echo of the Christian iconography discussed above, accepts the godhead as a spouse with whom she is united in eternal bliss. Stampa plays with and against these images of the pliable soul. In Poem Two she utilizes the image of the soul as "house" or refuge (*ricetto*) – as "nest" – for the illustrious *signore* whom she identifies as both beloved and "divine object," closely following Pico's paradigm. The divergences are significant, however. This soul's "uncleanness" (at least in the sexual sense) seems to be celebrated rather than abjured. And the soul remains linked to the body; the *signore* must reveal himself *in forma umana*, not as a wholly spiritual being. While Pico celebrates the moment of death – the soul "will desire to die in herself in order to live in her spouse, in whose sight surely the death of his saints is precious" (232) – Stampa's poem unequivocally celebrates birth.

The imagined *Conte*, in his many guises – as embryo, as tormentor, as muse, as "divine object," as lover – complicates the role of the poet, who creates for herself a series of changing identities. Stampa thus undermines the ancient tradition of woman as "mirror" for her male counterpart; the poet seems deliberately to disrupt the "specular duplication" that Luce Irigaray is still critiquing four centuries later:

> Now if this [male] ego is to be valuable, some "mirror" is needed to reassure it and re-insure it of its value. Woman will be the foundation of this specular duplication, giving man back "his" image and repeating it as the "same." If an *other* image, an *other* mirror were to intervene, this inevitably would entail the risk of moral crisis. Woman, therefore, will be this sameness – or at least its mirror

image – and, in her role of mother, she will facilitate the repetition of the same, in contempt for difference ...[16]

In her imagined incarnations, Stampa refuses to become the unitary "sameness" upon which the male ego is projected, the "material" upon which a patrilineal image is stamped. Even when she takes upon herself the role of nurturing mother, she refuses to obliterate the "sexual energy necessary" to the role, thus continuing to emphasize the difference between the sexes, pivotally important if woman is not to be subsumed into the model of man. Constantly shifting – a *chimera,* as she characterizes herself in a late poem (Sonnet 174) – she cannot be fixed in a single, mirroring identity. Although Stampa plays with roles that might be defined, in the terms of twentieth century feminism, as "essentialist," she redefines the possibilities within each role, as does Irigaray herself. Across four hundred years and a cultural chasm, the French philosopher seems to echo the Italian poet's sensibilities when she challenges the very notion of essential nature, "'I' am not 'I,' I *am* not, I am not *one*. As for *woman*, try and find out ..."[17]

In her revisions of various female roles, Stampa dares her reader to "try and find out" what "woman" might be. When she plays upon the paradigm of the "female soul," her intention seems to be to offer new possibilities rather than an overly simplified "essentialist" vision. Like Irigaray, it seems that Stampa would argue that "if 'God' has been conceived as a perfect volume, a closed completeness, an infinite circle as far as extension extends, it is certainly not as a result of women's imagination." In the "passion for an origin that curls around neatly, even at the risk of biting its own tail," the multiplicity of experience is lost (Irigaray, *Speculum*, 236). Circling back to the matrix of change, birth and creativity, and asserting her own power to re-imagine the canonical figures of religion and literature, Gaspara Stampa invents the language for a poetry "*in forma umana*." In so doing, she affirms her artistic identity, or perhaps we should say, her multiplicity of identities.

Sofonisba Anguissola: Conceptualizing the Mirrored Self

Though the radical representation of female self-conception found in Gaspara Stampa's work would not occur in the visual arts for another century (in the work of Artemisia Gentileschi), some subtler intimations of a reinterpretation of woman's place in the artistic universe may be found in her much longer-lived contemporary, Sofonisba Anguissola. This Italian painter and her gifted sisters were trained as artists through their father's instigation; Sofonisba fulfilled and even exceeded his expectations. Not only did she become a celebrated painter in her own country, she was appointed court painter to Phillip II of Spain and spent eighteen fruitful years in the austere Spanish court.

Chronicling her development as a woman and as an artist, Anguissola's series of self-portraits was begun in the year 1554 when she was probably about nineteen. The first of the surviving portraits shows the young woman holding an open book within which is inscribed, *Sofonisba Anguissola virgo se ipsam fecit 1554* (Sofonisba Anguissola, virgin, made this herself, 1554) (Fig. 2.1). Demonstrating that she could not only paint, but read and write basic Latin, the inscription also allies her with a specific (though long-dormant) female tradition. The inscription is "a conscious reference to the famous woman painter from antiquity called Iaia by Pliny and Marcia by Boccaccio. Both called her a *perpetua virgo*, who neither served Vesta nor any other priestess but renounced physical pleasure to dedicate herself fully to the arts."[18] The reference also allies her with a tradition of famous maidens who were celebrated for their chastity as well as for their more tangible accomplishments – going back to Athena herself, "coldly virginal ... defined not by sex but by intellect."[19] Thus insulating herself against any charge of lewd conduct, which was, of course, a real danger for any woman publicly revealing herself, Anguissola could also play upon the many resonances of the word *virgo*. But the artist also invokes an even more familiar figure when she identifies herself as *virgo*; here and even more vividly in a later self-portrait, she allies herself with the Virgin Mary. In emphasizing her own "making" of the image, Anguissola underlines her activity as an artist – indeed a questionable activity for a woman of the *Cinquecento* – as well as her own "pro-creative" activity.[20] Like the ancient artist Marcia, who is portrayed in a French edition of Boccaccio's text as painting a self-portrait while she gazes into a mirror (Fig. 2.2), Anguissola draws upon her female creativity to re-fashion herself, rather than to create a child. Self-defined by stainless chastity, like the Virgin, she can reproduce without taint of sin.

The distortion of the portrait itself seems to underline this idea in an unusual way: the excessively enlarged eyes and oddly proportioned face may appear this way because they were drawn from an image in a small, convex mirror. Joseph Koerner notes Albrecht Durer's deliberate portrayal of his struggle to represent himself while squinting into a convex mirror in his *Self-Portrait* of 1491.[21] Large mirrors were often prohibitively expensive even in the mid-sixteenth century, and the image in a round, convex mirror (like that we see in the background of Jan van Eyck's *Arnolfini Marriage Portrait*) was too small to be easily and accurately portrayed. Unlike Durer's much earlier work, Anguissola's *Self-Portrait* does not represent such a pivotal moment in the history of art; nevertheless it calls attention to the difficulties of its own creation in a similar, though less overt, fashion. What Koerner says of Durer may also be applied to his successor: "what occupies him is not a flawless rendition of his likeness, but rather ... the double activity of looking and representing" (5). Anguissola's exploitation of the mirror image is even clearer in a slightly later

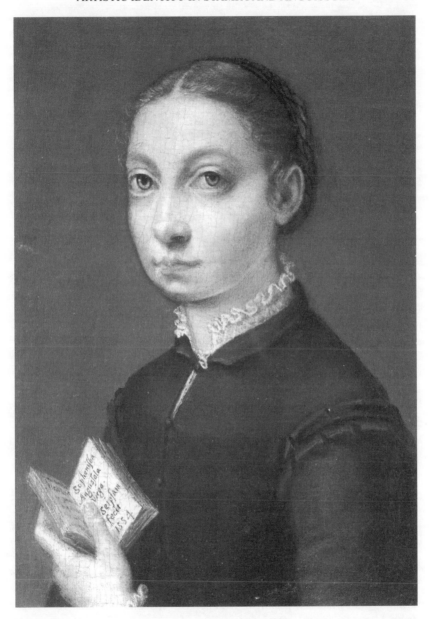

Fig. 2.1   Sofonisba Anguissola, *Self Portrait*, 1554

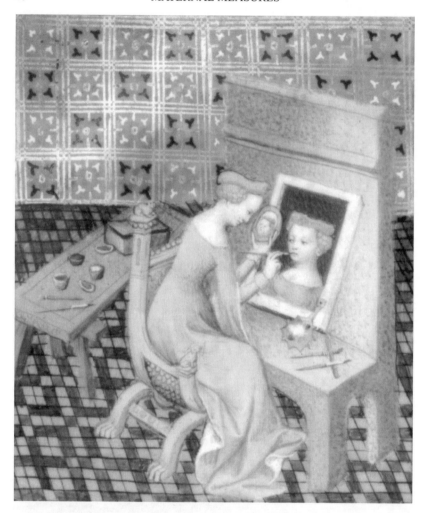

Fig. 2.2   Coronation Master (?), *Marcia Painting her Self Portrait*, 1403

self-portrait, which is also somewhat distorted (the unshadowed right eye appears larger than the left).[22] In this tiny miniature, the artist holds a medallion inscribed along its outer perimeter with the words, *Sofonisba Anguissola Virgo Ipsus Manu Ex Speculo Depicta Cremone* (The virgin Sofonisba Anguissola depicted with her own hand from a mirror at Cremona) (Fig. 2.3). Her fame at this point extended beyond Cremona, and this tiny miniature was probably intended as a gift – thus the inclusion the name of the artist's native city. The mysterious initials on the shield itself might represent the name of the recipient,

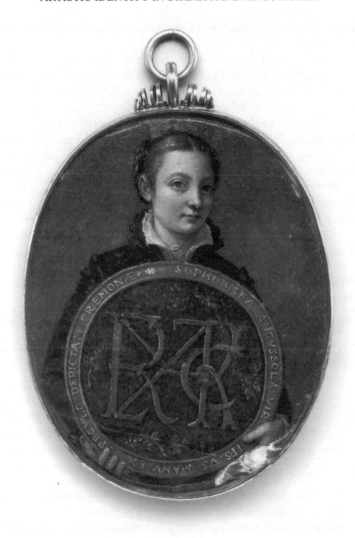

Fig. 2.3   Sofonisba Anguissola, *Self Portrait*, c. 1555

which would further play upon the mirror image, since he/she would gaze at the portrait and see his or her own name reflected there.[23]

Such a conscious representation of the mirrored image would also seem to emphasize this *virgo*'s connection to another *speculum sine macula* – the mirror without sin, an ancient metaphor for the Virgin Mary. The Virgin was also called the *speculum immaculatum*, the unspotted mirror, a designation which originated in *The Book of Wisdom*.[24] The iconographic depiction of the Blessed Virgin "surrounded by the symbols of the Litany to which the *speculum immaculatum* belonged" began in medieval France, and spread from there to Italy and Spain (Schwarz, 99, n.32). Anguissola played upon this iconography, both in the earlier self-portraits and, as I will argue below, in a later portrait where she "stands in" for the mythical portraitist of the Virgin: St. Luke. The use of such an image might imply that the artist was accepting a role of passive reflection; after all, the Virgin's perfection makes her the perfect mirror for God, the *speculum sine macula dei majestatis*, in yet another variation of the nomenclature (Schwarz, 99). Anguissola, however, employs these images with shrewd irony, emphasizing not only her own virginity, but the unique nature of her vocation. Like Stampa, she becomes, in Irigaray's terms, "the *other* mirror," intervening in a cycle of representation that ordinarily would produce an undifferentiated image of the divine. In *this* conception, the mirror reflects the female artist's image.

Moreover, this female artist employs an array of varying strategies to quietly emphasize her position. Speaking of the pagan model for Anguissola's self-representation, Joseph Koerner remarks that:

> Marcia's chastity was not imposed on her, by the pagan cult of Diana, say, but arose "through her own inner purity." Self-portraiture thus becomes the emblem of this personal virtue, which likewise is self-fashioned: the pictorial equivalent of a virgin birth. (124)

In an era when beauty alone mattered as a standard of female representation, the rather plain Anguissola justified her many self-portraits, indeed, her artistic production as a whole, by representing herself as an icon of chastity and moderation. With her somber dress and lack of ornament, the artist " presents herself 'like a man,' avoiding feminine signifiers that might link her with paragons of beauty or courtesans and emphasizing features associated with independence, self-possession and maturity."[25] Eschewing the feminine attributes that would objectify her, the artist brings the pictorial focus to her mastery of her art, to the process rather than the performer.

In depicting herself in this way Anguissola both accepts and defies the conventional assumptions of the period, which argue that only the male artist could endow a painting with *disegno*, the formative design which governs great works of art, and indeed that a woman "cannot conceive without man's invention but can only give body to his ideas."[26] When the young Sofonisba pictures herself in a creative role, dressed in a somber manner that imitates that of a male artist, she emphasizes her difference from ordinary women and her own unusual ability, a difference and ability remarked upon by contemporary commentators, Vasari among them. The great chronicler of the lives of the artists remarks with a certain breathlessness, "I must report that I saw this year (1566) in the house of [Sofonisba's] father at Cremona, a picture executed by her hand with great diligence (*tanta diligenza e prontezza*), portraits of her three sisters ... who appear truly alive (*vive*), and are wanting in nothing save speech."[27] So sure was Anguissola of her ability, that when Michelangelo himself reportedly commented upon her drawing of a young girl, saying that he "would have liked to see a weeping boy," she sent him the marvelous drawing, *Boy Bitten by a Crab*, which contains both a crying boy and his clearly amused sister.[28] The clear note of irony in the drawing, where a small, petulant boy howls and his older, more self-possessed sibling observes him, emphasizes the male figure's "ignoble position," and the artist's solid control of her medium (Garrard, "Here's Looking" 613).

It is worth noting that Sofonisba herself, in choosing to produce "offspring of the soul [rather] than those of the body" (she remained childless throughout her long life and highly successful career) was taking on a distinctly male role, one that Ficino characterized as "pursuing heavenly love."[29] This was, of course, the "higher" aspiration; the Neo-Platonism which infused the Italian Renaissance insisted upon the primacy of intellectual production over physical procreation. Even the far-seeing Leonardo, who argued against the "gendered" inferiority of painting, and extolled the ability of *colore* to show the "varying intensity and transparency of objects," at one point depicted reproduction as a male "conception."[30] When he sketched a depiction of the act of intercourse, Leonardo connected the brain to the seminal canal; explicating the drawing, Patricia Rielly writes, "[d]uring the act of procreation, the conception was transmitted from the mind of the male to the womb of the female ... the male's brain is integral to the act ... whereas the woman's need not even be present" (Rielly, 92).

In a painting executed around 1556 I believe that we can see vivid (though still quite understated) instances of Anguissola intentionally subverting the expectations of her viewers, as she did in the small drawing sent to Michelangelo mentioned earlier, *and* playing upon her 'less female' form of creativity. In her *Self-Portrait at Easel* (Fig. 2.4) the young artist depicts herself painting a Madonna, who, as Sylvia Ferino-Pagden notices, "conspicuously and tenderly hugs her child nestled closely against her" (24). The interaction between the Virgin and child goes further than this; they are very close to a nuptial kiss, and the Christ child is no infant, but a boy of three or four. We cannot know, if course, if Anguissola intended to play upon the various images of the Virgin as *sposa, madre e figlia* as Gaspara Stampa did in her sonnet two. It is clear, however, that here and in the much later *Madonna Nursing Her Child* (1588), the artist chooses to depict an unusual level of intimacy between mother and child. Of the latter painting, Naomi Yavneh comments that in the late *Cinquecento*, "a greater concern with nudity and decorum makes the subject ... problematic" for many artists; moreover, since Catholic theologians were emphasizing "Mary's sanctity and queenly

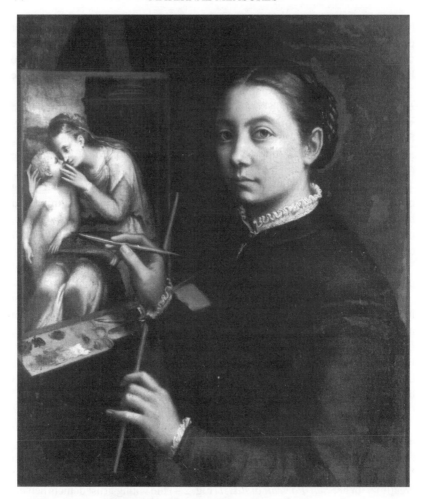

Fig. 2.4   Sofonisba Anguissola, *Self Portrait at Easel*, 1556

exaltation over [her] humanity," the church discouraged more homely
depictions of the Virgin (Yavneh, "To Bare or Not too Bare"). Nevertheless, in
Anguissola's painting we see an accurate depiction of "not only the physical
bodies and intimate relationship between the Madonna and her child, but
also the act of nursing ..." (Yavneh, "To Bare or Not too Bare"). Anguissola
obviously was willing to defy convention, and even possible censure, when
it suited her aesthetic purpose. Here and in the earlier *Self-Portrait*, she
naturalizes the Madonna, stressing the intimacy of her interaction with her son.
Neither painting depicts a 'queenly' icon; in fact, the *Self-Portrait at Easel*

further refines the mirror imagery we spoke of above, emphasizing the proximate relationship of artist, subject, and viewer.

Although this painting does not distort the artist's mirrored image as do the earlier self-portraits, specifically alluding to the mechanics of its production, it nevertheless incorporates some very old symbolism concerning the reflected image. Generally speaking, representations of an artist portrayed in the act of painting the Madonna allude to the apocryphal paintings of St. Luke, portraitist of the Virgin. Luke was not only the patron saint of painters but also that of glass and mirror-makers. When a painter depicted St. Luke in the act of painting the Virgin, he inevitably portrayed himself – as Henrick Schwarz contends, "[w]e may easily assume self-portraits in the various representations of St. Luke ... and interpret the mirrors also as allusions to and emblems of their profession" ("Mirror of the Artist," 99, n.33). In Anguissola's *Self-Portrait at Easel* we observe the unusual situation of a deliberate self-portrait of the Lucan artist, rather than an implied one, an understandable strategy, since Anguissola could not have assumed that her audience would understand a depiction of herself as a cross-dressed St. Luke.[31] But the painting is yet more complex. In the process of representing herself and the Madonna and child, Anguissola creates a sort of gallery of mirrors, where the artist is reflected in her work both within the painting and in the viewer's overall apprehension. Leonardo's famous comment is relevant here: *Ogni dipintore dipinge se,* "Every painter paints himself." Yet Anguissola's subtle gallery of mirrors – the artist mirroring St. Luke, reflected in the Virgin and in the Christ child – would seem to imply that the paradigm is not so simple for the female painter. She must both reveal and hide herself in a series of reflections, use an *appiagiamano*, a mahlstick, as she holds her "masculine" brush to the canvas.[32]

In all these mirrored and mirroring images, Anguissola seems to refuse a single fixed identity; just as the viewer tries to hold her fast, another distortion or reflection arises. Even in the portraits in which she ostensibly appears, Anguissola eludes what Mary Garrard calls the viewer's "confinement"; with her strategies of mirrored identities, she instead becomes representative of the shifting, mutable identity of the artist ("Here's Looking" 619). Like the *chimera* with which Gaspara Stampa identifies herself, Anguissola – even within her series of self-portraits – will not allow herself to be pinned to the canvas. Nevertheless, the artist does offer a complex "self-conceptualization," one that emphasizes the mutability of the very idea of self.

Thus, despite the power of the Aristotelian notion of conception and its influence upon religious and philosophical thought, these two women of the late Italian Renaissance did not hesitate to imagine an alternate paradigm. Within this paradigm, the fruitfulness of the Virgin Mary implies an 'essential' female productivity which becomes a prototype for the creative power of the female artist. Unlike the 'mater/ matter' model of the Aristotelian system, this alternate philosophical construction implies that female procreativity has an active spiritual and physical dimension, that maternity itself is a reflection of an inner creative fire. When Stampa, therefore, sees herself as the *Vergine bella*, or her terrestrial reflection, or Anguissola portrays herself as the Lucan artist basking in the Virgin's light, each is able to explore a multitude of paths to creativity, and imagine a multitude of selves.

Notes

1. Francesco Petrarca, *Petrarch's Lyric Poems: The Rime sparse and Other Lyrics.* Translated and edited by Robert M. Durling (Cambridge, Mass.: Harvard University Press, 1976), 38–9.
2. Patricia Phillippy, *Love's Remedies: Recantation and Renaissance Lyric Poetry* (Lewisburg, PA: Bucknell University Press, 1995), 71.
3. Here and throughout the rest of the article, the Italian text of Stampa's poems is from *Gaspara Stampa: Selected Poems*, edited and translated by Laura Anna Stortoni and Mary Prentice Lillie (New York: Italica Press, 1994); the English translation is my own.
4. John Frecerro, "The Fig Tree and the Laurel: Petrarch's Poetics," in *Literary Theory/Renaissance Texts*, ed. Patricia Parker and David Quint (Baltimore: The Johns Hopkins University Press, 1986), 32.
5. Nancy J. Vickers, "Diana Described: Scattered Women and Scattered Rhyme." *Critical Inquiry* 8 (Winter, 1981): 265–79; 109; Petrarch, *Rime*, 577.
6. Petrarch also refers to the Virgin as "feconda" (fruitful), but does not, of course, identify this fruitfulness with poetic creativity.
7. Gaspara Stampa, *Rime*, introduzione di Maria Bellonci, note di Rodolfo Ceriello (Milan: Bilioteca Universale Rizzoli, 1994). My translation.
8. Juliana Schiesari, *The Gendering of Melancholy: Feminism, Psychoanalysis, and the Symbolics of Loss in Renaissance Literature* (Ithaca, NY: Cornell University Press, 1992), 172.
9. See Poem 114. I refer to a brief suggestion in Stortoni and Lillie's introduction to *Gaspara Stampa: Selected Poems*.
10. Stampa seems to revise an earlier, more conflicted, vision of the Virgin as writer, one version of which may be seen in Sandro Botticelli's *Madonna del Magnificat*. See Susan Schibanoff's "Botticelli's *Madonna del Magnificat:* Constructing the Woman Writer in Early Humanist Italy," *PMLA* 109 no. 2: 190–206, for a thoughtful discussion of this painting and its implications.
11. Marina Warner refers to these figures in her chapter on the Virgin Birth in *Alone of All Her Sex* (New York: Knoph, 1976).
12. For a useful discussion of this tradition, which is both Biblical and iconographic, see Marina Warner's chapter "The Song of Songs" in *Alone of All Her Sex*, esp. 128–33.
13. St. Bernard, *In Assumptione Beatae Mariae Virginis* quoted in Warner, *Alone of All Her Sex*, 130.
14. Guido Ruggiero makes note of this in *Binding Passions: Tales of Magic, Marriage and Power at the End of the Renaissance* (New York: Oxford, 1993): "Across the Renaissance and on into the present, *uccello* in Italian has been a popular euphemism for the phallus;" he further speculates that "thus, the use of the hearts

of birds [in magic spells] had the potential to create resonances ... at two levels" (121–2).

15. Pico della Mirandola, "On the Dignity of Man" in *The Renaissance Philosophy of Man* (Chicago: University of Chicago Press, 1948), 232.

16. Luce Irigaray, *Speculum of the Other Woman.* Translated by Gillian C. Gill (Ithaca, NY: Cornell University Press, 1985), 54.

17. Irigaray, *This Sex Which Is Not One*, 120, quoted in Diana Fuss' *Essentially Speaking: Feminism, Nature and Difference* (New York: Routledge, 1989), 72. As Fuss notes, "[I]t is precisely Irigaray's deployment of essentialism which clarifies for us the contradiction at the heart of Aristotle's metaphysics ... the dominant line of patriarchal thought since Aristotle is built on this central contradiction: woman has an essence and it is matter; or put slightly differently, it is the essence of woman to have no essence ... [E]ssentialism represents not a trap [Irigarary] falls into but rather a key strategy she puts into play, not a dangerous oversight but rather a lever of displacement" (72). The last two lines could also apply to Stampa.

18. Sylvia Ferino-Pagden and Maria Kusche, *Sofonisba Anguissola: Renaissance Woman* (Washington, DC: National Museum of Women in the Arts, 1995), 16.

19. Margaret King, "Book Lined Cells: Women and Humanism in the Early Italian Renaissance" in *Beyond Their Sex*, ed. by Patricia H. Labalme (New York: NY University Press, 1980), 79–80.

20. I follow Fredrika Jacobs in using this term, which she develops extensively in her chapter, "(Pro)creativity" in *Defining the Renaissance Virtuosa: Women Artists and the Language of Art History and Criticism* (Cambridge: Cambridge University Press, 1997), 27–63.

21. Joseph Koerner, *The Moment of Self-Portraiture in German Renaissance Art*. (Chicago: University of Chicago Press, 1993), 3.

22. One could argue that Anguissola simply lacked the technical ability to accurately portray herself; however, the other beautifully proportioned, technically accomplished portraits she created at this time undermine this line of reasoning. See examples of paintings completed in the 1540s and 1550s in Ilya Perlingieri's *Sofonisba Anguissola: The First Great Woman Artist of the Renaissance* (New York: Rizzoli, 1992), 76–103.

23. Ferino-Pagden remarks on the mystery of the initials, which do not represent any of the Anguissola family as might be expected (23); the speculation about the possibility of the recipient's initials is my own.

24. (VII, 26). Noted in Henrich Schwarz, "The Mirror of the Artist and the Mirror of the Devout," 99.

25. Mary D. Garrard, "Here's Looking at Me: Sofonisba Anguissola and the Problem of the Woman Artist." *Renaissance Quarterly* 47, no. 3 (Fall, 1994): 556–622, 586.

26. Phillip Sohm, "Gendered Style in Italian Art Criticism from Michelangelo to Malvasia," *Renaissance Quarterly* 48 (Winter, 1995): 759–808; 787.

27. Giorgio Vasari, *Le Vite* ..., ed. Gaeano Milanesi (Florence, 1906), 6: 498–9. For a more complete discussion of Vasari's comments, and particularly of the 'domestication' inherent in his characterization, see Naomi Yavneh's essay, "To Bare or Not too Bare: Sofonisba Anguissola's Nursing Madonna and the Womanly Art of Breastfeeding" in this volume.

28. Tommaso Cavalieri (letter) quoted in Garrard, "Here's Looking," 611.

29. Marsilio Ficino, *Commentarium in Convivio Platonis*, 207, quoted in Patricia Rielly, "The Taming of the Blue," in *The Expanding Discourse: Feminism and Art History* (New York: Icon Editions, 1992), 92. Ficino also notes that this heaven-

inspired individual would "naturally love men more than women," since the former were understood to be more perfect than the latter.

30. *Paragone: A Comparison of the Arts by Leonardo da Vinci*, 104, quoted in Rielly, 89.

31. Anguissola's deliberate reference to St. Luke in the *Self-Portrait at Easel* is noted by Angela Ghirardi in her article on "Lavinia Fontana allo specchio" in *Lavinia Fontana* (Milano: Electa, 1994), 41.

32. Despite Michelangelo's efforts to associate painting with feminine activity, particular kinds of brushwork were considered masculine and vigorous, and Marco Boschini characterized the "painter's brush" as "manly" (Boschini, *La Carta del navegar pitoresco*, 1660, 678, quoted in Sohm, 798). It seems to me that the *appiagiamano*, or mahlstick, pictured in the *Self-Portrait at Easel* may be deliberately employed to underplay the assertion implied in Anguissola's representation.

Midwiving Virility in Early Modern England

Caroline Bicks

In 1651, a continuation of Sir Philip Sidney's unfinished *Arcadia* appeared in print. The author, a young woman named Anna Weamys, had taken great liberties with Sidney's earlier story lines, ignoring or rewriting sections of his original texts. In a poem commending Weamys and her pastoral romance, one writer mused:

> She's young, but yet ingeniously will tell
> You pretty stories, and handsomely will set
> An end to what great Sidney did beget,
> Yet never perfected; these embryons she
> Doth midwife forth in full maturity.[1]

The poet casts Weamys and her work as both inconsequential and indelibly authoritative: she is "young," and her stories are "pretty," words that suggest a quaint immaturity; at the same time, she "ingeniously" and "handsomely" crafts what she tells into a permanent "end" to the "great Sidney['s]" tale. By rewriting the great man's story, Weamys compromises Sidney's narrative virility with her own female touch: he begets imperfect embryons, while she "doth midwife forth" a mature finale.

Midwifery had long been used as a trope for the production of ideas; my argument here is that in the early modern period midwifery and its female practitioners embodied specific concerns about how the narratives that defined and underpinned male authority were produced. As Natalie Zemon Davis and others have argued, early modern childbirth provided a space within which typical gendered power relations were inverted.[2] Birth was generally an all-female affair throughout Europe in the sixteenth century, and in England well into the eighteenth.[3] State officials relied on the notion that a woman in the throes of labor would be likely to utter the truth about her child's father; consequently, they needed the testimony of birth attendants both to expose delinquent fathers and to quell the fears of anxious patriarchs in need of a legitimate heir.[4] The women of the birthroom, then, could compromise the physical and discursive sites of virility's production: they occupied the husband's marital bedchamber both during and up to a month after the birth, and reminded him of his inferior narrative powers when it came to telling stories about his wife and her offspring.

During the sixteenth century, female tales and the activities of the birthroom were becoming inextricably bound: "gossip," a formerly unisex term that designated a godparent or a confidant, came to mean both a female birth attendant and a female tattler.[5] Although there was a technical distinction between a midwife and a gossip – the latter being a friend or neighbor, but sometimes the child's deliverer as well – medical and literary texts often conflated these two figures and what they did together within the all-female birthroom. The gendered semantic shift of the term "gossip" and the conflation of gossips and midwives were part of a larger anxiety about the tales women scripted in this space, and specifically about the midwife's authorized yet troubling role as testifier to paternity and hence to female sexual behavior. Her stories could initiate a narrative about a man's virility that might not match his own. Whether or not they knew more than the husband or the state, birth attendants witnessed and testified to what few men could lay claim to having seen or known.

When Anna Weamys finished what the master started, she provoked an obstetrical poetics that embodied all of these concerns about the power of female narratives to tamper with male-authored genealogies of literary and monarchical figureheads – and perhaps to turn men like the "great Sidney" into a feminized, ineffective Astrophil who, at the start of Sidney's lyric sequence, is "great with child to speake, and helplesse in my throwes."[6] The poet who commends Weamys plays with language that initially diminishes but ultimately upholds her stories, hence enacting the ambivalence that characterized how early modern culture responded to the midwife's tales. In what follows, I will begin with the question of how "great" early modern men sought to control the terms of their progeny, focusing on Tudor England's midwifery regulations in conjunction with its precarious monarchical line; then I will turn to the early modern male subject more generally and examine a medical tale that explicitly connected a man's physical and rhetorical virility to the will of the midwives and gossips.

Midwives and Monarchs

The epistemological competition between male and female tales of paternity acquired particular significance in sixteenth-century England as the new Tudor monarchy sought to legitimize itself. Henry VIII famously invested much of his authority in redefining the rules of marriage and heredity – and, in so doing, creating his version of the Tudor family history – in his search for a legitimate male heir. In 1534 Johanne Hammulden, a Watlington midwife, and Mrs. Burgyn, a woman she had attended, were brought in for questioning before a quorum of justices at Reading: the midwife claimed that, while she was helping Burgyn to deliver, the woman had impugned Henry's new queen, Anne Boleyn. According to Hammulden, Burgyn had complimented her midwifery skills, telling her that she "might be mydwyff unto the queen of England if it were Quene Kateryn; [but] if it wer Queen Anne she was too good to be her mydwyf, for [Anne] was a hoore and a herlott."[7] Three months earlier, Parliament had supported Henry by passing the Act of Succession, invalidating his marriage to Catherine and naming Mary an illegitimate daughter, while validating Anne and her subsequent issue. Burgyn's claim that the new queen was a whore contradicted the official narrative of the royal family that Henry and his advisers had promoted. Hammulden allegedly had related this incident to a group of men that included the town constable, and the women were then brought in for a formal deposition.

The inherent instability of all these narratives, however, becomes explicit upon closer scrutiny of this story. The deposition exists only in the form of a letter from Sir Walter Stonor to Thomas Cromwell; as Stonor reports, "there is no reycorde of neyther of their sayings." Furthermore, the reliability of the midwife's testimony is tainted by her claim that "she wolde never have uttryed the words" if Burgyn had not threatened to do her harm. Burgyn "denyith that ever she spake any suche words" against the queen, but does claim to have heard that Hammulden had made treasonous comments about Boleyn to another of her laboring clients. Not only is Hammulden and Burgyn's testimony entirely hearsay passed from a knight to the king's secretary, it is infinitely elusive and revisable as the women utter and deny at will.

Stonor's report, however inconclusive, verifies the concerns of a monarchy and an age that sought to monitor and control both its women of child-bearing age and the spread of treasonous information. In the public medium of the deposition, Henry's judiciary machinery mobilized its defense of the king's word by outlawing what had originated as birthroom gossip and rendering it, like Catherine and Mary, illegitimate. At the same time, the birthroom in this narrative functions as a site of female-generated tales propagated at the expense of the monarchy: despite its attempts to cast doubt on the women's words, the letter provides an official space in which women gossip about the new queen's sexual behavior, opening up the possibility of revising Tudor family history and rescripting its genealogical future.

It is no coincidence that "gossip" as a term meaning a female birth attendant and a tattler was entering the English language at the same time that Hammulden and Burgyn's birthroom conference entered the public sphere of the courtroom. But the same institutions that sometimes railed against these female tales desperately *needed* the midwife's word, for she was the court-appointed ambassador of the birth chamber. Midwifery regulation and licensing was first instated in England roughly at this time.[8] A close reading of the midwife's oath reveals the ambiguous status of these specifically female deliveries. When Eleanor Pead took the first recorded midwife's oath in 1567, she had to swear the following: "I will not permit ... that any woman being in labor ... shall name any other to be the father of her child, than only he who is the right and true father thereof."[9] The oath makes explicit that paternity was fashioned by the words of two women: the mother and the midwife. And ultimately it was up to the midwife to deliver this genealogical news to a wider public.

This paradoxical definition of female narrative as both intrinsic and injurious to male authority subtends many early modern texts, from the consciously fictional to the purportedly objective. The result is a constant flux between female testimony that subverts and female testimony that affirms male-authored narratives of royal power and patriarchy. In Shakespeare's *The Winter's Tale*, for instance, an irate Leontes calls Paulina a "midwife" when she presents him with his Queen's daughter and insists upon his paternity.[10] Paulina was not present at Perdita's birth, but because her narrative contradicts the King's tale of an adulteress wife and a bastard daughter, the epithet and its hostile context suit her. Ultimately, the midwife's word trumps the King's: Paulina's testimony is validated by the gods themselves and by the scene of familial reunion with which the play concludes. As the title (and the "midwife") remind us, however, testimony and tales are often indistinguishable. Paulina points to this narrative instability in the final scene: "That she is living, / Were it but told you, should be hooted at / Like an old tale" (5.3.115–17).

Shakespeare underscored this epistemological uncertainty when he created Paulina's doppelganger a few years later, the Old Lady in *Henry VIII* (a play with the alternate and provocative title *All is True*). Henry first receives news of Elizabeth's birth from the Old Lady, and its delivery mocks the notion of narrative stability:

> *King.*   Now by thy looks
> I guess thy message. Is the Queen deliver'd?
> Say ay, and of a boy.
> *Old L.*   Ay, ay my leige,
> And of a lovely boy. The God of heaven
> Both now and ever bless her! 'tis a girl
> Promises boys hereafter ...
>
> (5.1.161–6)

The Old Lady's conscious manipulation of the midwife's testimonial language turns the great king into a victim of her syntactic games. "Ay, ay my liege, / And of a lovely boy" becomes its disappointing opposite, "'tis a girl," in the space of one contextualizing phrase; "promises boys hereafter" stands as a hollow genealogical promise that Shakespeare's Jacobean audience knew all too well had not been kept. The moment epitomizes what Phyllis Rackin has termed "women as anti-historians" in Shakespeare's plays: "historiography itself becomes problematic, no longer speaking with the clear, univocal voice of unquestioned tradition but represented as a dubious construct."[11] When Henry gives the Old Lady a hundred marks for her troubles (inadequate compensation in her eyes), she delivers a final blow to the King's already shaky tales of legitimacy and genealogy: "Said I for this, the girl was like to him? / I'll have more, or else unsay't" (174–5).

"If it be a man chylde"

Early modern concerns for the authority of male-authored narratives were central and troubling components of the Tudor family romance. At the same time, these fears that found such vibrant expression in the figure of the midwife went well beyond monarchs to encompass the fashioning of all European male subjects and their virility. Nowhere is this idea more clear than in the male-authored midwifery texts from the period that claimed to present objective and authoritative facts about birth. Men were not generally authorized to attend regular deliveries. With the exception of handbooks written by surgeons who would have attended emergency deliveries, the parts of their texts that presented birth scenes were often blatant fictions.[12] Medical men were usually one step removed from their material, whereas female midwives who talked and later wrote about their experiences had the advantage over most of their male colleagues of actually witnessing and handling deliveries.

One scientific belief that was developing at this time provides a fruitful opportunity for exploring this struggle for narrative authority both between midwives and medical men and between midwives and men more generally: the connection between the length of the umbilical cord and the length of a man's penis and tongue. Laurent Joubert wrote in 1578 that "Man is no sooner born than he undergoes surgery: the cutting of the navel string, which midwives remove after tying it off."[13] This operation had been in the hands of midwives for at least as long as medical texts had been in the hands of men: Aristotle and Hippocrates both singled her out as the cutter of the umbilical cord.[14] In early modern Europe the operation was considered such a central duty of the midwife that Rider's 1612 *Dictionary* gave the following definition: "Obstetrix, f. *Midwives that cut the navels of young children*."[15]

Although instructions for midwives cutting the umbilical cord appear in texts as ancient as Soranus' second-century *Gynecology*, the operation acquired added significance during the medieval period. A popular text attributed to the twelfth-century healer Trotula describes how the "*virga virilis*," the "virile wand," is made greater or smaller depending on how much of the cord was left after it was cut.[16] Medical writers meticulously documented and illustrated this idea, attributing the phenomenon to a ligament running from the bottom of the bladder to the navel.

Sometime during the sixteenth century, another tale about the umbilical cord regularly began to circulate within medical discourse. *The Byrth of Mankynde*, the first midwifery text published in English (1540), describes the following: "some say that of what length the reste of the navell is lefte / of the same length shall the chyldes tonge be / yf it be a man chylde."[17] Unlike the earlier link of the umbilical cord to the genitals, this theory connecting it to the organ of male speech remained unexplained by the medical community. Still, by the seventeenth century, many midwifery handbooks propagated both stories side by side. What is significant about the coincidence of these concepts in the early modern period is that a man's physical and verbal virility were imagined as being inextricably linked: at one moment, one *woman* determined the potency of England's future patriarchs.

These medical narratives that connected the male tongue, the "*virga virilis*," and the will of the midwife are clearly inflected by larger cultural concerns about female power over the virility of the early modern male subject. When we read such tales as part of a developing history that often placed gossip and female narrative in a problematically authoritative position, the stakes become even higher. Midwifery handbooks, many of them positioned as being written for women by men, provided an explicit forum for these implicit concerns about male authority versus female practice. The authors of these texts, publishing in the vernacular for the first time, publicly grappled to privilege the male word over that of the midwife, attempting to dispel the fears generated by the fact of her potentially superior knowledge in matters of paternity and sexuality. As Nicholas Culpeper asserts in his *Directory for Midwives*, "God speaks not now by voice to Men and Women as formerly he did; but he speaks in, and by Men, and tis no part of wisdom for Men and Women to stop their Ears against it."[18]

Tales of the tongue and the navel cord epitomized the problem of presenting a male midwifery text as an authorized narrative in the face of female experience and testimony. As the competition between medical men and mid-wives grew more overt over the course of the seventeenth century, discussions of the navel string began to appear alongside extensive disparagements of the midwife's judgement.[19] Male authors sometimes derided the beliefs, calling them "a mere Abuse"[20] and "a flagrant error."[21] It was not uncommon to attribute these theories to female-propagated lore, an attempt perhaps to mitigate the daunting vision of women toying with men's bodies. At the same time, the fact of the midwife's and the gossip's authority was potent enough to engender all-female scenes of genital and lingual reconstruction.

The enormously popular *Childe-Birth, or the Happy Deliverie of Women*, a 1612 translation of the royal surgeon Jacques Guillemeau's 1606 French text, ventriloquizes the voices of the birthroom women amidst its description of the navel string:

> Some do observe, that the Navell must be tyed longer, or shorter, according to the difference of the sexe, allowing more measure to the males: because this length doth make their tongue, and privie membres the longer: whereby they may both speake the plainer, and be more serviceable to Ladies. And that by tying it short, and almost close to the belly in females, their tongue is lesse free, and their naturall part more straite: And to speake the truth, the Gossips commonly say merrily to the Midwife; if it be a boy, *Make him good measure*; but if it be a wench, *Tye it short*.[22]

Putting the question of female newborns aside for the moment, Guillemeau here projects anxieties about male genital size and speech onto the all-female birth community. Carla Mazzio discusses this passage in her incisive analysis of "the imagined relationship between rhetorical and sexual performance" in the sixteenth and seventeenth centuries. In an essay that traces the culturally-inflected basis of this belief, she surprisingly concludes from Guillemeau's vision of the childbirth community that "this relationship was, for many midwives and 'gossips,' *a matter of fact*" (emphasis mine).[23] As Ann Jones has reminded us, however, "a woman represented in a text written by a man is a literary construction, not a historical woman."[24] Guillemeau's text is not a reliable record of women's beliefs and activities; but rather, it exemplifies how a cultural fiction could be mapped as a "matter of fact" onto communities that rarely documented themselves and their practices. Like Stonor's letter to Cromwell or Shakespeare's *Henry VIII*, Guillemaeau's *Happy Deliverie* is a male fashioning of female speech as unreliable gossip – a construction that ironically calls attention to the flimsy foundations of narrative authority itself.

In its translation, the text foregrounds even more clearly the gendered nature of this struggle for the last word: Guillemeau's French "*Dames*" become English "gossips." At the same time, his "*Sage Femme*" becomes the "midwife": her wisdom is lost in translation – what remains is her status "with-woman," the literal meaning of "midwife." In this English text in particular, then, the manipulative midwife and the gossips that egg her on are figures of female collusion, of sexual and verbal emasculation. Although the English translator may be attempting to control the status of these troubling beliefs by rendering them the ephemeral product of gossip (he remarks in a marginal note that this is "A common saying of women"), the text provides a pictorial and verbal space within which women ultimately do have the last word.

Some authors negotiated their discomfort with these domestic medical stories by displacing them onto foreign communities. John Bulwer attributes the extremely long penises of men from New Guinea to the actions of that country's midwives: "It may be these *Guineans* tamper not with Nature but have this prerogative from the subtle indulgency of their Midwives ... Now if the supposition be true, we are all at the mercy of the Midwives for our sufficiencie."[25] While purportedly exposing a bizarre foreign practice at the hands of indulgent, lustful midwives, Bulwer tellingly slips into the first person of an Englishman. Why are "we" all at the mercy of the Midwives if these women are safely overseas? As Bulwer's text demonstrates, there was a fine line, embodied in the navel string's own tenuous status, between virility and impotence. As *The Compleat Midwife's Practice Enlarged*, a compilation of advice from the most popular male-authored texts of the seventeenth century, warns: "the Midwives are from hence advertised, that they do not spoil the harvest of generation by cutting the sithe too short."[26]

Despite these many stories in which men's bodies are at the mercy of women, the midwife is rarely figured as a castrator. Her knitting hands threaten the sites of male sexual and narrative virility not by diminishing a man's sexual prowess or discursive gifts, but by manipulating them to serve female desire. Nicholas Culpeper writes in 1651 that midwives who cut the cords of male infants "would have the Instrument of Generation long, that so they may not be Cowards in the Schools of *Venus*."[27] Culpeper's vision, in which midwives force men to matriculate into a school headed by the goddess of Love, epitomizes the threat to male autonomy and control that these women and their communities posed. Over the century, writers built on and expanded each other's stories, adding their individual interests and fears to their culture's general concerns. Bulwer included Culpeper's phrase in his discussion of the New Guinea midwife, and in 1671 William Sermon lifted Guillemeau's passage *verbatim*, inserting his own disparaging view on the type of woman (or man) who would encourage this manipulation of the male body: "it doth make their Tongues and privy Members longer; by which means they will speak the plainer, and become the more serviceable to Ladies (or to such as delight in long things)."[28]

The midwife tampers with virility on a number of levels in all of these examples: as was generally believed at the time, extreme length made male seed inviable. By elongating the penis, she interfered with a man's lineal future: William Harvey speaks of the genitalia as being "by the string tyed to eternity" – the image is an apt one, recalling the fragility of genealogical narratives.[29] Helkiah Crooke explicitly places this power in the midwife's hands when he states that the penis "will be longer if the Navill-strings bee not close knit by the Midwife when the childe is new borne."[30] By falling victim to a grown woman's sexual desires, the man in these medical stories becomes significantly passive: he is, after all, an infant when the primal scene of bodily composition occurs.

Of primary interest here, men imagined the tongue, the organ of voiced narratives, as being reconstructed and redirected by the midwife and gossips to satisfy the women's own tales of seduction. Together, his speech and privy member service the entire woman – doubly effeminized, he becomes a slave to both her body and her narrative desires. Whereas plain speech was traditionally revered as a virile, effective style in the Renaissance, to "speak the plainer" in these texts marks a loss of a man's control over his sexual and verbal performance.[31] Like the long penis that inhibits procreative power but pleases women, the long tongue will say what women want to hear, but has no agency or potency outside of this restricted context. Paradoxically, the midwife gives him the power to speak in the most manly, "plain" way, but because that power depends upon *hers*, it is compromised – rendered potentially invalid at the very moment of its formulation.

In his treatise on the larynx, Julius Casserius, a Paduan physician writing in the late sixteenth century, warns against tampering with the organs of voice, connecting such corruption to a complete disruption of male power. He describes how the strength of a man's voice determines his ability to maintain his dominant position both at home and in the public domain: "our speech is taken from us if the larynx and the other instruments of voice are corrupted ...; we cannot rejoice in the intercourse of our fellows or share our ideas with others; nor do we have the ability to give our servants and maids their orders, to rule our household or to hold a good position either in private or public life."[32] Without speech, a man loses the ability to construct his position through the verbalizing of orders and ideas. Although Casserius does not directly blame anyone for instances where these "instruments of voice are corrupted," he later provides a telling image, likening the nerves that control the laryngeal muscles to "the little wheel, or instrument, by means of which spinning women roll up their thread."[33] This richly evocative moment recalls the age-old association of female story-telling and spinning, one that goes back to the Fates who cut the thread of life and so determined the longevity of each man's personal narrative. The locus of control over the instruments of voice lies mythically in the hands and the tales of women; the threads that they wind and the cords that the midwives cut occupy the same symbolic space.

Illustrations included with a text attributed to Casserius, *De formato foetu*, graphically foreground the gendered nature of these physiological tales. The male fetus is shown lying passive, still attached by the umbilical cord to a placenta that threatens to drag him down. The engraving emphasizes the male's reliance on an infantilizing and materially female world (Fig. 3.1). The female fetus, however, is actively sitting up. She pulls at her umbilical veins, one reaching toward the tongue, the other away from the genital area (Fig. 3.2). Whereas the male begins his life as a passive victim, the female appears to marionette her own sexual and verbal future.[34] This illustration of the female

TABVLÆ SEPTIMÆ
EXPLICATIO.

T Abula hæc septima vasa umbilicalia, & membranas, sive involucra fœtus explicat.

AAAA. Abdominis musculi, & peritonæum, ipsaque cutis crucis modo dissecta, & retrorsum flexa.

B. Hepar fœtus gibba sua parte prominens.

C. Vesica urinaria.

D. Rima seu fissura hepatis, in quam vena umbilicalis ingreditur.

E. Vena umbilicalis ipsa.

FF. Duæ arteriæ umbilicales deorsum ad iliacas arterias tendentes.

G. Vrachus ex vesica fundo prodiens.

H. Vasa umbilicalia extra corpus fœtus existentia quomodo conjuncta sint.

I. Membrana, quæ vasa umbilicalia extra ventrem involvit.

KKKK. Intestina fœtus.

LLL. Vasa umbilicalia à chorio ad fœtum extensa, & in modum funis longa, ac intorta.

M. Locus ubi rami vasorum umbilicalium in truncos collecti primum sunt.

NNNN. Ramus venæ umbilicalis per carnosam placentam chorii sparsus.

OOOO. Ramus arteriæ umbilicalis.

PPPP. Conjunctio ipsius venæ & arteriæ umbilicalis per placentam dissenimatæ.

QQQQ. Extrema ora venarum, & arteriarum umbilicalium desinentium in circumferentiam placentæ chorii.

RRR. Chorium.

aaaa. Vmbra, quam quatuor vasa umbilicalia in altum elevata in subjectis partibus efficiunt.

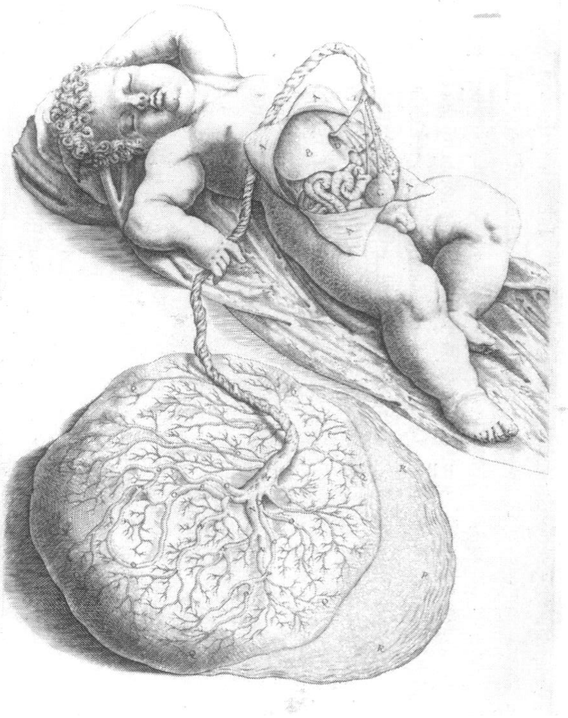

Fig. 3.1 Male foetus, from *De formato foetu*, in *Opera*, Sigelius, 1645

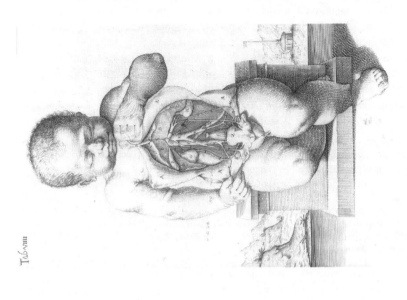

Tab. VIII

Tab. VIII

TABVLE NONÆ
EXPLANATIO.

Abula hæc nona continet muliebria omnia genitalia in fœtu.

AAAA. *Totum abdomen, hoc est quatuor tegumenta communia una cum musculis abdominis, & peritonæo cruci modo dissectum, reflexumque.*

B.   *Vena umbilicalis.*
CC. *Rima hepatis quam vena umbilicalis ingreditur.*
DD. *Sima pars hepatis.*
E.   *Rima ad sima hepatis usque pertingens.*
F.   *Vesica fellis.*
G.   *Dexter ren.*
H.   *Ren sinister.*
IIII. *Vtriusque renis vreteres.*
KK. *Vena emulgens sinistra.*
LL. *Divisio venæ emulgentis ante ingressum.*
MM. *Duæ venulæ, dextræ emulgentis vena vicem in hoc corpore gerentes.*

N.   *Arteria spermatica dextra.*
O.   *Vena spermatica dextra.*
QQQ *Truncus venæ cavæ.*
RRR. *Truncus arteriæ aortæ.*
SS. *Arteriæ iliacæ à quibus oriuntur arteriæ umbilicales.*
T.   *Alius ramus arteriæ aortæ.*
V.   *Ramus arteriæ iliacæ ad uterum pergens.*
XXXX. *Arteriæ umbilicales.*
YY. *Arteria spermatica sinistra.*
Z.   *Vterus.*
.   *Vena sinistra spermatica cum arteria se insurgens, & ad sinistrum testem defendens.*

a a. *Duo testes.*
b.   *Cervix uteri.*
cc. *Ligamenta uteri.*
d.   *Vesica, & ex ea prodiens urachus.*
f.   *Rectum intestinum.*
g g. *Gibba pars hepatis.*

Fig. 3.2   Female foetus, from *De formato foetu*, in *Opera*, Sigelius, 1645

59

fetus is a significant exception to Karen Newman's argument that "medical knowledge is visualized in early anatomy in and on a male body."[35] Unlike the open-torsoed female figures that typically appear in anatomies in their adult reproductive capacities, this figure of the female fetus displays a unique autonomy as it gestures toward an originary moment of female self-production.

These troubling images must have haunted the minds of men like Nicholas Culpeper, informing his explicit attacks on tales of virility resting in the hands of women. Culpeper wrote an extensive and anxious response to the belief in 1651, the same year that Weamys midwived Sidney's imperfect embryos:

> *Mizaldus* was in this point a little critical, and yet an honest man, and his Criticisms begat some errors in some modern writers, and in our Midwives at present: Hence (as I suppose) it comes to pass that Midwives (if *Spigelius* speak truth, or others who are but his Apes) leave a longer part of the Navel-string of a Male than they do of a Female, and their supposed Reason is this, Because in Males they would have the Instrument of Generation long, that so they may not be Cowards in the Schools of *Venus*: But in Females they cut it shorter, and that they think (forsooth) makes them modest, and their privities narrower: this *Spigelius*, and all our modern Writers jeer at.[36]

Here, Culpeper counters his female competitors with the authority of ancient and living medical writers, although, as Heather Dubrow suggests in her discussion of this passage, the rhetoric of these handbooks often volleyed between "firm assertions of authority and markers of uncertainty."[37] Culpeper suggests that the midwives are responsible for promoting this erroneous medical tale, while he and his male contemporaries "jeer" at it. Unlike Weamys's ingenious act of narrative midwifery, these midwives can only pass on the errors that Mizaldus "begat." At the same time, however, medical men had perpetuated the tale themselves in their own writings. By making room for it here, Culpeper himself gives it textual life.

By claiming that midwives sought to control the narrowness of the female genitalia as well as the size of the male organ, Culpeper and others imagined that gossips and midwives ultimately turned on their own kind, keeping them close-lipped and "modest," or "lesse free," to recall Guillemeau's translated text. In 1671, however, a midwife, Jane Sharp, did exactly the opposite when she published the first English, female-authored midwifery handbook for women. She positions her text as an all-female conference: "farther knowledge may be gain'd by a long and diligent practice, *and be communicated to others of our own sex*."[38] Sharp closely copies Culpeper's passage on the navel-string, but makes some notable changes that reveal, once again, the individual will behind medical narratives. Whereas Culpeper insists that "our Midwives at present can scarce agree," Sharp adds "Midwives *and physicians* can scarce agree" (emphasis mine),[39] and thus reconfigures the debate so that it no longer imagines disunity amongst female practitioners, but rather unity against male physicians. In another telling editorial decision, she leaves out Culpeper's claim that midwives want "the Instruments of Generation long so that men will not be Cowards in the Schools of Venus." Instead, Sharp diverts attention away from what the midwife may be doing to the male body, and focuses the activity of cutting onto the female subject: "Hence it is, if Spigelius speak truth, that Midwives cut the Females Navel-string shorter than they doe the Males, for Boys privy parts must be longer than womens." The sexually voracious female disappears in Sharp's text. In fact, Sharp reminds the reader that "Some men … have Yards so long that they are useless for generation." (p. 22).

Sharp makes no mention of the connection between the tongue and the midwife's cutting of the umbilical cord. Although she was clearly conscious of what it meant to have women address others of their own sex, she did not include the mythology of verbal emasculation that so haunted her male colleagues. Louise Bourgeois, a noted French midwife who wrote earlier in the century, similarly leaves out the scenes of lingual reconstruction that her contemporary, Guillemeau, so vividly portrayed and that Sharp's contemporary, William Sermon, similarly imagined. The belief that midwives controlled the size of a man's tongue indeed may have circulated only within male narratives scripted by authors for whom the midwife posed an authoritative threat. Sharp does, however, present her readers with a telling simile that may have been her wry contribution to the obstetrical fray: "If the Yard be of a moderate size, not too long, nor too short, it is as good as the Tongue is" (p.21). She ingeniously calls up the unsettling belief and then contains it within the realm of the midwife's poetic license.

Whereas Sharp talks around the issue of the tongue, she explicitly concurs with her male colleagues in stating that the midwife controls the male instrument of generation. She fashions this belief as fact, and bases it, not on the ancients or her contemporaries, but on the power of public opinion: "It is generally held, " Sharp writes, "that the length of the Yard depends upon cutting the Navel string; and this beside the general opinion, stands with so much reason, that all *Midwives* have cause to be careful to cut the Navel string long enough, that when they tye it, the Yard may have free liberty to move and extend itself, always remembering that moderation is best" (pp. 22–23). Sharp grants "free liberty" to the male organ, but she does so in such a way that we are reminded it is the midwife who spins and rolls up the thread of moderation.[40] "All Midwives have cause to be careful" stands as an ambiguous contribution to early modern narratives of genealogy and virility. By bringing this tale both into the realm of "reason" and uncontainable "general opinion," her words gesture toward innumerable and authorized narrative possibilities: like Anna Weamys or Shakespeare's Old Lady, it is up to each "midwife" to put her own end to what great men did beget.

Notes

I would like to thank Naomi Miller and Naomi Yavneh for their adroit comments on this essay. I am also grateful to Heather Dubrow for sharing her expertise on this topic, to the participants of the 1997 MLA convention panel sponsored by the Society for the Study of Early Modern Women for their feedback on an early version of this piece, to Jennifer Summit for directing me to the Anna Weamys text, and to Brendon Reay for his editorial assistance. Finally, I am indebted to Heidi Heilemann at Stanford University's Lane Medical Library Rare Books collection for her assistance in locating the illustrations from *De formato foetu*.

1. "On the Ingenious Continuation of Sir Philip Sidney's *Arcadia*, by Mistress A.W," in Anna Weamys, *A Continuation of Sir Philip Sidney's Arcadia*, ed. Patrick Colburn Cullen (Oxford: Oxford University Press, 1994), p. 5. Cullen suggests that the author of this poem, "W.P.M.," may be Henry Pierrepont, Marquess, but he adds that there is no evidence for this speculation. For a complete discussion of Weamys's work in its literary and historical context, see his introduction to this edition.

2. Natalie Zemon Davis was one of the first scholars to examine these power relations in her "Women on Top," in *Society and Culture in Early Modern France* (Stanford: Stanford University Press, 1975), pp. 124–51.

3. For a history of midwifery during this period, see David Cressy, *Birth, Marriage, and Death* (Oxford: Oxford University Press, 1997), pp. 35–79. For accounts of the regional and class differences within the profession, see *The Art of Midwifery: Early Modern Midwives in Europe*, ed. Hilary Marland (London: Routledge, 1993).

4. David Harley, examining court documents from Lancashire and Cheshire, illustrates how statements made to the midwife were considered more reliable than pre-labor depositions. "Provincial Midwives in England," in *The Art of Midwifery*, pp. 36–7.

5. The *OED* cites a line from Puck's first speech in Shakespeare's *A Midsummer-Night's Dream* as the first appearance of "gossip" to mean birth attendant.

6. Philip Sidney, *Astrophil and Stella*, in *Poems of Sir Philip Sidney*, ed. William Ringler, Jr. (Oxford: Clarendon Press, 1962), proem, line 12.

7. Sir Walter Stonor to Thomas Cromwell, in Sir Henry Ellis, *Original Letters, Illustrative of English History*, 3rd ser., vol. 2 (London: Richard Bentley, 1846), pp. 332–4.

8. For a detailed history of European midwifery regulations, see Thomas G. Benedek, "The Changing Relationship Between Midwives and Physicians During the Renaissance," *Bulletin of the History of Medicine* 51 (1977): 550–64.

9. John Strype, *Ecclesiastical Memorials ...* (Oxford, 1822), p. 391.

10. Leontes refers to Paulina as "Lady Margery, your midwife" (2.3.160). All citations from Shakespeare are to *The Riverside Shakespeare*, ed. G. Blakemore Evans, 2nd edn. (Boston: Houghton Mifflin, 1997). Gail Kern Paster uses this moment to argue, as I am doing here in my analysis of genealogical narratives, for "the inseparability of events within the birthing chamber from events outside of it." See her *The Body Embarrassed* (Ithaca: Cornell University Press, 1993), p. 271.

11. Phyllis Rackin, "Anti-Historians: Women's Roles in Shakespeare's Histories," in *In Another Country: Feminist Perspectives on Renaissance Drama*, ed. Dorothea Kehler and Susan Baker (London: The Scarecrow Press, 1991), p. 138.

12. For more on this history of surgeons and emergency deliveries in Europe, see Renate Blumenfeld-Kosinski, *Not of Woman Born* (Ithaca: Cornell University Press, 1990), pp. 32–47.

13. Laurent Joubert, *Popular Errors*, trans. Gregory David de Rocher (Tuscaloosa: University of Alabama Press, 1989), p. 173.

14. Aristotle, *Historia Animalium* 587a9; Hippocrates, *Muliebria* 1.68.

15. Francis Holyoke, *Riders Dictionarie, corrected ...*, 3rd edn. (Oxford, 1612).

16. Trotula, *De passionibus mulierum*, in *Gynaeciorum* (Strasbourg: Sumptibus Lazari Zetzneri, 1597), p. 49. For more on Trotula and the transmission of these texts during the medieval period see Monica Green, "Obstetrical and Gynecological texts in Middle English," *Studies in the Age of Chaucer* 14(1992): 53–88.

17. Richard Jonas, *The Byrth of Mankynde* (London, 1540), *fol.* 53.

18. Nicholas Culpeper, *A Directory for Midwives* (London, 1651), dedicatory epistle.

19. This increased competition between midwives and medical men, especially in England, has been well established. See Hilda Smith, "Gynecology and Ideology in Seventeenth-Century England," in *Liberating Women's History*, ed. Berenice A.Carroll (Urbana: University of Illinois Press, 1976), pp. 97–114. More recently, see Adrian Wilson, *The Making of Man-Midwifery* (London: University College London Press, 1995).

20. Francis Mauriceau, *The Diseases of Women with Child, and in Child-Bed*, trans. Hugh Chamberlen (London, 1710), p. 303.

21. Joubert, p.175.

22. Jacques Guillemeau, *Childe-birth, or the Happy Deliverie of Women* (London, 1612), p. 99.

23. Carla Mazzio, "Sins of the Tongue," in *The Body in Parts*, ed. David Hillmann and Carla Mazzio (New York: Routledge, 1997), p. 59.

24. Ann Rosalind Jones, preface to the special issue of *ELR*, Women in the Renaissance III: Studies in Honor of Ruth Mortimer, 24.1 (1994): 5.

25. John Bulwer, *Anthropometamorphosis* (London, 1654), p. 401.

26. *The Compleat Midwife's Practice Enlarged* (London, 1662), p. 48.

27. Culpeper, p. 175.

28. William Sermon, *The Ladies Companion, or the English Midwife* (London, 1671), p. 107.

29. William Harvey, *Lectures on the Whole of Anatomy*, trans. O'Malley et al. (Berkeley: University of California Press, 1961), p. 124.

30. Helkiah Crooke, *Microcosmographia* (London, 1615), p. 210.

31. For more on the plain style as virile in the early modern period, see Patricia Parker's "Virile Style," in *Premodern Sexualities*, ed. Louise Fradenburg and Carla Freccero (New York: Routledge, 1996), pp. 201–22.

32. Julius Casserius, *The Larynx, Organ of Voice*, trans. Malcolm H. Hast and Erling B. Holtsmark (Uppsala: Almquist & Wiksells, 1969), p. 14.

33. Ibid., p. 31.

34. These particular illustrations appear in Adriaan Spieghel's *Anatomica* (Amsterdam, 1645) and are included in a section *De formato foetu* attributed to Casserius in this collection. The copperplates were intended for an anatomical work by Casserius, but after Casserius' death in 1616, Spieghel (his pupil) carried on with *De formato foetu*.

35. Karen Newman, *Fetal Positions* (Stanford: Stanford University Press, 1996), p. 69. Although figure 2 is not identified in the Table as a male fetus, the few illustrations of female fetuses that do appear are explicitly labeled as "*muliebria*" or

"*foemineus*." As Newman argues, it was conventional to use male bodies as the generic anatomical model.

36. Culpeper, p.175.
37. Heather Dubrow, "Navel Battles: Interpreting Renaissance Gynecological Manuals," *ANQ* 5.2 (1992): 67–71.
38. Jane Sharp, *The Midwives Book* (London, 1671), p. 3.
39. Culpeper, p. 174; Sharp, p. 213.
40. The 1662 *Compleat Midwife's Practice Enlarg'd* uses a similar phrase, but the syntax does not place the midwife in a comparably active position: "if the Navel-string be left at a longer distance, the Urachos is enlarged, and consequently the Yard hath more liberty to extend it self" (p. 48).

CHAPTER FOUR

To Bare or Not Too Bare: Sofonisba Anguissola's Nursing Madonna and the Womanly Art of Breastfeeding

Naomi Yavneh

In 1588, Sofonisba Anguissola created a realistically depicted image of the Virgin Mary nursing Jesus (Fig. 4.1). Although nothing in the limited historical record of the reception of *La Madonna che alatta il bambino* suggests that it created any uproar,[1] the work is unusual in a variety of ways. First of all, while the *Madonna lactans* had been an extremely popular subject for Italian art during the fourteenth and early fifteenth centuries, by the sixteenth century its use was extremely limited. Although the increased naturalism in the representation of mother and child that we find in high Renaissance images serves to enhance the intimacy so central to the depiction of the nursing dyad, it likewise creates greater anxiety about the use of this particular theme, especially as the erotic breast comes to be more commonly depicted.[2] Moreover, as late-Cinquecento theologians attempted to distance themselves from the iconoclasm and saint-rejection of the Protestants, they privileged Mary's sanctity and queenly exaltation over the humility which earlier had served to make her more accessible to the common worshiper. Thus, homely themes such as the *Madonna lactans* were all but completely replaced by the Immaculate Conception, Assumption and Coronation, emphasizing the Virgin's unique purity and distinction from all other women. Finally, *any* painting by Sofonisba Anguissola must perforce be considered extraordinary by virtue of its creation and reception: her status as highly celebrated as well as highly respectable woman artist makes her – almost like the Virgin herself – virtually "alone of all her sex."[3] But the particular choice of subject is in itself unusual, for although religious works are not unknown among her *oeuvre*, Anguissola is primarily known as a portraitist.

How, then, are we to understand the *Madonna che alatta il bambino*? Why

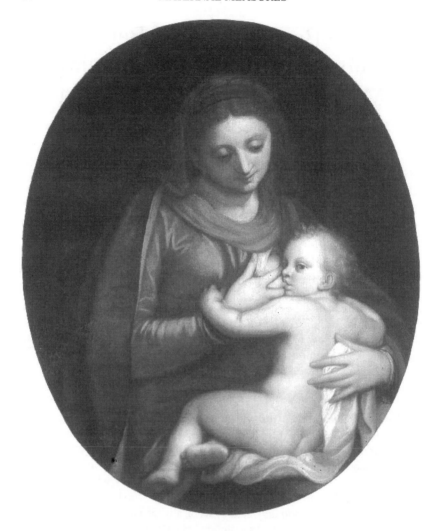

Fig. 4.1   Sofonisba Anguissola, *The Madonna Nursing the Christ Child*, 1588

do we find this almost uniquely naturalistic representation of a breastfeeding Virgin painted by a major woman artist at a time when the subject had largely fallen out of use and developments in the post-Tridentine Church emphasized Mary's glory rather than her humility?

In order to respond to these questions, we must first examine the role of the nursing Madonna at the height of its popularity, distancing ourselves from preconceived notions about the representation of a naked breast. As Megan

Holmes has noted, the topic of Mary's "nudity" has received considerable attention from scholars who question "whether the Virgin's breast, bared for the Christ Child to suckle, was understood by contemporaries in terms of established religious doctrine, or whether it had the potential to trigger erotic associations."[4] Holmes follows Margaret Miles in emphasizing the remarkably unrealistic and thus desexualizing depiction of the Virgin's "one bare breast" in the fourteenth and early fifteenth centuries; as in Fig. 4.2, such a breast "is partially covered with the Virgin's veil and drapery; it is displaced to the level of her collarbone, detached from her body and distorted in size and shape."[5] This active avoidance of the sexualization of the breast suggests a conscious attempt to avoid any inference of an already existing erotic significance.

Part of the critical problem in understanding the *Madonna lactans* stems from the incredible anachronism created by late twentieth-century perceptions of breastfeeding and exposed breasts; in American society, the erotic aspect of the breast has been so privileged over the nutritive that numerous states have had to pass legislation legally defining the act of breastfeeding in public as *not* obscene. But perhaps more significantly, while we cannot (and should not) deny the sexual connotations of breasts for the late-Medieval and early-Renaissance viewer (Dante, after all, denounces the exposed nipples of fashionable Florentine women, while, as Marilyn Yalom points out, French narratives of courtly love from as early as the twelfth century leave no room for lactation in their praise of firm, white, apple-like breasts)[6], we must also remember that the Virgin is not merely baring her breasts but using them to feed her child. And in a breastfeeding culture, the primary association of a breastfeeding breast is food.

In the days before refrigeration and formula, access to fresh breast milk – whether from a wet nurse or the child's own mother – was quite literally a matter of life and death. Although early modern medicine was not familiar with the almost miraculous immunological and species-specific nutritive qualities of human milk, doctors, theologians and lay-people were quite aware of the dangers posed by feeding a baby the milk of a goat or some other animal. According to humoral theory, milk is but a whitened form of the blood that nourished the child *in utero*;[7] just as that blood has formed the fetus, influencing the baby's corporeal and emotional development before birth, so the milk continues to shape the child both physically and morally after, so that he takes on the qualities of whoever nurses him. Goat's milk, accordingly, is likely to leave the child looking "stupid and vacant and not right in the head"[8] but the milk of an immoral wet nurse is equally threatening. In Tuscany, these perceived as well as other real dangers posed to the child by the increasingly popular practice of wet-nursing among the upper and middle classes became of central importance during a period of demographic catastrophe such as the Trecento, when repeated seasons of famine in the first half of the century were

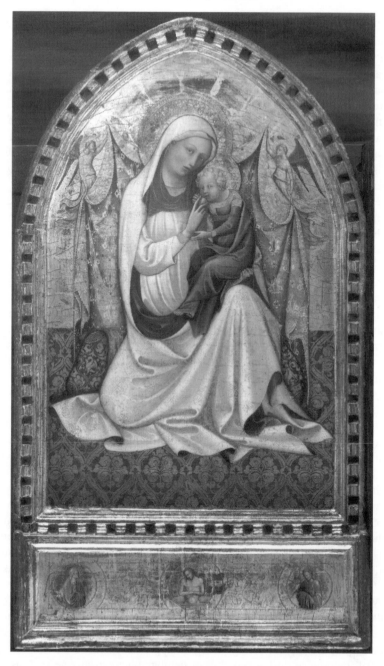

Fig. 4.2   Lorenzo da Monaco and Assistant [Bartolomeo di Fruosino?], *Madonna of
             Humility*, c. 1410

followed by the utter devastation of the black death starting in 1347. As Margaret Miles has demonstrated, to a more than decimated population, the image of the Virgin feeding her own obviously robust child would have been striking indeed. If the blessed Mother of God condescends to nurse her Son, who are her worshipers not to follow her example?

This persuasive function of the *Madonna lactans* is dependent upon the exemplarity which is one of the outstanding features of Marian devotion in the late Medieval-early Renaissance period. In Catholic doctrine, the Virgin Mary holds a unique position as mediatrix between her son and his people. Accordingly, although not divine herself, she is the object of *hyperdulia*, a form of adoration below the *laetria* offered to the Trinity, but above the *dulia* owed to God's saints. Yet beyond the technicalities of doctrine, the mother of God was the single most important female in the Church, the second Eve whose chastity and humility redeem the fault perpetrated by her ancestor. She is distinguished both by her conformity to and distinction from the lived experience of the Christian, for while she herself may have been conceived without sin[9] and given birth effortlessly and virginally, she is first and foremost a mother who nurtures, nourishes and finally buries her child.

For the fourteenth century especially, her exemplarity lies in the humility which, paradoxically, exalts her. In Dante's terms, Mary is "umile e alta più che creatura" (*Par. XXXIII*, 2); chosen by God to bear God, she willingly submits to the Lord's will and nurses her child – a task that in the early modern period is not only unfashionable, but of some risk to the mother's health and appearance.[10]

If we view the fourteenth century *Madonna lactans* as pro-maternal lactation propaganda, the *bambino* of Ambrogio Lorenzetti's *Madonna del latte* (c. 1340; Fig. 4.3) is quite a convincing poster Child: while the typical *puer senex* of the period – the "little old man" style of Baby Jesus whose wisdom belies his years (see, for example, Fig. 4.2, Lorenzo da Monaco and Assistant [Bartolomeo di Fruosino?]'s *Madonna of Humility* or Giotto's *Ognissanti Madonna* [1305]) – underscores the former term in the Incarnation miracle of *God* made man, this Jesus insists that not only was God made man, but a real *baby*. In contrast to the rather flat and iconic presentation of the body of the Virgin, whose almond eyes, semi-profile and plate-like halo create a Byzantine effect, Jesus is a large and robust toddler with curly blond hair and large, round eyes, who pushes with his foot against his mother's arm in a homely gesture familiar to anyone who has nursed an older baby. Lines in his arms suggest the fat-folds of a well-fed child, while the modeling in the folds of the shawl in which the Virgin has wrapped him, and from which he has freed his chunky left leg, suggest a real substance to his body, as does the Virgin's right hand, which realistically grips the buttocks of a seemingly heavy and active baby.

Although the Madonna's gaze is directed at his face, her son's direct glance at the viewer, designed to render the spectator a participant in the painting's action, has special significance for this particular subject: the Virgin is not only mother to her son but *Mater* and therefore (in Anselm's terms) *nutricula nostra*, nurse of the faithful. And Christ's suckling of the whitened blood which is his mother's milk is a recollection of the Eucharist, reminding us of our own obligation and blessing to feed off the body and blood of Christ.

But the *Madonna del latte* is more than an allegory of Communion; what is noteworthy in Lorenzetti's representation of the subject is the artist's surprising naturalism. While Jesus turns his face to the viewer, he leaves his body turned toward the Virgin and her nipple in his mouth. According to Millard Meiss, this combination of movements is "one of the most remarkable innovations of early Trecento Italian art,"[11] emphasizing an intimacy between figure and viewer which parallels that between the figures themselves. What creates that intimacy as well as the intense humanity conveyed by both the mother and son of God is not just the formal effect of the dynamic contraposto connecting the baby's body to his mother and his gaze to the viewer, but the familiarity of the scene: Jesus' turned head is not only a gesture of invitation but a recognizable realistic detail which underscores the somewhat advanced age of this baby whose own mother continues to nurse him.[12]

That outward glance – like the circular lines of the painting, the mother's downward gaze, the curved line of the baby's back, and the realistically-lifted leg – serves to direct our gaze back to the mouth suckling the breast: the work's focal point. Although Margaret Miles uses this painting as an example of the unrealistic depiction of the bare breast which is the focus of her article, the Virgin's rounded breast, with the pink suggestion of a nipple, is certainly more life-like than, for example, the fifteenth-century anonymous painting of the intercession of Christ and the Virgin, reproduced in Miles, where the breast seems to be completely detached from the Virgin's body, or the Madonnas of Lorenzo da Monaco (Fig. 4.2, c. 1410) and Carlo da Camerino (1380), reproduced in Holmes. Certainly, the right side of the Virgin's dress is flat, but the lines of her decorative veil, along with the baby's hand position, demonstrate the curve of the part of the left breast which remains covered. Rather than the same element of detached displacement evident in the other three works, we find another of Lorenzetti's attempts at realism: the modest Virgin keeps her body covered by her cloak and veil as she discreetly reveals her breast to both her son and his worshipers.

Again, this naturalism is in keeping with other such attempts in the painting. Despite the Byzantine qualities of the Virgin's face already noted and her flat body which serves primarily as the dark background to project her son's nude and solid body, the artist attempts to create depth by placing the gold halos of both mother and child in front of the purple band that borders the painting. Like

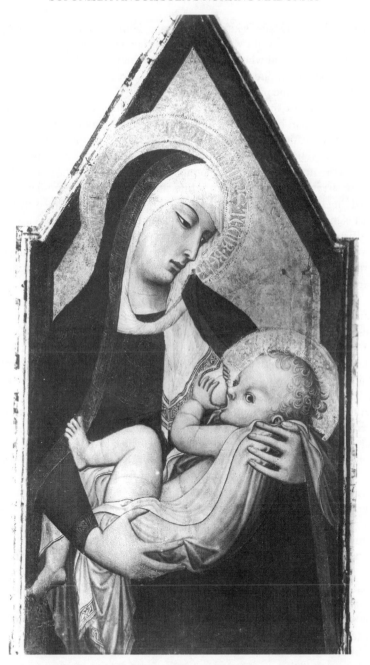

Fig. 4.3   Ambrogio Lorenzetti, *Madonna del Latte*, c. 1340. Church of San Francesco, Siena, Italy

the curved lines, the baby's knee and his gaze, both Jesus' projecting halo and the Virgin's, with the veil (whose whiteness again creates a stark contrast with her dark garments and whose decorative edge draws our attention) that leads from it to the breast, direct our gaze toward the breast – as we have seen, the central element in the painting.

Why this intense focus upon the breast? The realistic details and attempts at naturalism are part of a move in fourteenth-century religious practice towards greater identification of the devout with Jesus, Mary and the other exemplary characters of religious narrative. But the Virgin's humanity not only serves to render her more accessible to the common worshiper, it also guarantees that of her son. Breastfeeding, mother and child share a ubiquitous quotidian act, and in so doing insist upon their own flesh and blood – i.e., incarnate – selves. The breast is the point at which the miracles of both the Incarnation and Virgin birth are affirmed, where God and Virgin mother meet as humans.

According to Leo Steinberg, that Jesus eats is a sign of his humanity, affirming the miracle of the Incarnation. But the critic's convincing arguments regarding what he terms the sexualization of Christ in the high Renaissance may lead him to efface the significance of Christ's mother in the preceding century. For what he misses is that Jesus is not merely eating here, he is suckling at his mother's breast. Once again to quote Dante, Mary's is "la faccia che più somiglia a Cristo" (the face which most resembles Christ); she is the source of his human substance, both before birth, when his body is formed from the blood within her sin-free womb, and after, when he drinks the milk itself formed from that blood.

Although there is no evidence that the artist was familiar with the work by Lorenzetti we have been considering, Sofonisba Anguissola's nursing Madonna and Child of 1588 resembles the *Madonna del latte* in several ways. As in the painting created some 250 years earlier, mother and child emerge from a black background as the only figures in the painting. A demure young matron rather than a Byzantine icon, this Mary nevertheless gazes down at her large, naked, nursing son, whose body is turned toward his mother, even as his head, still attached to her nipple, turns to look at the spectator. Just as the Virgin's embracing arms serve in the earlier work both to demonstrate the real substance of the child she holds and the intimate relationship between the pair, here, the use of the oval format emphasizes the encircling arm of the mother, whose protective and nurturing embrace is echoed in the plump baby arm similarly grasping the maternal arm whose fingers guide her nipple to the baby's mouth. Again, naturalistic details like the baby's wispy curls and tucked-under foot create the sense of a real mother and child with whom we can identify.

The naturalistic appearance and affectionate intimacy are, in the late sixteenth century, nothing new to the representation of the Madonna and her child. But the specific choice of the *Madonna lactans* makes the work unusual, for, as mentioned above, while the subject had not disappeared entirely from Cinquecento Italy, it had passed out of favor for a variety of reasons.

First, the greater focus on and eroticization of the breast in sixteenth-century Italian art combined with the previous century's transition to a more naturalistic style in painting made the representation of the Virgin's breast far more vexed. This is not to suggest, however, that the Madonna and Child no longer served to underscore Christ's humanity. Rather, the emphasis shifts from mother to child. Beyond the *ostentatio genitalium* which, as Steinberg has argued, demonstrates the Incarnation doctrine that God has become man – and not just man, but often baby boy – in *all* his parts,[13] high Renaissance depictions accentuate the miracle of the Incarnation through the naturalistic representation of the physical embodiment and affectionate relationship of an adorable real-life baby boy and the beautiful mother whom he resembles: the *dolcezza* and affective intimacy of the myriad *Madonne* and children produced by Raphael and his studio are not mere sentimentality churned out in greedy response to market demands, but a theologically-significant commentary.

Raphael's *Madonna della sedia* (Fig. 4.4) typifies and perfects this lesson of humanation. Against a black background, the seated Madonna tightly embraces the chubby toddler seated facing her on a pillow on her lap, while San Giovannino, hands folded in prayer, leans into the picture plane to gaze in adoration at mother and child. As in the later Anguissola, the tondo format echoes the encircling arms of the mother and the curve of the two central figures toward each other; at the top of the painting, the line of the Virgin's head so clearly conforms to the edge of the painting that it cuts off most of her halo – a bare filament rather than elaborate gold, yet the only indication (aside from convention and the presence of John the Baptist) of the divinity of this loving and exquisite pair.

The baby may no longer be nursing, but his humanity is nevertheless accented by his interaction with the mother in whose protective arms he is tightly nestled. Although, as in the Lorenzetti, Jesus looks directly at the viewer, the stranger anxiety so common to his age group is clearly demonstrated by the way, hand tucked under her shawl, he draws back toward his mother, spreading his toes in a bobinski reflex. Again, naturalism is given a theological twist in the sad irony of this child's ultimate human – if not his divine – fate.

But while the child has become more human, in the sixteenth century the mother becomes less so. For the Catholic Church, the rejection of the Blessed Virgin's divinely privileged status was among the most troubling of the Protestant heresies. Whereas to Catholics, Mary's sanctity reaffirmed that of the son born from her virgin womb, to Protestants its assertion detracted from Christ's unique redemptive power. They thus opposed the doctrine of the Immaculate Conception, for how, they questioned, could someone be conceived

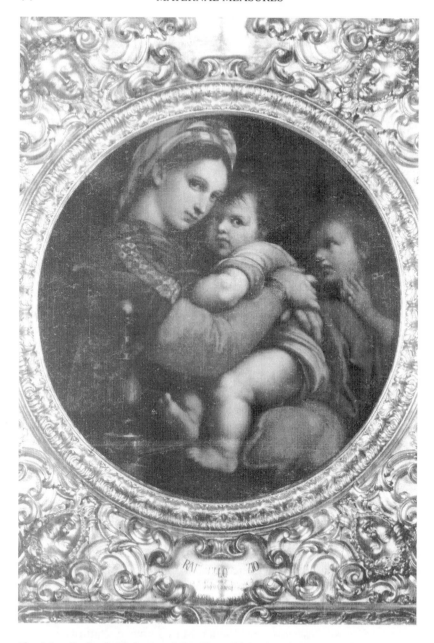

Fig. 4.4   Raphael, *Madonna of the Chair*. SOO49157, K98758, Galleria Palatina,
Palazzo Pitti, Florence, Italy

without sin *before* the Crucifixion?[14] The Virgin, like all postlapsarian humans, is redeemed only by the death of her son. According to Luther, "If you believe in Jesus Christ, you have as much sanctity as she."[15]

Historically, Marian worship has always been most devout when under attack; the iconoclast heresy of the eighth century, for example, had been a catalyst to the development of the Virgin's cult.[16] The strength of the Virgin's powers against heresy was again accented in the second half of the sixteenth century, when the attacks on her sanctity and sovereignty served to intensify her worship in the Catholic Church as virgin Mother of God and Queen of Heaven, and while the Doctrine of the Immaculate Conception did not become actual dogma until 1854, the Council of Trent affirmed that Mary was both conceived without Original Sin and Eternally virgin, and re-emphasized her powers as intercessor. We thus see a concomitant move in the multitudinous artistic depictions of the Virgin away from representations which emphasize Mary's humanity and similarity to other women, such as the *Madonna lactans*, towards images such as the Assumption and Immaculate Conception, which stress her divinely privileged difference.

Beyond their special interest in the status of the Virgin, Tridentine theologians were concerned with the function of religious images in general, and the particular problem of the erotic effect of nudity. One of the final directives of the Council was the order to paint drapes and veils over offending (i.e., naked) figures in Michelangelo's *Last Judgment,* and although the canons and decrees of the Council's final session (on the role of sacred images) are brief, numerous treatises were subsequently written in explication thereof, declaiming against both nudity and doctrinally inaccurate representations.[17]

While the *Madonna lactans* is not specifically censured in the Italian tractates, this greater concern with nudity and decorum makes the subject again problematic, although not unheard of. Titian, for example, nearing the end of his life, painted a devotional *Nursing Madonna* (c. 1570; National Gallery, London; Fig. 4.5), who, like the aged Virgin of the artist's *Pietà* (c. 1577; Academia, Venice), displays none of the "obvious and traditional trappings of sanctity."[18] According to Rona Goffen, these final Madonnas reflect a spiritual turn in the artist as he approaches the end of a long and successful artistic career.

But Titian's choice is unusual, and can hardly be considered a model for an artist such as Anguissola, known primarily for her innovations and skill as a portraitist. After all, a *gentildonna* – and for many years, Lady-in-Waiting as well as artist and teacher to the pious queens and infantas of Spain – could not respectably paint lurid histories or nudes. Yet the suggestion of Ilya Perlingieri that the subject would appeal to the woman artist as her unique opportunity to paint a nude[19] seems to fall short of the mark.

In my view, however, the artist's chaste reputation does in fact play a role in her choice of this particular subject, reflecting a conscious effort to shape her identity as an artist. In a compelling consideration of Anguissola's numerous self-portraits suggestive for our discussion, Mary Garrard demonstrates that at a time when a woman who was free with her tongue (or paintbrush) was usually presumed to be free with other body parts as well Sofonisba prided herself on and cultivated a chaste and almost austere reputation by – at least in her self-portraits – dressing in black or other dark colors, styling her hair in a demure fashion and severely limiting her use of jewelry and other ornaments.[20] Moreover, before her marriage at the very late age of about forty, she signed as many as eight of her paintings with the descriptor *virgo*, a term which suggests not only her virginal status and "impeccable morals ... but the implication of independence and self-possession, a broader metaphoric dimension that may have appealed to this female artist" (Garrard, 580).

Anguissola's self-fashioning can be seen not only in her signature and appearance, but in the very structuring of her canvases. In a process of negotiation which recalls the efforts of contemporary Italian women poets such as Gaspara Stampa to create a uniquely feminine (and feminist) version of the masculine language and subjectivity of *petrarchismo*, Sofonisba reframes the norms of sixteenth-century art. For example, as Garrard argues, the choice to represent herself in the act of playing the virginals signals a departure from the sexualizing tradition apparent in such works as Titian's *Venus and Cupid with an Organist* (c. 1550) which draw upon the analogy between the keyboard and the female body as instruments to be played upon, for not only does Anguissola convey the concepts of "self-possession and self-management," but "extend[s] the range of the synecdoche so that the virginals represent not only body but also mind, talent and abilities." (595).

Although Garrard is only concerned with Sofonisba's self-portraits, the artist's representation of the breastfeeding virgin may be another such feminine transformation, particularly when considered in the context of Anguissola's positive construction of chastity, as well as the somewhat suspect position of any female artist. Prior to her departure for Spain in 1559, Sofonisba was one of the very few women to be included in Vasari's *Lives of the Artists*. Vasari praises the especially life-like quality of her figures – particularly in the celebrated painting of her sisters playing chess – which are created "con tanta diligenza e prontezza, che paiono veramente vive, e che non manchi loro altro che la parola" (with such diligence and spontaneity that they seem to be truly alive, and that they lack nothing but speech).[21] Yet this laudatory tribute is countered by a remark seemingly designed to domesticate the marvelous *virtuosa*, for the artist-critic continues, "Ma se le donne sì bene sanno fare gli uomini vivi, che maraviglia che quelle che vogliono sappiano anco fargli sì bene dipinti" (But if women know so well how to create living men, why should we marvel that those who wish to also know how to depict them so well; 6:502). Sofonisba is praised as a creator, but with the implication that, as Garrard puts

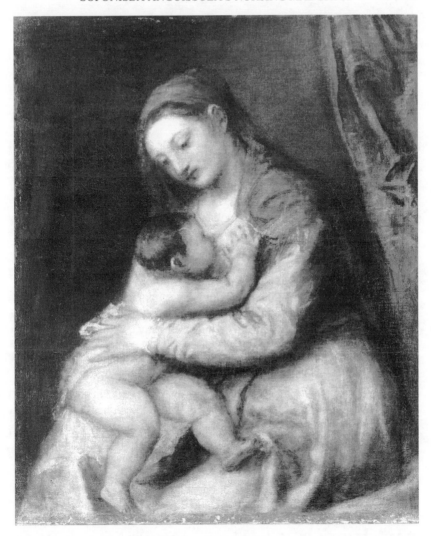

Fig. 4.5   Titian, *The Madonna and Child*, c. 1570

it, "women's art-making is a natural anatomical function" and thus less creative than the cerebral art-making of men.[22] The use of the verb "vogliono" similarly denigrates her unique abilities by suggesting that other women could, in fact, be equally skillful if they chose to direct their energies not toward the role of motherhood which Sofonisba has *not* fulfilled but rather to the less miraculous creativity of art which she has embraced instead.

But if this somewhat back-handed compliment ascribes Anguissola's prodigious talent to the ubiquitous and natural female reproductive abilities in which the artist – for whatever reason – does not participate, her accordingly "virgin" conception would seemingly parallel that of the Virgin herself, whose physical and human substance, her "sangue purissimo,"[23] forms that of her son both before and after birth. Accordingly, the depiction of Mary actively nursing her child would have special significance for this artist: not only is the Virgin the model for the moral conduct so central to her self-definition, but for her act of creation as well.

The parallel between the role of the artist painting the Virgin and the Virgin's shaping of her son seems underscored by the attention paid to the delineation of the actual process of suckling. Although Titian's *Nursing Madonna*, with which Sofonisba was probably not familiar, is extremely naturalistic in its portrayal of the strong affective bond between mother and child, the activity of nursing is not accurately depicted. While Titian's is not the displaced, detached bare breast of the fourteenth century, it is obscured by the painterly style typical of the Venetian's final works. In contrast, Anguissola realistically portrays not only the physical bodies and intimate relationship between the Madonna and her child, but also the act of nursing: both the Virgin's bare and covered breasts are naturalistically shaped and the fingers of her right hand position the nipple for her baby in a manner instantly recognizable to any nursing mother,[24] while simultaneously drawing our attention to the baby's suckling mouth.

As in the earlier Lorenzetti, the attention to realistic detail does not appear casual. The active role of the Virgin suggested by the work's title ("the Madonna who nurses the Christ-Child") is similarly reflected in the fingers that aid the flow of milk from her breast. The Virgin here, with her downcast eyes and gradual emergence from the solid black background of the oval, is an appropriately self-effacing model of humility; the light which appears to come from a position just in front of the work's upper right primarily shines upon her child – her work of art and the light of the world. But it does illuminate her forehead and nose, and correctly-positioned hand, leading us to her breast, as does her own glance and the outward gaze of the suckling baby, whose chubby, healthy body signifies the success of the Virgin's lactation.

As we have seen, the *Madonna lactans* celebrates the humanity of both the Virgin and the Incarnate God whom she miraculously bears. If Sofonisba has not borne the children expected of the early modern woman, she is nevertheless responsible for wondrous offspring which guarantee her own self-definition as *virtuosa*. Like the exemplary analogy drawn between the humble Virgin and her faithful in the traditional *Madonna lactans*, Anguissola's Madonna becomes a model for the successful female artist, exalted precisely by her chaste creation of living – indeed, robust – beings.

Notes

1. The oil painting, measuring 77 × 63.5 cm and attributed to Anguissola., was donated to the Szepmuveszeti Muzeum, Budapest, in 1912. It was attributed to Luca Cambiaso from 1958 until 1967, when cleaning revealed the authentic inscription "...onisba Lomelina" (Anguissola p. 1588). See the discussion in *Sofonisba Anguissola e le sue sorelle* (Exhibition Catalogue; Leonardo Arte, 1994), p. 266.

2. For a consideration of the effect of the fifteenth-century emphasis on naturalism on the representation of the Virgin's breast, see Megan Holmes, "Disrobing the Virgin: The *Madonna Lactans* in Fifteenth-Century Florentine Art." In *Picturing Women in Renaissance and Baroque Italy*, ed. Geraldine A. Johnson and Sara F. Matthews Grieco (Cambridge and New York: Cambridge University Press, 1997), pp. 167–95.

3. Sofonisba Anguissola, the oldest child of a learned gentleman, was born about 1528 in Cremona; unlike other women artists of her time, who were educated at home, she studied with Bernardino Campi, and became one of the very few women to be mentioned by Vasari in his *Vite*. In 1559, she became Lady-in-Waiting and Court Painter to Queen Isabella of Spain, instructing the queen in art and painting numerous portraits of her, the king and the *infante*. After the death of Isabella, Sofonisba remained close to the *infante*, but was granted a dowry by the king and left Spain in about 1569 to marry a Sicilian. She was left a widow approximately five years later, and marrying a Genoese sailor, returned to Northern Italy, where she lived until her death in 1625, still celebrated for her skills in portraiture. Anguissola has only recently begun to receive serious attention from critics; for recent discussions of her biography, see *Sofonisba e le sue sorelle* (op.cit.) and Ilya Sandra Perlingieri, *Sofonisba Anguissola: The First Great Woman Artist of the Renaissance* (New York: Rizzoli, 1992).

4. Holmes, p. 167. On the significance of the Virgin's exposed breast, see Caroline Walker Bynum, *Jesus as Mother: Studies in the Spirituality of the High Middle Ages* (Berkeley: University of California, 1982), "The Body of Christ in the Later Middle Ages: A Reply to Leo Steinberg," in *Renaissance Quarterly* 39 (1986), pp. 399–439, and *Holy Feast and Holy Fast: The Religious Significance of Food to Medieval Women* (Berkeley: University of California, 1987); Leo Steinberg, *The Sexuality of Christ in Renaissance Art and in Modern Oblivion* (2nd edition, Chicago: University of Chicago, 1996) and probably most influentially, Margaret Miles, "The Virgin's One Bare Breast: Female Nudity and Religious Meaning in Tuscan Early Renaissance Culture," in *The Female Body in Western Culture*, ed. Susan Suleiman (Cambridge: Harvard University Press, 1986), pp. 193–208.

5. Holmes, p. 169.

6. "sarà ... interdetto / a le sfacciate donne fiorentine / l'andar mostrando con le poppe il petto" (Purg. 23, ll. 102ff); Marilyn Yalom, *A History of the Breast* (New York: Knopf, 1997), p. 39.

7. See, for example, Galen's *Hygiene*, "Hitherto, while in the uterus, we are wont to be nourished by blood, and the source of milk is from blood undergoing a slight change in the breasts. So that those children who are nourished by their mother's milk enjoy the most appropriate and natural food" (trans. Robert M. Greene [Springfield, IL: Thomas, 1951], p. 24).

8. Paolo da Certaldo, *Libri di buoni costumi* (1327?); cited in Miles, p. 198.

9. Although the doctrine of the Immaculate Conception does not become dogma until 1854, it was widely held throughout the early modern period. See note 14, below.

10. In a discussion of breastfeeding which might as easily apply to the fourteenth as the seventeenth century, Gail Kern *Paster* remarks that "the number of pages in … medical and midwifery treatises devoted to care of the breasts and nipples implies a high incidence of breast infections and indicates the number of painful and potentially disfiguring diseases breasts and nipples were prone to. Breasts became marked by infections and abscesses, nipples scarred over because of infected cuts or might even be completely lost … Though the complete loss of the nipple may have been unusual, the painful experience of nursing with cracked or bleeding nipples cannot have been" (*The Body Embarrassed: Drama and the Disciplines of Shame in Early Modern England* [Ithaca: Cornell University, 1993], p. 203).

11. Millard Meiss, "The Madonna of Humility" (1936) in *Painting in Florence and Siena after the Black Death*, p. 146. He continues, "The Child is presented at a moment when involved in two opposed interests and movements. And these movements, turning in divergent directions in space, are organically integrated in such a way that they suggest a sudden, temporary shift of interest, responsive to an individual will" (146–7).

12. Remarking on Meiss' analysis, Leo Steinberg argues that the older critic "misses the demonstrativeness of the action, the urgency of its appeal, the sense of a message conveyed, as if to say, 'I live with food like you – would you doubt my humanity?'" Certainly, the humanization of Christ is an essential element of such depictions. But what Steinberg misses is just how human this action really is. Commenting on the inability of other critics to perceive the message he identifies, he quotes another scholar who, Steinberg declares, "mistakes its grave summons for a momentary distraction: 'La Madonna sta offrendo il seno al bambino distratto e rivolto verso di noi …'" What Steinberg, in turn, misses is that the distraction is part of the message as well. Just as, as Steinberg argues, we have lost sight of the original meaning of Christ's revealed genitals in Renaissance paintings, so, too, our "bottle culture" often misses the significance of the nursing baby. We no longer recognize the signs, in this case, not because our society's particular obsession with sexuality obscures a theological point but because what should be a homely, immediately-recognizable interaction between mother and child has become defamiliarized.

13. See Steinberg, *passim*.

14. The doctrine of the Immaculate Conception – that is, that Mary was herself conceived without the Original Sin that has tainted all humans since the Fall – was highly contested by many Catholics as well as Protestants. Wishing to avoid further strife, the Council of Trent decided not to make this a definite dogma. Nevertheless, as a majority of the Council did in fact believe in the Immaculate Conception, they did not want to implicate Mary in Original Sin, and hoped to leave the possibility for the doctrine to become dogma at a later date. The decree concerning original sin, made in 1546 at the Council's fifth session, contained the following reservation: "The Sacred Synod declares that it is not its intention to include in the passage treating of original sin, the blessed and Immaculate Virgin Mary, the mother of Jesus Christ, nor does it intend at present to go in any way beyond the decree of Sixtus IV of happy memory" (cited in Jedin, p. 155). In 1547, Canon 23 of the sixth session, on Justification, declared: "If anyone saith that a man once justified can sin no more, nor lose grace, and that therefore he that falls and sins was never truly justified; or, on the other hand, that he is able during his whole life, to avoid all sins, even those that are venial – *except by a special*

privilege from God, as the Church holds in regard to the Blessed Virgin ; let him be anathema" (cited in Warner, p. 384, my emphasis).

15. For a discussion of Protestant attacks on Mary, as well as the Catholic response in the sixteenth and seventeenth centuries, see Emile Mâle, *L'art religieux après le Concile de Trente*, pp. 20ff. For a discussion of the status of images in general and virgin martyrs in particular during and after Trent, see Naomi Yavneh: "Dal rogo alle nozze: Tasso's Sofronia as Virgin Martyr Manque" in *Renaissance Transactions: Essays on Ariosto and Tasso*, ed. Valeria Finucci (Duke, 1999), pp. 270–94. For a readable and informative history of Marian worship, see Marina Warner, *Alone of All Her Sex* (New York: Pocket Books, 1976).

16. For a discussion of the iconoclast heresy and the cult of the Virgin, see Warner, pp. 108–9.

17. see Yavneh, *op. cit.*

18. Rona Goffen, *Titian's Women* (New Haven and London: Yale University Press, 1997), p. 4.

19. Perlingieri, 176.

20. Garrard, "Here's Looking at Me: Sofonisba Anguissola and the Problem of the Woman Artist." *Renaissance Quarterly* 47 (1994), pp. 566–622. In this regard, we might consider the slightly younger Artemisia Gentileschi (1593–1653), whose notoriety as rape victim serves to enhance the popularity of her dramatically-depicted images of *femmes fortes* such as Judith and Lucretia.

21. Vasari, volume 6, p. 498 (all translations my own). Of her painting of her father Amilcare with her sister Minerva and brother Asdrubale, Vasari remarks, "anche questi sono tanto ben fatti, che pare che spirino e sieno vivissimi" (these, too, are so well-made they seem to breathe and be alive; 499).

22. Garrard, p. 574.

23. While the Cardinal Gabrielle Paleotti does not address in his treatise on sacred images (1588) the depiction of the nursing Madonna, it is significant for our discussion that he denounces as heretical the representation in the Annunciation of a little fully-formed baby descending toward the Virgin's womb. Such images, he argues, erroneously imply "che Cristo Signor nostro avesse portato il corpo suo eterreo dal cielo e non fosse stato formato del sangue purissimo della madre" (277).

24. *La Leche League* now recommends a "c-hold" (cupping the breast with the entire hand), rather than this "v-hold," but the "v-hold" is still universally recognizable.

"But Blood Whitened": Nursing Mothers and Others in Early Modern Britain

Rachel Trubowitz

I begin this essay with the following sixteenth-century Salesian folktale:

> A Jew offered to buy milk from a Christian wet nurse who instead sold him the milk of a sow. He then got a poor peasant who owed him money to execute his orders on the promise that his debt would be erased. He brought him to the foot of a gallows, made him cut off the head of the hanged man's corpse, and had him place it in a receptacle filled with the milk. Afterward the Jew ordered the peasant to put his ear to the head and asked him, "What do you hear?" The peasant responded, "The grunting of a herd of pigs!" "Woe is me!" the Jew then cried, "the woman tricked me!" The next day all the pigs within a radius of eight kilometers gathered at this spot and killed one another.

The story ends with a question: "What would have happened if the good Christian had obtained human milk for the Jew?"[1] This exemplum is one of many enduring anti-Semitic tales of Jewish duplicity, sorcery, and heinous crimes against Christians, which circulated throughout Europe during the early modern period. Claudine Fabre-Vassas includes it in her fascinating recent study of Christian discourse on the pig and on Jewish dietary prohibitions against eating pork to underscore the instruction that it, and the myriad of tales like it, provides on the relationship between Jews and pigs. "In every case," she writes, "the pig is introduced as a substitute, serving to denounce the Jew."[2]

I single out this story for a somewhat different reason: to underscore its encapsulation of the intimate relations between mothers' milk, wet nurses, and Jews as forged in the cultural imagination of early modern Christian Europe; it is these triangulated relations that this essay explores. I use this folktale as a point of entry into a discussion of gendered and racialized "boundary panic," to borrow Janet Adelman's apt phrase, as recorded in, mostly, English texts from the late sixteenth- and first half of the seventeenth century.[3] In this turbulent historical moment, England's geographical and political borders underwent rapid and repeated revision through the dynastic shift between the Tudor and Stuart states, accelerated imperial expansion, and, at mid-century, revolution and civil war – breeding mounting anxieties about England's cultural and racial (in)coherence. The "texts" I examine within this temporal space are generically quite distinct – domestic guidebooks, travel narratives, pamphlets, engravings, Shakespeare's plays, among others – but they betray similar preoccupations with breast milk, blood, and the racialized construction of English national identity. This essay, in short, considers texts that both assess and help to shape and stabilize the maternal body, the foreign body, and the body politic in conditions of rapid social change and cultural fragmentation. I concentrate, more specifically, on representations of nursing mothers, wet nurses, and Jewish men as a trinity of culturally constructed types, in which the wet nurse occupies an intermediate position between, on the one hand, the idealized Christian mother, feeding her child with the milk from her own virtuous white body and, on the other, the dark demonized/criminalized figure of "the Jew" hungering for the blood and bodies of Christian children.

i

One of the resonant narratives submerged in the bit of Salesian folklore with which I began is a cautionary tale about the commodification of human breast milk through wet nursing. By offering maternal milk as a marketable good, the wet nurse creates, as the story's concluding question suggests, the potential for corrupting this "purest" – at once most natural and spiritual of foods – into a deadly Jewish potion inciting fraternal and civil warfare. This tale narrates, in short, a crucial linkage between unpolluted breast milk – that which is lovingly and freely offered by "good" mothers – and the health and welfare of the Christian *polis*. It also demonstrates how wet nursing might weaken this vital tie by turning human milk into potentially deadly currency, and hence subjecting it to the worldly vice and corruption associated with Jews, who, in the lurid anti-Semitic "imaginary" of early modern Europe, dirtied Christian money through usury and befouled Christian bodies through ritual mutilation and murder, a subject to which this essay returns.

Cautionary tales about wet nurses that link non-maternal breast milk and social instability also find culturally resonant articulation in early modern didactic literature about the English home, especially that literature printed during the historical frame this essay considers. Cutting against the upper-class norm for infant and child care, domestic-guidebook writers, like Robert Cleaver, John Dod, and William Gouge, uniformly celebrate maternal breast-feeding over wet-nursing by exalting nursing mothers and by delineating the various ways in which the unregulated and "strange" milk purchased from wet nurses could endanger the physical health and moral integrity of both children and families. Some of the twenty-three arguments Gouge offers in his much-reprinted *Of Domesticall Duties* (which went through twelve printings over the course of the seventeenth century) on the benefits of maternal breastfeeding are strictly medical in emphasis – babies breast-fed by their mothers are less susceptible to disease and death, for example. But, more often than not, he and other writers of texts attempting to account for and offer advice on breast milk and breastfeeding register concerns that are as much moral as medical, that medicalize morality and moralize the medical. Guidebook advice on domestic "manners" and mores is in this regard akin to the accounts of reproduction written by early modern physicians, like Edward Jordan (James I's doctor), in which as Gail Kern Paster notes "no stable semantic demarcations separated ethics from physiology."[4]

One key medical/moral concern was that breast-milk physically transmitted the moral and bodily character of the nurse to her charge, ideally complement-ing, but more often compromising or even eradicating the familial identity the child had inherited from its parents. "We may be assured," maintains James Guillimeau in *The Nursing of Children*, "that the Milke (wherewith the child is nourish'd two yeares together) hath a power to make the children like the Nurses, both in bodie and mind; as the seed of the Parents hath to make the children like them."[5] The guidebooks' perception of nurse-milk's competition with and perversion of parentally transmitted identity surfaces as well in Shakespeare's plays, especially at heightened moments of familial conflict. Hence, in *The Winter's Tale*, Leontes demands that Mamillius be removed from the powerful shaping influence of what he jealously presumes is Hermione's corrupt and hostile foreign body. He laments that "[t]hough he does bear some signs of me," his son has too much of her adulterous, female, and hence, innately unstable and illegitimate, "blood in him." His only solace is: "I am glad that you did not nurse him" (II.i.57–8, 56).[6] When Lord Capulet disowns Juliet for refusing to marry Paris, he but formalizes the familial estrangement and loss of hereditary identity that his daughter has experienced not only through her love for Romeo but also through the likeness she bears to the bawdy Nurse – and the Nurse bawdy/body – who suckled her.[7]

As these examples suggest, children put out to wet nurses or breastfed by unfit mothers not only were thought more likely to die than those offered "tender" maternal care and nourishment – "The number of nurse children that die every yeare is very great" – but they were also believed to experience a social "death" unknown to their properly suckled counterparts.[8] To the extent that they were transformed and remade by the base or noxious qualities of unfamiliar breast milk, they were forever estranged from their families. "Such children as have sucked their mothers breasts, love their mothers best," writes Gouge, "yea we observe many who have sucked others milke, to love these nurses all the daies of their life."[9] David Leverenz's summary of the ethical divide in the guidebooks between "tender" mothers and "strange" milk is especially apt: "Tender mothers and tender children go together. Mothers should not be surprised if children deny them later in life, ran the warnings, when they deny children the breast early in life. Strange milk would lead to strange manners."[10]

The affective ties between nurse and child thus had the potential to generate strangeness and strangers, to interrupt the genealogical transmission of identity, and so to tarnish a family's good name and disrupt the hereditary transmission of properties and titles – hence, the emphasis in the guidebook literature on creating synonymity between maternal love and maternal breast milk. "How can a mother better express her love to her young babe, then by letting it sucke of her owne beasts?" writes Gouge.[11] For Dod and Cleaver, women acquire "the sweet name of Mother ... full of incredible love" by breastfeeding, their first and most important maternal duty.[12] "Incredible" love and milk, affective ties and familial bonds, maternal duty and desire, all cohere at the idealized breast of the nursing mother, which in turn guarantees the spiritual and physical "prosper[ity]" and intact identity of children. "Daily experience confirmith," writes Gouge, that children tenderly breastfed by their mothers, "prosper best. Mothers are most tender over them and cannot indure to let them lie crying out, without taking them up and stilling them, as nurses will let them crie and crie againe, if they be about any businesse of their own."[13] Indeed, as Fabre-Vassas notes, the deprivation of milk and motherly love through wet nursing or an overly abrupt weaning process from the maternal breast is associated in French folklore with a potentially fatal depletion of appetite, desire, happiness, to which children are especially vulnerable. This melancholic "sickness of lack," which in French (particularly in the Pyrenean dialects), is termed, *anaigament*, is etymologically linked to liquefaction and deliquescence. The illness, which results from and implies deprivation of the affective relation with the mother and her nourishing, vital fluids, manifests itself by sapping the child of all energy and dissolving him or her into liquid, a symptomatic insignia of the slow leakage of origin and identity.[14]

It is precisely the beloved duty and dutiful love which maternal breastfeeding bespeaks that underpins guidebook definitions of maternal breastfeeding as a spiritual vocation "the most proper work of [a mother's] speciall calling," even as guidebook writers simultaneously attempted to rationalize nursing motherhood by redefining maternal nurture as governed by natural law. As Cleaver and Dod maintain, "We see by experience, that every beast and every fowle is nourished and bred of the same that beare it: onely some women love to be mothers, but not nurse. As therefore every tree doth cherish and nourish that which it bringeth forth: even so also, it becometh naturall mothers to nourish their children with their owne milk."[15] The desire to nurse one's own baby is defined as a biological drive or law of nature to which even trees correctly respond. This slide from "sacred" to "natural," and back again, points to an important conceptual paradigm shift that, as Stephen Greenblatt has recently argued, finds its beginnings in the sixteenth and seventeenth centuries. For Greenblatt, it is precisely at this moment that "the natural" comes to replace "the sacred" as the conceptual category that governed early modern English attempts to think through and chart the boundaries between England and the radically different cultures it increasingly encountered through trade, missionary work, and colonial conquest. Indeed, that maternal breastfeeding is defined as at once a natural drive and a sacred calling reflects this moment of conceptual transition. Greenblatt's comments are most illuminating: "the sixteenth and seventeenth centuries also saw the beginning of a gradual shift away from the axis of sacred and demonic and toward the axis of natural and unnatural ... but the natural is not to be found, or at least not reliably found, among primitive or uncivilized peoples ... The stage is set for the self-congratu-latory conclusion that European culture, and English culture in particular, is at once the most civilized and the most natural."[16] In guidebook formulations, the "naturall" nursing mother shores up this "self-congratulatory" construction of English cultural identity by interpellating her suckling children into the natural order and thus, in the same gesture, also into the English state as civilized subjects. By contrast, the wet-nurse undermines the intact identity of the nation-state by rendering children unnatural and uncivilized or, in other words, not English.

Closely allied to these concerns about lactation, civilization, savagery, and England's national identity was the widely embraced notion of breast-milk as white blood – "nothing else but blood whitened" as Guillimeau notes.[17] "Experience teacheth, that God converteth the mothers bloud into the milke where with the child is nurse," write Cleaver and Dod.[18] If nurse milk can, through the powerful affective ties it creates, pervert or eradicate familial identity and social bonds, it is also a blood carrier of color-coded character – a conception that generated concerns about the pollution of bloodlines through morally and physically tainted human milk. "Now if the nurse be of an evill complexion," write Dod and Cleaver, "... the child sucking of her breast must needs take part with her."[19] The emphasis on "evill complexion" is striking, given the nuances that "complexion" newly acquires in this historically specific moment, when the term, which refers to "moral character," begins to allude for the first time to hair and skin color.[20] As deployed in the passage from Dod and Cleaver, "evill complexion" encapsulates an easy slide from an ethical to a proto-racialized notion of identity that paints both the spirit and body of the wet nurse in diabolically dark hues. To return to Guillimeau's formulation, "Milke ... hath a power to make the children like the Nurses, both in bodie and mind." Embedded within these medical and moral perceptions of breast milk as "blood whitened" are concerns about safeguarding white English complexions from the darkening powers of "unnatural" lactation. To the extent that they affiliate human milk and body color, the guidebooks help to document the cultural construction of whiteness in the early modern period.

This cultural project becomes particularly pressing during the first few decades of the seventeenth century, when much of the guidebook literature is first printed or reprinted. This is, as noted, the historically specific moment in which English foreign trade, travel, and colonization accelerate and intensify, breeding racialized "boundary panic" about the distinctions between English-ness and otherness. As Kim F. Hall argues, "it is England's sense of losing its traditional insularity that provokes the development of 'racialism.'"[21] England's "discovery" of racialized differences between the intact national home and uncharted foreign worlds, I suggest, silently inflects the guidebooks' preoccupations with "white blood" and the tainted milk of morally, and physically, dark-complexioned women. To put this another way, newly racialized anxieties about England's global presence and national integrity are displaced onto the familiar and more easily regulated site of the maternal breast and its identity-sustaining milk/blood, as represented in and circulated by the domestic guidebooks and affiliated texts, such as early modern drama. But such attempts to monitor the maternal breast tended less to cure the "boundary panic" that generated racialized difference in the early modern period than to restate this "panic" about race and national identity in gendered terms. While serving as an affecting icon of English domesticity, the idealized white-blooded maternal breast always threatens to lapse into the reviled, morally dark-complexioned breast, despite the guidebook writers' energetic efforts to dichotomize them.[22]

It is this inevitable conjunction between "good" breast and "bad," reverence and repulsion that the guidebooks attempt to sort out by characterizing wet nurses as strangers and expelling them from the English home. To put this another way, the wet nurse evokes the subversive threat of the requisite alien who must be expelled in order to achieve social and personal cohesion. Such a threat, however, had long attached itself, in the Christian "imaginary," to anti-Semitic perceptions of "the Jew" as unintegrable and, therefore, deportable.[23] It is, as such, possible to read guidebook vilifications of the wet-nurse as encrypted rehearsals not only of longstanding Anglo-Christian constructions of Jewish difference but also of prevailing English anxieties about hidden "judaizing" tendencies within the nation, anxieties that persisted long after the large-scale deportation of Jews from England under the Expulsion Act of 1290. It is to these concerns about the absent presence of Jews in early modern England and to the specter of "the Jew" in English discourse on breastfeeding that this essay now turns.

ii

The fraught relations between "others," nursing mothers, and wet nurses, as reflected in the guidebook literature, can be discerned in many of the period's travel narratives, such as those of Samuel Purchas, which I shall investigate in this second part of my essay. While their detailings of the so-called exotic peoples and traditions of Asia, Africa, and the Americas might seem to be literally at a distance from the English household, travel narratives can be seen as allied with the domestic guidebooks of Gouge, Guillimeau, and others in their efforts to help their readers establish a clear sense of their Englishness and to secure their personal and national boundaries. Just as the domestic guidebook is perhaps most interesting in its proximity to the travel narrative, i.e. when it reveals its fascination with and anxieties about places and people outside the familial and national home, so too the travel narrative is especially revealing when read as a kind of domestic guidebook that defines the white English domestic "norm" in opposition to the "deviance" visible in dark, foreign worlds. I am particularly interested in travel-narrative depictions of Jews, especially Jewish men, who, as suggested earlier, I believe can be glimpsed in the guidebook's racialized formulations of wet nurses and nursing mothers. In my reading, it is "the Jew," as glimpsed in the travel narrative, (and elsewhere) who shadows the guidebooks' idealized representations of maternal nurture and who is shadowed in the dark figure of the wet nurse and her unfamilial milk.

Let me underscore that while, "officially," no Jews lived in England within the temporal frame this essay considers, unofficial Jews, i.e. secret Jews or Marannos, Jewish-Christian hybrids, Jewish converts to Christianity, continued in fact to populate the nation, as is well documented by Shapiro's important study. Stepped-up colonial expansion and foreign travel and trade also brought an increasing number of Englishmen into more frequent and closer contact with Jews outside of England, and hence it is to the travel narrative that I turn to find early modern records of English impressions of Jews. These impressions are key, since they chart the ways in which, by gathering first-hand observations of "real" Jews outside of England, English travelers tried to document the "fact" of racialized Jewish difference, occluded by the unofficial presence in England of Jews who passed for English; in this way, the travel narratives helped to stabilize England's own rapidly shifting and newly color-coded boundaries.

Travel-narrative attempts to clarify the differences between Jewishness and Englishness are, however, complicated by the unacknowledged intimacies between these two officially distinct identities. While the Jews were expelled from England in 1290, "the Jew" continued to reside quite openly in England as a familiar scriptural and legendary type or "shadow" – a presence, however spectral, that shapes the cultural construction of not only Jewish identity but

English national identity as well, especially during this moment of intensified "boundary panic." The imaginary English Jew is, as such, inseparably intertwined with the foreign "real" Jews encountered and depicted by English travelers. The travel narratives hence "document" the confused interface between real and imagined, familiar and strange, white and black that frames English perceptions of Jews as much as they report on the lived experiences of actual Jews in the early modern period.

Perhaps most relevant for my purposes here is that "the Jew," witnessed by Purchas and other English travelers plays an important role in the "racialism" that Hall believes is discovered at this historically specific moment, since this part-real/part-imagined figure not only confirms Jewish difference but is embedded as a precursor figure, or "type," of the foreign peoples given newly racialized representation in the travel literature. Emergent formulations of racialized difference were, as Shapiro argues, "almost always skewed by what [English travelers] had first read about the Jews."[24] The Jew, as constructed by the dominant culture, thus implies and is implicated in English travelers' first-hand accounts of black, "tawny," red, and other variously colored non-white, non-English people. This essay urges that the stranger-figure of the wet nurse, found in the domestic guidebooks and elsewhere during the same temporal frame in which the travel narratives were first printed and circulated, be counted among these racialized/Judaized "others." I would also add that it is in relation to the part-real, part-imagined Jews who emerge in the travel literature and in other early modern texts that the wet nurse's intermediate position between mother and "other" becomes most clearly visible. Just as she, in practice, stands in for the maternal breast, she metaphorically acts and speaks for "the Jew."

Perhaps the most striking instance of the affinities I detect is the conflation that Samuel Purchas creates between wet nurses and Jewish men in *Purchas His Pilgrimage*. One of his text's most bizarre bits of exotica – against which he establishes the domestic "normality" of England – is a detailing of Jewish male breastfeeding. "If you believe their *Gemara* (can you choose?)," Purchas writes, "a poor Jew having buried his wife and not able to hire a nurse for his child, had his breasts miraculously filled with milk, and became nurse himself." Purchas also alludes to the figure of a breastfeeding Mordecai represented in a Midrashic interpretation of the Book of Esther.[25] Purchas's examples demonstrate the fuzzy boundary between the "breasts" of Jewish men and wet nurses – note that the poor Jew "became *nurse* himself" (my emphasis), not mother. Here, the "mirac[le]" of lactation and breastfeeding is less sacred than profane.

To be sure, Galenic physiology implied biological likeness between men and women, especially in relation to sex and reproduction. As Thomas Laquer has argued, in Galenism's one-sex, one-flesh model of human anatomy, male and female genitalia were understood as inversions of one another and identical in function. Both men and women were thought to have "seed," or sperm, for example, and breasts, for that matter.[26] Gender differentiation was, in the early modern period, much more clearly a function of the enculturation process, in which guidebook literature, conduct books, and travel narratives played a key role. Marking distinctions not only between men and women, but between "true" men and "false" is thus a key part of the work that Purchas's image accomplishes. Evoking long-standing anti-Semitic perceptions of Jewish manhood as impaired and degenerate, and hence as "female," the image is deployed as a gendered sign of Jewish difference. This kind of "female" encoding of Jewish men was reinforced by the commonly held assumption that Jewish men menstruated. Jewish male bodies, like those of women, were thought of as leaky vessels, which discharged a monthly flow of unclean blood. Thus, the Spanish physician Juan de Quinones wrote "a special treatise to prove the claim that male Jews have a tail and, like women, a monthly flow of blood."[27] Samuel Purchas's observations about Jewish male breastfeeding can be read as an extension of this theory of Jewish male menstruation, since mothers' milk was believed to be formed from menstrual blood.[28]

Most important for my purposes here is that Purchas's image not only aids in the cultural work of differentiating men from women (and "false" men), but it responds as well to the "boundary panic" that seems to rule this historical moment by gendering the difference between Englishness and Jewishness, even though these racial/national/religious categories had, in fact, been impossibly blurred by forced and voluntary conversion, intermarriage, and the formation of small Portuguese Marrano communities in and outside of London. It is important to note, however, that if it vividly underscores the differences between the normative English "self" and the marvelous/repellent "other," Purchas's account of Jewish male wet-nursing cannot completely sustain the gendered racial, national, and religious differences it appears so indelibly to inscribe. In the distinction he implies between nurses and mothers, Purchas suggests that mothers resemble Christian Englishmen more than they do Jews – a resemblance reinforced by the key role maternal milk plays in the transmission of hereditary identity, both familial and national. The "good" Christian mother, in short, is closer to the normative English "father" and Stuart fatherland than she is to the aberrant wet-nurse or infidel Jew.

The leakage of blood/milk thus places Jews in close proximity to wet-nurses as a "female" threat to social and familial stability – a perception strengthened by anti-Semitic attitudes toward circumcision, a subject to which I shall return. Such leakage was also perceived as both symptom of and explanation for what was thought to be Jews' insatiable thirst for Christian blood. This blood-thirst, which points to a lack both physical and spiritual, was believed to drive Jews to abduct, forcibly circumcise, and ritually murder young gentile boys and drink their blood. This signature Jewish crime – the so-called "blood libel" – also finds a point of origin in the cluster of presumed ritual murders in medieval and Renaissance Europe, all following the same pattern. The most famous include Richard de Pontoise (1163), Dominguito de Saragoss (1255), Hugh of Lincoln (1255), Werner d'Oberwesel (1287), and Simon of Trent (1472).[29] The enduring strength of English belief in the "reality" of these Jewish "crimes" cannot be over-estimated: as Shapiro points out: "Not even the Holocaust put to rest such allegations [of Jewish ritual murder] in England."[30] These enduring anti-Semitic assumptions about blood, sucking, and Jews also form an important, if lurid, subtext for the guidebooks' and other idealized images of the Christian mother suckling her (male) child with her "white blood."

Perhaps the most notorious of these was the murder of the two-and-a-half-year-old Simon. In a colored German engraving of 1480, the standing figure of the small beatified boy is shown surrounded by seven vicious Jewish tormentors, all with carefully inscribed Hebrew names. The figures closest to Simon make incisions in his body with sharp needles and chisels, while one, tellingly named "Israel" collects the blood in a small bowl, while another, "Moses," operates on the boy's genitals to circumcise him as part of the death ritual. This engraving and the "event" itself can be read from a number of different perspectives, but what is most important to my argument here is that the supposed ritual murder of "Simonet" and other "cases" linking Jewish men and Christian children through the drinking of blood (the consumption of bloody animal flesh is, of course, strictly prohibited by Jewish dietary law) and death invert the idealized mother-child dyad created and circulated by the domestic guidebooks and other texts. The "blood-libel" mythology helps to generate grotesque images of Jewish men drinking the blood of a dead gentile child that inversely, and perversely, shadow model constructions of the Christian mother whose "white blood" is suckled by her vital infant. This inversion is key since it makes legible the differences between white Christian mothers and dark Jewish men, while concealing the similarities between their secret rites and rituals (both the birth room and the synagogue were closed to Christian men) and, as such, the unmarked filiation between Anglo-Christian domesticity, both familial and national, and unregenerate Jewish strangeness.

Inversion, as Stuart Clark notes, functioned in the early modern period, "as a universal principle of intelligibility as well as a statement about how the world was actually constituted."[31] Not unlike "the world turned upside down" created by, for example, folkloric rites, festival celebrations, and the court masque, the blood-libel cases and other legends of Jewish crimes against Christians engender an inverse world of essentialized disorder and vice, (mis)ruled by the devil-Jew, in which the perverse bond between blood-thirsty Jew and dead gentile child at once threatens and legitimizes the primal bond between the idealized nursing Christian mother and child. This same demonized Jewish counter-world is conjured up almost as a cultural necessity during the festive moment of Easter to reinforce the radical break between Jew and gentile that occurred during the Crucifixion and Passion, the founding events of Christianity celebrated by the rituals of Holy Week. It is not accidental that the ritual murders of Simon of Trent, William of Norwich, and other supposed "child-crucifixions" were thought to occur at Easter, an association reinforced by the belief that Jews needed Christian blood for ritual use during the Passover seder, specifically for making matzah.

Equally important is that Easter also commemorates the Crucifixion's guarantee of gentile freedom from, and erasure of, the ritual mark left by circumcision, the sign of God's covenant with Israel as mandated in Genesis 17:10–14: "This *is* my covenant, which ye shall keep, between me and you and thy seed after thee; Every man child among you shall be circumcised ..." (Authorized KJV). In Milton's poem, "Upon the Circumcision," Christ's circumcision, the sign of his Hebraic manhood, is, in fact, typologically linked to his Crucifixion, the sign of his Christian divinity: he "now bleeds to give us ease" (l. 11).[32] It is precisely this linkage between circumcision and crucifixion that is profaned by the dramatic events played out through the blood-libel cases, in which the charge that Jews circumcised their victims before "crucifying" them was a standard feature Thus, we see in the engraving depicting Simon of Trent's ritual murder that "Moses" circumcises the young boy's penis while the other Jews collect his blood from various limbs and bodily organs, notably his heart and breast, thereby creating, as it were, *faux* stigmata. The young English boy, Hugh of Lincoln, was also thought to have been circumcised before being eviscerated. Purchas himself "documents" this kind of imagined Jewish crime, noting especially its "devilish" parody and inversion of the "original" events commemorated by Easter, and hence its desecration of Christianity's foundational moment as well: "One cruel and (to speak the properest phrase) Jewish crime usual amongst them every year toward Easter, though it were not always known ... [is] to steal a young boy, circumcise him, and after a solemn judgement, making one of their own nation a Pilate, to crucify him out of their devilish malice to Christ and Christians."[33] The salvific "progress" from circumcision to crucifixion, which Milton traces in his poem, is thus transformed by Jewish ritual murder into a diabolical descent into barbarism. The blood-libel case, in short, reduces entangled Jewish–gentile relations to an (over-)simple binary, in which Judaism represents the realm of the "savage," Christianity that of the "civilized" – a categorical distinction reminiscent of that between the natural nursing mother and the unnatural wet nurse, and one that affiliates Jews with so-called primitive, non-European "others," whom English colonists and travelers, such as Purchas, encountered especially in the New World.[34] Although it falls outside the scope of this essay, I would nevertheless like to suggest that "the cannibal," the standard early modern icon of American wilderness and primitivism, might be fruitfully read in relation to anti-Semitic European perceptions of Jewish hunger for Christian blood and bodies.

In the English cultural imagination then, Judaism, in some very specific contexts, implies the primitive and pagan, and hence the idolatrous worship of material objects and graven images rather than Christianity's transcendent Trinitarian deity, of whom objects and images are simply material symbols and signs. This literalizing pagan preference for matter/flesh over spirit implicit in "the Jew" is made explicit by the blood-libel cases, which both de-allegorize the typological connection between circumcision and Crucifixion and carnally reverse Christianity's miraculous supersedure of the old Hebraic covenant, of which circumcision is the bodily sign. Most relevant to my purposes here is that by emptying the Crucifixion of its spiritual and allegorical content and hence by denying Christianity its foundational miracle, "the Jew," as both the circumcised and the circumcisor, perfects his most standard stereotypical role as devil or anti-Christ, who inverts and negates Christian origin and identity – the very entities preserved by the idealized gentile mother and transmitted through her milk to her suckling child.

Martin Luther's revealing comment about himself and his wife underscores precisely the fraught interconnectedness of circumcised penis and maternal breast: "I hope I shall never be so stupid as to be circumcised. I would rather cut off the left breast of my Catherine and of all women."[35] To the extent that in Luther's text the circumcised penis implies and can be substituted for the cutting off of a maternal breast and its identity-forming milk, the two severed body parts achieve an imagined synonymity. Their figurative linkage carries tragic, and one might even say traumatic, resonances since it metonymically evokes the devastating loss of both mother and father and the terror of being orphaned. As such it signifies the near-death consequent to deracination, homelessness, and diaspora, all of which are subsumed and performed by anti-Semitic typifications of Jews as wanderers or literally errant, i.e. "the wandering Jew." Given the insistent threat of homelessness, (im)migration, and loss of insular national identity that early modern English "boundary panic" bespeaks, it seems unsurprising that Jewish "vice" and "villainy" haunt English texts written during the period, especially those like the guidebooks and travel narratives that attempt to remedy England's "identity crisis" and to renegotiate the relations between home and world, mothers and others.

Luther's affiliation of circumcised Jewish penis and female Christian breast was no doubt facilitated by Christian perceptions of circumcision as a metaphor for castration and emasculation, one that was thought in certain instances to be literally acted upon. To return to Purchas's image, if circumcision turned Jewish men metaphorically into women or feminized men, then this hermaphroditic transformation might "naturally" result in their growing of breasts and becoming wet nurses for their children. The alliance between Jewish men

and wet nurses is further strengthened by the strikingly parallel threats that
forcible circumcision and nurse milk present to inherited familial identity. Like
nurse milk, forcible circumcision marks and threatens forever to alter (change
and make "other") the identity of children. Just as the affective attachment of
child to nurse can never be weakened or redirected – "yea we observe many
who have sucked others milke, to love these nurses all the daies of their life" –
so too the mark of forcible circumcision forever makes a child "one of their
own nation," thus denoting a tie to Judaism that can never be erased –
even when, in the case of the Jewish convert, the spirit was willing. Some
Jews who converted to Christianity employed gentile doctors to reverse their
circumcisions surgically and thereby erase the telltale sign of the Judaism
they had renounced. The sixteenth-century French doctor Laurent Joubert
describes the procedure as follows: "To remake a foreskin, one must cut the
skin of the virile member against its roots all around. When it has thus lost its
conduit, one pulls it little by little from below, as one strips a branch of willow,
to make a trunk, until the head is covered with it."[36] But by a strange irony,
the procedure did not erase but in fact doubled the Judaic mark of circumcision.
As Fabre-Vassas points out, "the *langue d'oc* term that designates someone
who has undergone this operation is clear: *re-talhat*, twice castrated. For
Christians, then, Jews cannot escape their destiny."[37] To the extent that forcible
circumcision attempts to bequeath this inescapable destiny to gentile children,
it, like the dark-complexioned nurse-breast vilified in the domestic guidebooks,
threatens permanent alteration both of normative gentile European identity and
of the "natural" and hence "civilized" white European, and, more specifically,
English body. Cleaver and Dod's morally dark-complexioned wet nurse and
Purchas's "devilish" Jew move toward convergence as racialized types in the
English cultural "imaginary," despite the rather different generic and cultural
contexts in which their stories find expression.

Christian eyewitness accounts of the circumcision ceremony contain
perhaps the most striking expressions of the imagined convergence of
circumcised Jewish penis and gentile female breast, and it is to the early
modern travel narrative that we once again must turn to find these reports.
Driven by post-Reformation interest in Hebraic rituals and customs and
desirous of touring hitherto closed exotic worlds, English travelers happily
accepted invitations to witness circumcisions. Perhaps the practice that seemed
most surprising to these "tourists" was the *metzizah*, the (not always enacted)
part of the ritual in which the rabbi or *mohel* sucks the blood off the infant's
circumcised penis. In his journal entry for January 15, 1645, John Evelyn notes
of a circumcision he witnessed in Rome that when "the circumcision was done
the priest sucked the child's penis with his mouth."[38] The Elizabethan traveler,
Thomas Coryate underscores "the strange manner, unused (I believe) of the
ancient Hebrews" in which the *mohel* "did put his mouth to the child's yard, and

sucked up the blood."[39] Alluding to the circumcisions witnessed by Evelyn, Coryate, and Frynes Moryson, yet another English traveler, Shapiro notes the homoerotic implications that *metzizah* must have had for these witnesses: "Apparently, this innovative practice, introduced during the Talmudic period, though not universally practiced by Jews, must have seemed to these English observers to have sodomitical overtones."[40] I would add that *metzizah*, (the Hebrew word for "sucking") might have also seemed to English travelers (busily engaged in measuring the "normality" of the English home against examples of foreign "deviance") to be a shocking inversion of idealized maternal breastfeeding, that celebrated "sucking," which, as we have seen, provides didactic texts on English domesticity with their most affecting icon. When the "exotic" circumcision ceremony is read against the domestic ritual of maternal breastfeeding, a reading that English travelers would have been likely to perform, the vice evoked by *metzizah*, and elliptically suggested by Coryate's phrase, "strange manner," is, I would argue, not sodomy but wet nursing, the "strange" and "unnatural" sucking that forever shadows idealized maternal breastfeeding as its "evil" double. Rather than sodomy, the "deviance" presented by the Jew-as-wet-nurse, (a version of Purchas's lactating Jewish men) summoned in Anglo-Christian accounts of *metzizah*, suggests incest and pedophilia; *metziah*, that is, ritually performs, in these accounts, the carnal and perverse (re)inscription of precisely that spiritual and natural love of child which Cleaver and Dod, among others, equate with "the sweet name of Mother."

Like Coryate and other travelers, Montaigne also witnessed a circumcision, and his depiction of the ceremony he attended in Rome is notable for its resonant account of the practice of *metzizah*: "As soon as the glans is uncovered, they hastily offer some wine to the minister, who puts a little in his mouth, and then goes and sucks the glans of the child, all bloody, and spits out the blood he has drawn from it, and immediately takes as much wine again, up to three times." After the child's penis is bandaged, the circumcisor is given another glass of wine: "He takes a swallow of it, and then dipping his finger in it he three times takes a drop of it with his finger to the boy's mouth to be sucked … He meanwhile still hath his mouth all bloody."[41] Montaigne's description of the "minister['s]" bloody mouth and of the "blood," as wine, that metaphorically drips from the boy's mouth after he sucks the (phallic) finger of the *mohel* or rabbi must have confirmed gentile impressions of Jewish blood-thirst and perverse sexuality. But the wine/blood on the boy's mouth in Montaigne's account also recalls with uncanny exactitude the domestic guidebooks' depictions of the "white blood" that adheres to the mouth of the idealized nursing child. The resemblance between these wine- and milk-stained children's lips acquires further precision when considered adjacently with the scene of blood and violence that ever-threatened to interrupt and overturn the idealized scene of nursing maternity celebrated by the guidebook authors. "[Ambrois]Pare" as Audrey Eccles notes, "considered it a great dispensation of nature that the blood turned white, otherwise people would be shocked by 'so grievous and terrible spectacle of the childes mouth so imbrued and besmeared with blood.'"[42] To the extent that Montaigne's description of the practice of *metzizah* evokes this "grievous and terrible spectacle" of the child's blood-besmeared mouth and the blood-spurting lactating breast, it underscores the striking alliance between gentile suckling and Jewish "blood sucking" constructed by early modern texts. If, as Kathryn Schwarz incisively argues, "nursing threatens to produce the image of the bloody child" and, I would add, the bloody breast, it also evokes and is evoked by gentile depictions of the bloody child and the circumcisor's knife.[43] To put this another way, at the point at which women's breasts fail to live up to the idealized maternal breast imagined in the guidebooks and affiliated texts, they threaten to "turn Jew."

iii

This is precisely the threat, however veiled, suggested by Purchas's image, if we can return once more to that resonant bit of text. If Jewish men can be miraculously (and demonically) transformed into wet nurses, then perhaps, wet nurses might "turn Jew," or at least carry in their breast milk the traces of the Jew and other infidel "exotics," for whom, as we have seen, Jews served as either substitutes or precursors. Such is the fear indirectly conveyed in *The Winter's Tale*, in which Hermione, as we have seen, is thought by Leontes to transmit infidel(ity) to Mamillius just by the close proximity and affective ties between their bodies. The threat that unfit mothers and nurses might foster infidel children emerges as well in texts, such as the guidebooks, that delineate household programs for the education of children. David Leverenz has shown that Puritan mothers served as the primary educators of their children during their early years, a responsibility that was linked specifically to their intertwined duty and desire to breastfeed their children.[44] As Robert Pricke proclaims in *The Doctrine of Superiority*, mothers are charged with the "tender care of noursing & bringing [children] up in their younger & more tender years."[45] At birth and while the child was in swadling bands and still nursing, "the care especially lieth upon the mother." As the child grew older, mothers were expected to provide some religious instruction along with their love and nourishment. Cleaver, in fact, maintains that Christian education be concurrent with breastfeeding or at least immediately follow upon the weaning process. St. Paul, he writes "would have them sucke in religion, if not with mothers milke, yet shortly after as-soone as they are capable of it."[46] Religion, in Cleaver's Pauline formulation, is, in short, almost identical to "mothers milke." The Word is literally sucked in at the maternal breast – a perception that underscores the crucial role that lactating motherhood is mandated to play in the transmission of official discourse. To put this another way, maternal breastfeeding, as represented in the didactic literature on the English home, secures the shifting parameters of English national identity by interpellating children into the state as normative speaking subjects.

Understood in these terms, the figure of the nursing mother, as constructed by the official culture, can be allied to such ideological state apparatuses as the Church, among others, in which discourse is used to repress or eradicate cultural and religious difference.[47] It is not surprising, given the parallel role that the lactating maternal breast and the Church are shown to play with respect to the dissemination of official discourse, that ministers of sixteenth- and seventeenth-century Puritan churches conventionally depicted themselves as lactating mothers who could provide spiritual milk, in the form of scriptural truth, to their congregations. Thus Cotton Mather could state at the very end of this long rhetorical tradition: "*Ministers* are your *Mothers* too. Have they not *Travailed in Birth* for you, that a CHRIST may be seen *formed in you*? Are not their *Lips* the *Breasts* thro' which the *sincere Milk of the Word* has pass'd unto you, for your Nourishment?"[48] In relation to this conjoining of maternal (and paternal) breast to scriptural text, mothers' milk to divine Word, non-maternal nurse milk is implicated as an infidel source of linguistic fallibility and insurgence. Wet nurses, in other words, could be said to bear the potential to provide children with a counter-language through which they might eventually articulate unofficial and subversive political and religious truths. Just as she, in practice, stands in for the nursing mother, so the wet nurse represents a substitute or supplemental form of discourse, which gives speech to those (like Jews) disenfranchised by official English language, culture, and nationhood. It is precisely these concerns about language, culture, nation that Spenser voices in *A View of the Present State of Ireland*, when he dictates against the English colonial practice of hiring Irish wet nurses: "for the first the childe that sucketh of the [Irish] nurse must of necessity learn his first speech of her, the which being the first that is enured to his tongue is ever after most pleasing unto him, insomuch as though he afterwards be taught English, that the smack of the first will always abide with him, and not only of the speech, but of the manners and conditions."[49] That these same concerns about breast milk, language, and identity can, outside the Irish context, acquire distinctive anti-Semitic valences is exemplified by the story of the Expulsion that the sixteenth-century Jewish historian Samuel Usque narrates in *Consolation for the Tribulations of Israel*. The most salient part of this tale for my purposes here is that which concerns a group medieval English monks who attempt to convert a group of Jewish children by first stealing them from their parents. Their aim was to make the children forget "their ancient Law" by depriving them of the "nourishment of the Jewish milk they had imbibed," and by filling them instead with "Christian doctrine and faith," or, in other words, *the sincere Milk of the Word*,"to repeat Cotton Mather's highly suggestive phrase.[50]

It is important to note, especially in light of Fabre-Vassas's important study, that "Jewish milk," as alluded to in the passage above, was habitually linked in the gentile "imaginary" of medieval and Renaissance Europe to pig's milk, or, more specifically, the milk of the *Judensau*, as depicted by, to take but one example, Renaissance German engravings of Jewish men suckling the teats of a sow. As Fabre-Vassas's study makes clear, this perception of Jews' filial relationship to the pig, rendered by the engraving's noxious debasement of the Jewish mother–child relationship, is central to the ways in which Jewishness is racialized as redness, the color of porcine "skin." Red hair, freckles, measles, burns, skin inflammations, leprosy, fevers, among other kinds of red markings and "red" sicknesses that manifest themselves on the skin or elsewhere on the body were associated with Jews, most notably, the red-bearded Judas, the archetypal Jewish Christ-killer. The relevance of Fabre-Vassas's highly suggestive linkage between Jews and redness, as made through the pig, to the issues upon which my essay has focused is further underscored when the "red Jew," to borrow her apt term, is read adjacently with the nursing scenes and sites depicted in the guidebook literature and other early modern texts.[51] "Grievous and terrible" redness, as we have seen, is ever-implicit in the bloody act of breastfeeding, or, to restate Kathryn Schwarz's incisive argument, "nursing threatens to produce the image of the bloody child." I would add that the nursing's latent image of blood-spurting breasts and blood-splattered infants can be affiliated with the racialized and diseased redness that is associated with Jews, even as the horrific red specters potentially evoked by both nurse and Jew are simultaneously repressed by the conversionary act of idealized gentile maternal breastfeeding, which changes red blood into white and, by extension, Jews into Christians.

In all of the texts this essay considers, gentile perceptions of Jews seem fixated on perverse forms of redness, blood, and sucking as signs or symptoms of the so-called diseased, demonic, and unnatural Jewish body and character. Given these preoccupations, it is not surprising that anxieties about Jewish and other forms of racialized difference enter English discourse through the suckled, gentile female breast. This "boundary panic" feeds, and is fed by, the cultural reconstruction of nursing maternity into a political mechanism through which children can be interpellated into the state as normative subjects – a governing reinscription of motherhood that necessitates the demonizing or, more precisely, the Judaizing of wet nurses and other "deviant" maternal figures. It is this same cultural pathology that underpins early modern English attempts to conjoin nation-building and maternal breastfeeding as interlocking social projects, both designed to secure the always-permeable borders between nursing mothers and "others."

Notes

1. Cited by Joshua Tractenberg, *The Devil and Jews: The Medieval Conception of the Jews and His Relation to Antisemitism* (New Haven: Yale University Press, 1945), 145.
2. Claudine Fabre-Vassas, *The Singular Beast: Jews, Christians, and the Pig*, trans. Carol Volk (New York: Columbia University Press, 1997), 145.
3. Janet Adelman, *Suffocating Mothers: Fantasies of Maternal Origin in Shakespeare's Plays, Hamlet to The Tempest* , (New York: Routledge, 1992), 29.
4. Gail Kern Paster, *The Body Embarrassed: Drama and the Disciplines of Shame in Early Modern England* (Ithaca: Cornell University Press, 1993), p. 169.
5. James Guillimeau, *The Nursing of Children. Wherein is set downe, the ordering and gouernment of them, from their birth*; affixed to *Childbirth, or the Happie Deliverie of Women* (London, 1612), sig.Ii4.
6. All quotations from Shakespeare's plays are taken from *The Complete Works of Shakespeare*, updated fourth edition, ed. David Bevington (New York: Longman-Addison Wesley Longman, 1997) and are noted in the text. Janet Adelman reads these lines in relation to "the fantasy of male parthenogenesis" in *Suffocating Mothers*, p. 225. Gail Paster discusses nursing and orality from a psychoanalytical perspective in *The Body Embarrassed*, pp. 260–80.
7. For illuminating analysis of wet-nursing and maternal surrogacy in *Romeo and Juliet*, see Paster, pp. 220–31.
8. William Gouge, *Of Domesticall Duties. Eight Treatises*, (London, 1621), p. 518.
9. Gouge, p. 512.
10. David Leverenz, *The Language of Puritan Feeling: an Exploration in Literature, Psychology, and Social History* (New Brunswick: Rutgers University Press, 1980), p. 72.
11. Gouge, p. 509.
12. Robert Cleaver and John Dod, *A Godly Form of Household Government: For the Ordering of Private Families, according to the Direction of God's Word* (London, 1621, 1st edn., 1614), sig. S4v.
13. Gouge, p. 289.
14. Fabre-Vassas, p. 57.
15. Cleaver and Dod, sig. P4r.
16. Stephen Greenblatt, "Mutilation and Meaning," in *The Body in Parts: Fantasies of Corporeality in Early Modern Europe*, ed. David Hillman and Carla Mazzio (New York: Routledge, 1997), pp. 230, 236–7.
17. Guillimeau, *The Nursing of Children*, Preface, I.i.2.
18. Cleaver and Dod, sig. P4r.
19. Cleaver and Dod, sig. P4v.
20. See "complexion," (entry 4), *Oxford English Dictionary*, which dates the term's first reference to "the natural colour, texture, and appearance of the skin, *esp.* of the face" to 1568.
21. Kim F. Hall, *Things of Darkness: Economies of Race and Gender in Early Modern England* (Ithaca: Cornell University Press, 1995), p. 3.

22. Illuminating commentary on the "good" breast/"bad" breast dichotomy from perspectives different from my own can be found in Peter B. Erickson, "Patriarchal Structures in *The Winter's Tale*," *PMLA* 97 (1982), 819, and Kathryn Schwarz, "Missing the Breast: Desire, Disease, and the Singular Effect of Amazons," in *The Body in Parts*, p. 157.

23. Mary Janell Metzger argues that prevailing notions of Jews as "resistant and finally integrable," epitomized by Shylock, also led to the construction of "deserving" Jews, i.e. Jessica, who might be "truly convertible" in "'Now by My Hood, a Gentle and No Jew': Jessica, *The Merchant of Venice*, and the Discourse of Early Modern English Identity," *PMLA* 113 (1998): 52–63.

24. Shapiro, p. 171.

25. Samuel Purchas, *Purchas His Pilgrimage* (London, 1626), p. 182.

26. Thomas Laqueur, *Making Sex: Body and Gender from the Greeks to Freud* (Cambridge: Harvard University Press, 1990), esp. pp. 25, 37, 38, 171–4. Laqueur's study is contested by, among others, Gail Paster (*The Body Embarrassed*, esp. Chapter 2 and 4.)

27. Quoted in Shapiro, p. 38.

28. On early modern perceptions of breast milk as a derivative of menstrual blood, see Adelman, p. 7, and Audrey Eccles, *Obstetrics and Gynaecology in Tudor and Stuart England* (Kent, Ohio: Kent State University Press, 1982), pp. 49–50.

29. Notable studies of the myth of Jewish ritual murder include Trachtenberg, R. Po-chia Hsia, *The Myth of Ritual Murder* (New Haven: Yale University Press, 1988), Shapiro, pp. 100–111, Fabre-Vassas, pp. 129–36.

30. Shapiro, pp. 101.

31. Stuart Clark, "Inversion, Misrule, and Witchcraft," *Past and Present*, 87 (1980), 110.

32. References to Milton's poetry are taken from *Complete Poems and Major Prose*, ed. Merritt Y. Hughes (New York: Odyssey Press, 1957) and noted in the text.

33. Purchas, *Pilgrimage*, p. 152.

34. Achsah Guibbory discusses the commingling of "Heathenisme" and "Judaisme" in Herrick's "sacrifice" poems in *Ceremony and Community From Herbert to Donne: Literature, Religion, and Cultural Conflict in Seventeenth-Century England* (Cambridge: Cambridge University Press, 1998), pp. 95–105, and in "The Temple of *Hesperides* and the Anglo-Puritan Controversy," in *"The Muses Common-weal": Poetry and Politics in the Earlier Seventeenth Century*, ed. Claude J. Summers and Ted-Larry Pebworth (University of Missouri Press, 1988), p. 142.

35. Cited in Leon Poliakov, *A History of Anti-Semitism*, 3 vols. (New York: Vanguard Press, 1974), I, p. 223, and Shapiro, p. 113. Neither provides the source for this quotation. The quotation also implicitly elevates a wife made Amazonian by mastectomy over a gentile man judaized by circumcision.

36. I borrow this translated passage from Fabre-Vassas, p. 119. The original French text appears in *Erreurs populaires* (Paris, 1578), p. 205.

37. Fabre-Vassas, p. 119.

38. Cited in Shapiro, p. 260–1.

39. Thomas Coryate, *Coryate's Crudities; Reprinted from the Edition of 1611. To which Are Now Added, His Letters from India* (London, 1776), vol. 3, sig. U7r–U8v.

40. Shapiro, p. 116.

41. Michel de Montaigne, *Montaigne's Travel Journal*, trans. Donald M. Frame (San Francisco: North Point Press, 1983), pp. 81–2. That the passage was recorded

by one of Montaigne's servants charged with compiling the journal may account for its almost complete occlusion of Montaigne's own Jewish lineage, which complicates any reading of this "testimony."

42. Eccles, p. 51.

43. Schwarz, "Missing the Breast," p. 156.

44. Leverenz, p. 73–5. I follow Leverenz's argument very closely here, even though my aims fundamentally diverge from his. While Leverenz argues that the confluence between Christian education and maternal breastfeeding helps to weaken traditional norms of masculinity, I argue, on the contrary, that sucking in the Word, as it were, reinforces official discourses and identities.

45. Robert Pricke, *The Doctrine of Superiority, and subiection, contained in the Fift Commandment* (London, 1609), section K.

46. Robert Cleaver, *A Briefe Explanation of the Whole Booke of the Proverbs of Salomon* (London, 1615), pp. 352–3.

47. My thinking about language and lactation has benefitted from Mihoko Suzuki's theorizing of the (gendered) public sphere and women's political subjectivity in *"Subordinate Subjects": Gender, Class and Nationhood, 1588–1688* (in manuscript), and I would like to thank her for allowing me to see a draft of her study.

48. Cotton Mather, *A Father Departing* ... (Boston, 1723), pp. 22–3.

49. Edmund Spenser, *A View of the Present State of Ireland*, ed. W.L. Renwick (Oxford: Clarendon, 1970), p. 67

50. Samuel Usque, *Consolation for the Tribulations of Israel* (Ferrara, 1553), trans. from the Portuguese by Martin A. Cohen (Philadelphia: Jewish Publication Society of America, 1965), pp. 181–4. Shapiro counts the threat of Jewish contamination as one of the "more striking aspects of Usque's story," while my focus is on the imagery of "Jewish milk" and breastfeeding, both spiritual and material.

51. Fabre-Vassas, on the *Judensau*, pp. 108, 126, 135; on "The Red Jew," pp. 105–9; the section on "The Mark of Judas," pp. 109–12 is also pertinent.

PART II

NURTURE AND INSTRUCTION

Language and "Mothers' Milk": Maternal Roles and the Nurturing Body in Early Modern Spanish Texts

Emilie L. Bergmann

Pure Blood, Pure Milk, Pure Language

In 1615, an Andean chronicler, Felipe Guaman Poma de Ayala, wrote to his monarch to protest the corruption and abuses of Spanish colonial administration in Peru. Central to his critique was the disruption of Andean community life resulting from the practices of immoral clergy and colonial officials. Throughout his 1200-page manuscript Guaman Poma repeats the lament, "y los yndios se acaban," a simple phrase that reflects a complex historical process: "the Indians are finished / it's finished for the Indians." In addition to the slaughter of individual Indians in the Spaniards' military campaigns, their economic, political, religious and social policies were wiping out indigenous culture, lineage and population through forced labor in the mines and sexual exploitation of indigenous women. The mixture of races, or *mestizaje* that resulted was not only that of Europeans with indigenous Andeans but also Africans and mulattoes with Indian "blood." Almost negligible in comparison with the catalogue of Spanish sexual abuses of Indian women is a brief passage in which Guaman Poma attributes the bad character of Peruvian-born Spaniards to their wetnursing by women of other races:

> ... los dichos criollos que se crían con la leche de las yndias o de negras o los dichos mestizos, mulatos, son bravos y soberbios, haraganes, mentirosos, jugadores, auarientos, de poca caridad, miserable, tranposos, enemigo de los pobres yndios y de españoles. Y ancí son los criollos como mestizos, peor que mestizos ... (566)

> (the said *criollos* (Peruvian-born Spaniards) who are raised on the milk of Indian or African women or the said *mestizos* [and] mulattoes, are aggressive and arrogant, lazy, lying, gambling, greedy, uncharitable, stingy, swindlers, enemies

of the poor Indians and Spaniards. Thus the *criollos* are like *mestizos*, or worse
than *mestizos* …) [translation mine]

This aspect of Guaman Poma's critique of the abuses of colonial administration
dominated largely by *criollos* is constructed upon the early modern concept of
milk as a form of blood, and the ethnicity and character of the nurse as
transmissible through her milk to the upper-class infants she nurtures.

There is, however, another socially disruptive process to which Guaman
Poma does not refer directly, the changes in gender relations resulting from
Indian women serving in the homes of the *criollos*. Irene Silverblatt argues that
in pre-Inca Andean societies, the agricultural, textile and childrearing labor of
women was valued equally with that of men as an essential contribution to
the wellbeing of her *allyu* (community) (Silverblatt, 8–9). Before Spanish
colonization, the Inca empire had already imposed gender hierarchies, and
Spanish rule brought new categories and disruptions of traditional Andean
social structures. In her study of domestic labor in colonial Peru, Elinor Burkett
found that the labor of Indian women caring for the first generations of
Peruvian-born Spanish infants in colonial households had a significant impact
on traditional social structures (111). Women domestic servants had access to
information about their colonizers that was unavailable to their male
counterparts, and these women's earning power gave them another significant
advantage over the men in their families. Guaman Poma's reference to
contamination by the nurturing female body deploys a figure familiar to his
monarch and his ministers in order to protest the destruction of a body politic so
different from the Spanish model that his monarch and his ministers might well
not recognize it as such without the familiar figure of milk as blood.

The most disruptive intersections of colonization and the maternal body
were related not to the practice of wet-nursing but rather to the alienation of
women from their communities through the violence of rape, the exploitation
of concubinage, or the betrayal by men desperate enough to try to buy their
freedom from forced labor in *mitayas* by offering the women in their families to
colonial officials. The brief passage regarding wetnursing, however, connects
sixteenth and seventeenth-century Spanish colonial society with the multi-
cultural medieval history of the peninsula. Among his discussions of *mestizaje*
elsewhere in the *Nueva crónica*, involving indigenous mothers and European,
African, or mulatto fathers, Guaman Poma makes specific mention of the
"mancha" or taint inherited by the children of a Jewish father. By this he means
a father of Jewish descent, or rather a descendant of Spanish "new Christians,"
Jews who converted to Christianity before 1492. He disregards the Jewish
perspective on this question. Instead of tracing Jewish identity through the
mother's line, Guaman Poma's concern is with the Jewishness of *mestizo*
children of Indian mothers.

The preoccupation with maintaining ethnic communities through purity of "blood" has a long history in Hispanic cultures. The medieval phenomenon of a multi-ethnic and trilingual culture in much of the Iberian peninsula left its mark on discourses of the maternal. Although advice literature regarding wet-nursing in early modern Spain shares many characteristics with other didactic texts addressed to mothers in English and Italian, there are significant differences arising from the eight-centuries of transculturation among Christians, Muslims and Jews. Throughout Europe, medical and moral discourse of wet-nursing can be traced to their common Greek, Latin and Italian sources: among them Galen, Soranus, Alberti and Juan Luis Vives. The most obvious of these shared characteristics is the contradiction between the moral and medical admonitions against wet-nursing and the practical advice on choosing wet nurses that almost invariably follows them.[1] Perhaps less contradictory, because it is based upon practice rather than theory, is the advice that the nurse be well-spoken, acknowledging that the earliest linguistic influences on infants come from the women who nurture them.[2] This advice dates back to Greek and Latin sources, but it takes on a particularly problematic aspect for Spanish-born parents in Peru or Mexico, where despite advice to the contrary, infants were likely to have nurses whose mother tongue was Nahuatl, Quechua, or Yoruba.

The eight centuries of transculturation among Muslims, Christians and Jews in Spain did not end in 1492 with the expulsion of Jews and Muslims; rather, the culturally and genetically internalized others became focal points of Christian culture, haunting presences in the language and in everyday cultural practices. The preoccupation with ethnic purity, imagined culturally as purity of blood, was common to all three groups in the medieval period, and the milk-as-blood model placed wet-nursing in a contested position. Heath Dillard in her study *Daughters of the Reconquest* observes a new, "harsher climate of intolerance" evident in thirteenth-century laws that separated women of the dominant Christian group from their Jewish and Muslim counterparts by prohibiting cross-cultural wet-nursing, among regulations regarding domestic activities (206–207). Iberian conduct manuals and misogynistic satire lent the image of Jewish and Muslim otherness to the potential dangers of negligent or unhealthy wet nurses.

Despite the awareness that virtually all the children of the literate and political, economically and culturally dominant groups were nurtured by women other than those who gave birth to them, the metaphor of maternal breastfeeding was commonplace in discussions of the vernacular as "mother tongue." This metaphor is deployed as an authorizing discourse by two Hispanic humanists whose positions with regard to Castilian ethnic, religious and territorial hegemony were significantly problematic. Juan de Valdés's *Diálogo de la lengua* (c. 1535) is an affirmation of his native Castilian as the language of empire. The self-taught *mestizo* humanist Inca Garcilaso de la Vega wrote his *Comentarios reales* (1609) as a chronicle of the Inca empire, and he bases his historiographical authority on his familiarity with Quechua, the language he can literally call his mother tongue or *lengua materna*.[3] The setting of Valdés's dialogue is Naples, and the characters are Valdés himself and a group of Italian students interested in learning the language of power, since Naples and Sicily were under the crown of Aragon. Valdés positions himself in the dialogue as a representative of power, but his Erasmian religious ideas placed him on the social margins and forced him into exile. The Inca Garcilaso authorizes his voice as *mestizo* chronicler of pre-conquest Andean history and culture, son of a conquistador and an aristocratic Inca mother, a *palla*. He "drank in" his knowledge of Quecha "with his mother's milk," listening to tales of lost glory told by his maternal relatives. The Inca frames his linguistic corrections of the colonizers' representation of Quechua place names and cultural terms in humanistic rhetorical and philological discourses. Both writers' use of the naturalizing metaphor of culture and language as "mothers' milk" challenges the conceptual separation between maternal culture and patriarchal language. Valdés literalizes the term "mother tongue" as the specifically oral form of the vernacular spoken by the mother while at the same time pursuing a profoundly contradictory project, that of legitimizing the replacement of Latin with Spanish, and colloquial, spoken Spanish in particular, as the language of power:

> todos los hombres somos más obligados a ilustrar y enriquecer la lengua que nos es natural y que mamamos en las tetas de nuestras madres, que no la que nos es pegadiza y que aprendemos en libros. (44)

> (We are all more obliged to glorify and enrich the language that is natural to us, and that we suckled at our mothers' breasts, than the language that was stuck onto us, the one we learned in books.)

Valdés practices the spoken style he prescribes in his use of the colorful colloquial terms "tetas" (the more Latin-derived term would be "pechos") and "pegadiza." While Latin continued to be the language learned at school by those boys being prepared for positions of political and intellectual authority in the early modern period, a vernacular language, the specifically Castilian pronunciation and usage advocated and explained by Valdés, was constituted as the language of power throughout the Spanish empire. In addition to the religious outsider Valdés's equivocal position as one of the empire's "others," his naturalizing image of the maternal breast is compromised by his readers' awareness that in the privileged ranks of society to which they belonged or aspired, the practice of wet-nursing effectively severed the authorizing discursive lineage through the mother's body.

Valdés's legitimization of the "mother tongue" as basis for the written style of learned men can be traced to a concept of archaic purity in maternal usage, as María Rosa Lida points out in her discussion of Cicero's representation of Cornelia, mother of the Gracchi, as exemplary teacher to her sons who grew up to be renowned for their eloquence (42). This classical depiction of admirable archaism in women's language was, not surprisingly, exploited by Renaissance writers as a justification for excluding women from advanced education. Juan Luis Vives, in *De officio mariti* (1528) (On the duties of the husband) transforms Cornelia's linguistic legacy into exemplary silence (Lida 243–4). Vives conceptualizes the maternal body as a passive receptacle for the family's and the state's treasure, an archaic tradition of eloquence that is "soaked up" rather than learned systematically by the women of antiquity as if it were a liquid similar to the milk with which they are proverbially depicted as imparting language and eloquence to their sons. As with Valdés's metaphor of maternal language, Vives's discourse concerning the careful choosing of well-spoken wet nurses in *De institutione feminae Christianae* (1523) (On the Education of the Christian Woman), and his readers' familiarity with the practice of hiring wetnurses casts doubt on his model for the "natural" absorption of language and values from mother to son.

More than half a century after Valdés and Vives, the Inca Garcilaso continued to use humanist discourses of knowledge and language to authorize his historiographic project, and to use the verb "mamar" (nurse, suckle) to appropriate the traditional metaphor of the connection between the mother's body and language learning: "que yo protesto decir llanamente la relación que mamé en la leche" (I, xix, 46) (I declare that I am telling plainly the narrative that I suckled with [my mother's] milk); "la lengua que mamé en la leche" (the language I sucked in with milk); "aquestas fábulas y verdades, como yo las mamé" (II, x) (these narratives and truths, just as I drank them in) (Garcés 1991: 127). The Inca represents as his mother tongue the language in which he learned the history of the Inca empire (I, xvii, 42) in contrast to the Castilian that was his father's legacy and the Latin he taught himself, although he cites an uncle as the maternal relative who supplied the oral sources for the historical narrative.

In Cervantes's *El coloquio de los perros* (The Dogs' Colloquy), published in 1613, only a few years after the publication of the Inca Garcilaso's historical narrative of pre-conquest Peru, the dogs Cipión and Berganza invert the association of the "mother tongue" with linguistic authority and historical truth. Instead, these canine pícaros attribute to the maternal a legacy of malice and gossip: "El hacer y decir mal lo heredamos de nuestros primeros padres y lo mamamos en la leche" (We inherit the tendency to do and speak evil from our first parents and absorb it with our mothers' milk) (Cervantes 315, cited in Garcés 1993: 304). Interestingly, Berganza includes nurses in his primal linguistic scene: "Y casi la primera palabra que habla [el niño] es llamar puta a su ama o madre" (Almost the first word the child utters is to call his nurse or his mother whore) (Cervantes 315, cited in Garcés 1993: 304). The abjection of the maternal is clearly delineated in Berganza's account of his encounter with

Cañizares, a self-identified witch who claims to have witnessed his birth as a human and his transformation into a dog. Berganza's interlocutor, Cipión, tries unsuccessfully to temper his "backbiting" satire, an exaggeration of picaresque misogyny.

Physical revulsion toward the female body pervades the fifteenth-century Valencian poem often cited as a precursor of the picaresque, Jaume Roig's *Espill o llibre de les dones* (ca. 1460) (Mirror or Book of Women). The third of the four books that constitute the *Espill* is the "Lliçó de Salamó" (Sermon of Solomon) a ventriloquized diatribe against women that the narrator claims to have heard in a dream.[4] Among the moral and social vices on Solomon's long list he includes a satirical depiction of wet nurses. Later advice literature refers to the dangers of unhealthy or negligent wet nurses in more abbreviated form and offset by descriptions of the ideal wet nurse's temperate habits and character. Roig's satirical purpose, however, is served by his horrifyingly detailed list of bizarre cases that illustrate the medieval concept of correspondences: a hermit who inherited his taste for wilderness and solitude from the doe who nursed him, a young woman who acquired from the dogs who suckled her the disgusting habit of re-ingesting food she had vomited, and a boy who loved to roll in the mud because he was fed with sows' milk.[5] For Vives and later authors of conduct manuals, the mud-loving boy sufficed. Roig accuses wet nurses of endangering infants' lives by giving them harmful drugs to make them sleep (a practice still in use in the eighteenth and nineteenth centuries in other countries) and maliciously concealing their inadequate lactation and serious illnesses. The infants who survive the nurses' deceit suffer from a long list of illnesses and deformities: insanity, ugliness, left-handedness, crossed eyes, hunched backs, hernias and pigeon-toes. Roig assimilates the Old Testament figure of Solomon into the ranks of Old Christians; his ventriloquized admonitions include a warning against hiring Jewish wet nurses, whose milk could cause a child to grow up timid ("medroso") (90). Roig's warnings reflect an attitude reflected in laws throughout medieval Europe segregating Christian women from Jewish and Muslim women (Fildes 39–41). "In 1258 the Cortes of Valladolid prohibited Christian women from becoming nurses to Jewish and Muslim children and barred women of the minorities from nursing Christians, an order repeated by the same body at Jerez ten years later" (Dillard 207). In medieval Spain, a double standard had long before imposed severe penalties on sexual relations between Christian women and Jewish or Muslim men, while "no stigma attached to the Christian man who consorted or cohabited with Jewish or Muslim women" (206–207).

Valerie Fildes observes that "[a]ttacks on wet nursing only really began in England after the Reformation, when Puritanism was becoming a major religious and behavioural force" (68), but the bitterness of Roig's medieval satire is matched by other fifteenth-century misogynistic works. Grotesque visions of the maternal body continue to surface in two sixteenth-century Spanish conduct manuals, Vives's *Institutione Feminae Christianae* and Fray Antonio de Guevara's *Relox de príncipes* (1529). Both compare human mothers disparagingly to their sister animals, using metaphors of mammalian behavior to claim the justification of nature as a superior guide (Bergmann 1992). Vives cites Columella's treatise on agriculture as the source for his example of ideal maternal behavior: "de canibus … sic scribit Columella: 'Nec unquam eos, quorum generosam volumus indolem conservare, patiemur alienae nutricis uberibus educari, quoniam semper et lac et spiritus longe magis ingenii atque incrementa corporis auget." (Vives 1745 [1964], 258) (When we wish to conserve the noble lineage of dogs, we do not allow them to be nurtured or raised at the breasts of other nurses. Their bodies and character grow much more when they receive the milk and spirit of their own mothers. [Paraphrase mine]). Columella refers not to "natural" maternal instincts among canines but to the practices of purebred dog-breeders. In his Castilian translation of 1528, Juan Justiniano omits the reference to dogs and wisely replaces Columella with a much longer citation from Aulus Gellius's *Noctes Atticae*, a more commonly cited authority on family life among humans (Vives 1995, 319–21).

The garrulous and sometimes fanciful counselor to Charles V, Antonio de Guevara, creates an array of grotesque anatomical and zoological images, contrasting overcivilized, "monstrous" human mothers to the "natural" practices of other mammals, and simian mothers in particular, whom he claims to have observed himself (Bergmann 1996). His readers can prove for themselves by observing how these ideal mothers never let go of their nursing offspring for a single moment from the moment of their birth until they are weaned: "Hallarán por verdad todos los que leyeren esta escritura, y si quisieren lo verán como yo lo vi por experiencia, que desde la hora que la mona pare a sus hijos jamás hasta que están destetados los dexa de sus braços" (507). Donna Haraway designates as "monsters" the primates whose behavior is observed and analysed in social science fieldwork, and groups them together with women and cyborgs as "odd boundary creatures who play a destabilizing role in the great Western evolutionary, technological, and biological narratives. These boundary creatures are, literally, *monsters*, a word that shares more than its root with the word, to *demonstrate*. Monsters signify" (2). "Nature," she reminds her readers, is always a contested term in philosophical and scientific discourse. Guevara displays primate mothers, exemplars of "natural" maternal behavior in contrast to the cautionary narratives of famous miscarriages and matricides of antiquity that resulted from such urban excesses as tight-waisted dresses and overindulgence in diet, dancing, and attendance at crowded parties.

Guevara's virtuoso performance of the maternal grotesque also deploys the examples of wolves, pigs, and swans, who are attributed with the desire to hold and nurse their avian offspring if only they were human, but it approaches

Rabelaisian proportions when he lists a series of appendages from which infants might be produced. The reiterated "naciessen" could lend the emphatic solemnity of a sermon (and Guevara was best known as a preacher) but in this context the anatomical fragmentation of the passage is hysterically comical:

> si los hijos naciessen de las uñas, o naciessen de los codos, o naciessen de los dedos, o naciessen de las muñecas, parece que no sería mucho darlos a criar a amas estrañas, pero yo no sé qué corazón de muger basta a lo sufrir, que el hijo que nace de sus mismas entrañas le osse fiar de manos agenas. (506)

> (If children were born from the fingernails, or were born from the elbows, or were born from the fingers, or were born from the wrists, it would not seem like much to give them to strangers to nurse, but I do not know what woman's heart can dare to allow that the child born of her own belly be entrusted to the hands of strangers.)

In early modern Spain the criteria for choosing wet nurses generally conform to the classical models of Galen and Soranus cited by Valerie Fildes. Bernardus Gordonius's fourteenth-century medical treatise, known in Spain as *Lilio de la medicina* was a popular source of practical advice for midwives on women's medical problems and childbirth in particular. Gordonius reminds the employers of nurses to warn them of the risk of serious injury and fatalities caused by "overlaying," but acknowledges the affective bonds that make it difficult for the nurse to deny the infant's desire for the warmth and comfort of sleeping next to her (Martínez Blanco 213–14). His detailed instructions for choosing wet nurses include the traditional low-tech test of the consistency of breast milk by observing the behavior of a drop placed on a fingernail (Martínez Blanco 213; Fildes 20–22). It is worth noting that another medieval version of this test is clearly gender-marked in its recommendation that the milk be placed on the blade of a sword (Fildes 32, citing *Practica Puerorum* [12–15th C.] 24), perhaps reflecting the dominant paternal role in the recruitment of nurses for the children of the elite, and adding the question of class to that of infant care and feeding. Male or female, noble or peasant, thumbnails are virtually universal, while a sword would be an easily accessible gauge for the quality of milk handy only to those men whose noble lineage gave them the privilege of wearing one.

The Milky Way to Social Privilege

There is more abundant documentation on wet-nursing practices involving foundlings and royal infants than on the history of maternal practices among the middle ranks of Spanish society during the early modern period. Since the appearance of Valerie Fildes's research on foundling hospitals in England and Christiane Klapisch-Zuber's work on wet-nursing in Florence, Joan Sherwood,

Claude Larquié, and María del Carmen Simón Palmer have published pioneering research on the Inclusa in Madrid and other foundling hospitals from the seventeenth to the early twentieth century. Heath Dillard's work on medieval Spanish women includes significant material on legal recognition of wetnurses. Simón Palmer's *Cocina de palacio* includes lists of rations provided for the royal *amas de lactancia* and the daunting diet of solid food that immediately replaced the nurse's milk as soon as royal infants were weaned.[6]

Advice literature intended to regulate the nurturing of heirs to privilege can be traced at least as early as Alfonso X the Learned's codification of medieval Spanish law in the *Siete partidas* (1256–1265). As were other Castilian treatises on wet-nursing the *Partidas'* criteria for choosing nurses for royal infants were based on Avicenna's version of Soranus. The ideal royal wet nurses are described as healthy, with virtuous habits and good lineage, and care is to be taken that they not be "muy sañudas" (ill-tempered): "si el ama 'non fuere sañuda, criarlos ha más amorosamente, e con mansedumbre, que es cosa que han mucho menester los niños, para crescer ayna" (2.6 cited in Dillard 156, and 2.7.3 cited in Voltes, 82) (if the nurse "is not ill-tempered, she will raise them more lovingly, and with gentleness, of which children have a great need, in order to thrive.) Dillard notes that "Castilian royal nurses, unlike their counterparts in the towns, were hired for ten or twenty years as governesses, and their importance to royal children is attested by the gifts of land many received at their retirement in recognition of devoted service (157). The importance of wet nurses in nurturing royal infants is made clear in the Catalonian chronicle of the adventures and military campaigns of Ramón Muntaner (1256–1336). The *Crónica* narrates Muntaner's strategy of locating and deploying nurses for the infant Jaume II, thus successfully delivering the future king of Mallorca to his grandmother in 1315 (Voltes 81).

The benefits accruing to wet nurses who served the royal court included not only land but in some cases the privileges of knighthood (*hidalguía*), among which exemption from taxes and billeting soldiers were particularly valuable. Dillard notes the household personnel of a knight were also exempted from municipal taxation, and that the *Partidas* extend the knight's privileges to his widow and children regarding "certain essential agricultural employees," among whom wet nurses are the only women specifically listed (156). The historical records of the Biblioteca de Palacio and the Archivo General de Palacio in Madrid document two cases of privileges of knighthood bestowed on a former palace nurse by the king. In the first of these examples, dated 1189, the transaction is between women: the king, Alfonso VIII, acts on the request of his daughter Berenguela's request.[7] The document confirms that the donation was given, along with other possessions, by Doña Elvira and her husband Don Diego Piédrez to the monastery of San Pedro de Arlanza in the province of Burgos, where the Cid Campeador, Ruy Díaz de Vivar, left his wife and daughter in the care of monks in the previous century. Fildes, citing Dillard, notes that while gifts might be made to the nurse and her husband, "the principal beneficiary was always the nurse" (37).

By the time of the second document in 1792, the beneficiary had changed. In this eighteenth-century document regarding an honorary title rather than land, Charles IV directly grants the privilege of *hidalguía* (knighthood) to the husband of a former royal wet nurse "en atención a haver tenido D. Ysavel Martinez de San Miguel, Muger legitima de vos Don Pedro Garrido, Vecino del Lugar de Salduendo en Castilla la Vieja, el honor de dar el Pecho a la Ynfanta Da. Maria Teresa, mi mui cara y amada Hija" (In recognition of Doña Isabel Martínez de San Miguel, the lawful wife of yourself, Don Pedro Garrido, inhabitant of the town of Salduendo in Old Castile, having had the honor of giving the breast to the Infanta Doña Maria Teresa, my very dear and beloved daughter).[8] The privileges are granted to Don Pedro Garrido and to his sons and direct descendants on the male side ("vos el dicho Dn. Pedro Garrido y vuestros hijos que al presente teneis y los que tuvieren adelante y que descendieren de ellos varones y hembras legitimos y naturales por linea recta de varon") to enjoy "in perpetuity and forevermore," without requiring any further service in return. The historical context of revolution circumscribes the Spanish Bourbon's promise of privileges held "in perpetuity" at a time when his relatives' royal privileges, not to mention their lives, were being terminated in France.

The historical records of the Biblioteca and the Archivo General de Palacio document the expeditions sent to the province of Burgos, home of the medieval epic hero the Cid Campeador, in search of nurses suitable for the royal household.[9] In 1651 two meetings were held among the palace physicians concerning the criteria and recruitment of royal wet nurses.[10] Unlike the medieval nurses contracted for ten to twenty years, these nurses were sent home once the infants were weaned, or the nurses' milk was no longer adequate or had declined in quality.[11] In order for the nurses to be sent home, they had to be paid, and that final transaction proved difficult to complete during the frequent economic crises. Documents from the eighteenth century allow a glimpse of the restless *amas de lactancia* continuing to live in the palace and in the homes of courtiers while the palace accountants desperately juggled the books in search of funds from other sources to pay their travel expenses:

> 1713. 24 setiembre. Las amas del Príncipe D. Luis e Infante D. Fernando piden se las paguen sus haberes como antes de la suspensión de pagos.

> (The nurses of the Prince Don Luis and the Infante Don Fernando ask that they be paid their salaries as they were before the suspension of payments.)

> 1715. A.M. dispone que del dinero que tiene D. Ricardo Lepreux, se paguen los gastos para el avio de las amas.

(His Majesty allocates funds from Don Ricardo Lepreux's account to pay for provisions for the nurses.)

1729. Que se paguen a las amas despedidas de los Señores Infantes: y que sean mejor y más puntualmente asistidas las demás amas de SS.AA. que están de repuesto en Madrid.

(That the nurses who have been dismissed from service to the Infantes be paid and that the other nurses of their majesties in Madrid be better and more punctually attended.)[12]

The palace archives continue to document the Spanish preoccupation with ethnic purity well into the nineteenth century. The documents regarding nurses chosen for the Infanta Francisca de Asís in 1824 include an affidavit of baptism and purity of blood (*limpieza de sangre*) for two peasant women from the province of Burgos, signed by the parish priest.[13] While the northern region of Asturias, not coincidentally known for its dairy cows, was the nineteenth-century bourgeoisie's preferred source of nurses, the province of Burgos, home of the Cid, was ideal hunting ground for royal wet nurses from the seventeenth to well into the nineteenth century. A mid-eighteenth century search party, however, ventured into La Mancha, perhaps to find descendants of Dulcinea del Toboso. Nurses are often are described as having dark brown hair and eyes, "good color," meaning either olive or "robust" complexion, and good and abundant milk. One of the women listed in the 1824 document, Angela Castillo from the town of El Cid del Bivar, had a two and a half-month-old child; the other, María Santos Gómez, from Cardeña Ximeno, had a twenty-five-day-old child, and the sketchy information does not include the fate of those infants.

Nurses on the Move: Geographic and Economic Mobility

The research of Heath Dillard on the medieval period and Carmen Sarasúa on the eighteenth and nineteenth century shows that wet-nursing was relatively well paid, offering unique opportunities for women in the labor market. Although wage scales varied throughout Castile, Dillard notes that "[t]he Cortes of Jerez in 1268 set the day wage of a woman labourer in Andalusia at six maravedís, half that of a man, although as a wet nurse she would earn ten" (164). Medieval Iberian legal codes imposed severe punishment for injury to a woman's breast, in recognition of the loss of income this could entail for professional wet nurses and the danger to the children of other women (Martínez Blanco 212). Among surviving documents regarding wet-nursing are the records of salaries paid from municipal treasuries to nurses who took in abandoned infants (212).

Carmen Sarasúa's study of the role of domestic service in the labor market in eighteenth and nineteenth-century Madrid reveals a highly mobile work force, including women working as wet nurses, moving between city and countryside. The nurses whose employment she studied were equally willing to provide their services as domestic servants living in wealthier households or keeping infants in their own homes in Madrid or in small towns within a day's journey of the capital. These women paid others to care for their infants or left them in the foundling hospital in order to earn the desirable wages for nursing the children of other women (142). The demographic studies of Sarasúa, Larquié, and María F. Carbajo Isla have found that wet-nursing was a seasonal occupation. Since wet nurses tended to neglect their charges during the harvest, mortality rates were high during August. In the winter months, peasant women sought employment as nurses to supplement the family income, and emigration to Madrid peaked in inverse proportion to declining peasant income during March and April. In times of economic crisis, peasants went to Madrid in search of work but did not solicit nurselings to live in the villages (Sarasúa 155). Anastasio Rojo Vega's research in the provincial archives of Valladolid reveals the range of salaries for *amas de leche*: in 1543 the annual salary for nursing a newborn girl was 2,244 maravedís, in 1555 it was 4,488 and in 1564, 5,000 maravedís. The nurse for the children of the Count of Lemos earned 150,000 maravedís annually; the nurse for the son of a military officer, 14,000 (157). Rojo Vega cites prices ranging from 11 to 22 maravedís for a loaf of bread during this period, and wages for laborers working in carpentry and agriculture from 34 to 51 maravedís per day.

At the lowest end of the economic and social scale, infants left in foundling hospitals were nursed by the poorest women. These women's wages were considerably lower than those of other nurses, since they were paid by charitable institutions with scant resources. Sherwood's and Larquié's research on the nurses of the foundling hospital in Madrid, the Inclusa, offers a grim picture of high rates of mortality, with only a handful among the hundreds of infants abandoned in the courtyard of the filthy, poorly-ventilated hospital surviving past their first year of life. The Inclusa could not afford to recruit nurses who fulfilled the criteria of moralists and medical practitioners, and Sherwood finds in the hospital's records evidence of boisterous and neglectful crowds of wet nurses, well aware that they were indispensable. The conditions of employment required that nurses who intended to take the infants to their homes had to travel to Madrid to pick up the infants and return each year to collect their salaries. Almost all of the nurses came from communities within fifty kilometers, no more than a day's journey, from Madrid, and the Inclusa's accounts record advances for many of the nurses, especially in certain months and in drought years. The work of Sherwood, Sarasúa and Larquié shows significant demographic shifts and delineates the limits of survival among peasants, artisans and the urban poor. Larquié notes the shift in occupations, from farmers and artisans to urban laborers, among the husbands of wet nurses employed by the Inclusa in the seventeenth century. The supplemental income from nursing infants from the foundling hospital helped the families of artisans and peasants in relatively comfortable circumstances, but for the poorest families, a nursing infant added an excessive burden to households where mothers were too poorly nourished to provide milk for another infant (1983, 238). In addition, once infants were weaned, caring for the child paid only a third of the salary for nursing (1983, 237).

Colonial Spanish culture in the Americas provides another, very different perspective on the economic and social effects of the practice of wet-nursing. Elinor Burkett's study of the status of indigenous women in sixteenth-century Peru shows that there was "a classic market situation wherein the scarcity of white women increased the value placed on Indian women" (123). The only contracts that specified the responsibilities and obligations of female servants were those of nursemaids or wet nurses, whose salaries were at the top of a scale for women's paid labor that ranged from six to thirty *pesos corrientes* (111). While the domestic employment of indigenous women in Spanish households, including wet-nursing, "strengthened their position within Hispanic society, it nonetheless broke down the relationships between these females and indigenous males, tying the women into a sex-based, rather than a race-based, social network" (122–3). The domestic labor available to women in Peru in this period is a key to understanding how a situation could develop that was so "radically different from contemporary social ideals of the position of nonwhite females in societies dominated by white men." With a new generation of Peruvian-born colonizers, the demographic balance of the sexes was re-established among the dominant caste, and the mobility and relative economic privilege of indigenous women was curtailed (123).

In addition to the protests of Guaman Poma in his *Nuevo gobierno*, the dominican Lizárraga (c. 1600) criticizes both interracial nursing and education: the children of Spaniards in Peru are spoiled by their parents and nursed by Indian or drunken African women who raise them in filthy surroundings. A *criollo* child plays with "indiezuelos" (Indian children; the suffix has potentially derogatory connotations), and after the age of five, when bad influences could be overcome by education, he is allowed to continue with "las inclinaciones que mamó en la leche." (the bad habits he drank in with [the nurse's] milk) Lizárraga paraphrases a proverbial expression, "hará lo que hace aquel con quien pace" (he does the same as the one with whom he grazes), picturing the nurse's body as a "pasture" for any number of young animals to assimilate bad cultural influences.

The difference is obvious between prescriptive treatises that warned against "impure blood" and the practice of hiring available women, who were as likely to be indigenous, African or of mixed heritage in the American colonies as they were of *converso* lineage in Spain. As Merry Wiesner puts it succinctly,

"wealthy women were pressured to produce many heirs, and people seem to
have been aware of the contraceptive effects of lactation; [women] were taught
that sexual intercourse would corrupt their milk and that their first duty was to
their husbands" (71), that is, to produce heirs to their husbands' property and
privilege. Yvonne Knibiehler points out that fathers who placed their newborn
infants with wet nurses were demanding a sacrifice from their wives, but that
the practice also created a kind of equality: being unable to nurse the infant
himself, she argues, he prevented his wife from nursing as well and thus
reduced lactation to a subaltern function, transforming a gendered relationship
into one based on class (103). The practice of wet-nursing created a unique
labor market and inspired a moralizing discourse of motherhood that could not
change the practice because the moralists' criticisms were aimed at the wrong
target. The decision and the ideology behind the practice of sending infants to
wet nurses were in the hands of the fathers, a figure of speech that brings
to mind Guevara's curious digital fantasy of childbirth. The moralists and the
medical practitioners, however persuasive their preaching might be, could not
compete with the economic interest of producing male heirs through the
optimum maternal fertility achieved through suppressing lactation, nor could
they offer anything comparable to the economic advantages and the geographic
and, in some cases social mobility the practice afforded to the nurses
themselves.

Notes

1. I thank Julia Hairston for allowing me to read Chapter 2 of her unpublished
   doctoral dissertation, "The Economics of Milk and Blood in Alberti's *Libri della
   famiglia*: Maternal versus Wet-Nursing," in which she presents a comprehensive
   discussion of these contradictions.
2. See Fildes's discussion of the preference among the Roman upper classes for
   Greek nurses. She cites the recommendations of Soranus (fl. 98–117CE) (16–17).
3. Margarita Zamora addresses the Inca Garcilaso's historiographic self-authoriz-
   ation in the *Comentarios* through his maternal ancestry.
4. Vidal i Alcover notes that Solomon's misogynistic speech in Roig's dream was
   inspired by Jean Lefèvre's *Mathèolus*, in which no less a figure than God serves
   as the author's mouthpiece, and by Bernat Metge's *Lo somni* (1399) in which the
   narrator argues against a misogynistic argument presented by Tiresias (v). Vidal
   i Alcovar argues convincingly that the *Espill* belongs to medieval misogynistic
   literature rather than to the picaresque since the protagonist is no *pícaro*, and
   the intervention of the patriarchal figure of Solomon is alien to the structure and
   perspective of picaresque narratives. He also points out the very limited diffusion
   of the *Espill* in contrast to such better-known misogynistic works as Boccaccio's
   Corbaccio, the Arcipreste de Talavera Alfonso Martínez de Toledo's *Reprobación
   del amor mundano* or *Corbacho* (1498), and Francesc Eiximenis's *Llibre de les
   dones* (c. 1390).
5. Fildes refers to the "universal belief that the physical and mental characteristics of

the nurse were imbibed by the child through her milk" (20), referring to her *Breasts, Bottles and Babies* (Edinburgh, 1986): 15, 30, 189–90.
6. I am grateful to Dr. Simón Palmer for generously sharing her bibliographic expertise at the Consejo Superior de Investigaciones Científicas and to María Luisa López-Vidriero, Carmen Morales and the staff of the Archivo and Biblioteca de Palacio in Madrid for their invaluable assistance with my research.
7. Biblioteca de Palacio ((II / 713): folios 46r–47v), identified in the catalogue as an eighteenth-century copy of the lost original, a "Privilegio" signed by Alfonso VIII at the request of his daughter the Infanta Berenguela, on behalf of "Doña Elvira, Nutriz de dicha Ynfanta." The library document indicates that the original manuscript was included in a 1713 inventory but in 1741, when the library was being reorganized, the manuscript had been lost.
8. Ejecutoria Real, March 11, 1792. Biblioteca de Palacio II / 3325.
9. Archivo General de Palacio, Madrid, Sección de Historia, "Amas de lactancia" (henceforth referred to as AGPM) Caja 1, expt. 21, includes a list of expenses dated August 1631 for a journey in search of wet nurses, at the request of Philip IV.
10. AGPM Caja 1, expte. 22, March 18, 1651.
11. AGPM, Caja 1, expt. 19, dated January 22, 1626: four "amas de respecto" are being sent home with their travel expenses paid by the palace, "porque se busca leche más fresca su Alteza. La suya ya no es apropósito" (because his Majesty seeks fresher milk and theirs is no longer appropriate).
12. AGPM, Index to Caja 1.
13. AGPM, Caja 1, expte. 37.

Works Cited

Bergmann, Emilie L. "The Exclusion of the Feminine in the Cultural Discourse of the Golden Age: Juan Luis Vives and Fray Luis de León," in *Religion, Body, and Gender in Early Modern Spain*. Alain Saint-Saens, ed. Mellen Research University Press, 1992. 124–36.

—— "Monstrous Maternity in Fray Antonio de Guevara's *Relox de príncipes*." *Brave New Words: Studies in Spanish Golden Age Literature*. Edward H. Friedman and Catherine Larson, eds. New Orleans: University Press of the South, 1996. 39–50.

Burkett, Elinor. "Indian Women and White Society: The Case of Sixteenth-Century Peru." *Latin American Women: Historical Perspectives*. Asunción Lavrin, ed. Westport, Connecticut: Greenwood Press, 1978. 101–28.

Cervantes Saavedra, Miguel de. *El coloquio de los perros Cipión y Berganza. Novelas ejemplares*. Vol. I ed. Harry Sieber. Madrid: Cátedra, 1981.

—— *Two Exemplary Novels*. trans. C.E. Jones. London: Penguin, 1972.

Fildes, Valerie. *Wet Nursing: a History from Antiquity to the Present*. Oxford: Basil Blackwell, 1988.

Garcés, María Antonia. "Lecciones del Nuevo Mundo: la estética de la palabra en el Inca Garcilaso de la Vega." *Texto y Contexto*. (Bogotá) 17 (Sept.–Dec. 1991): 125–50.

—— "Berganza and the Abject: The Desecration of the Mother," in *Quixotic Desire: Psychoanalytic Perspectives on Cervantes*. Ruth Anthony El Saffar and Diana de Armas Wilson, eds. Ithaca: Cornell University Press, 1993: 292–314.

Garcilaso de la Vega, el Inca. *Comentarios Reales de los Incas*. Ed. Aurelio Miró Quesada. Caracas, Venezuela: Biblioteca Ayacucho, 1976.

Guaman Poma de Ayala, Felipe. *Nueva crónica y buen gobierno*. Ed. John V. Murra, Rolena Adorno and Jorge L. Urioste. 3 vols. México: Siglo XXI, 1987.

Guevara, Antonio de. *Relox de príncipes*. Emilio Blanco, ed. [Madrid] ABL Editor, Conferencia de Ministros Provinciales de España, 1994.

Haraway, Donna J. *Simians, Cyborgs, and Women: The Reinvention of Nature*. New York: Routledge, 1991.

Klapisch-Zuber, Christiane. *Women, Family, and Ritual in Renaissance Italy*. Transl. by Lydia Cochrane. Chicago: University of Chicago Press, 1985.

Knibiehler, Yvonne. "Madres y nodrizas." *Figuras de la madre*. Silvia Tubert, ed. (Madrid: Cátedra / Instituto de la Mujer, 1996): 95–118.

Larquié, Claude. "Les milieux nourriciers des enfants madrilènes au XVIIe siècle." *Mélanges de la Casa de Velázquez*. XIX: 1 (1983): 221–42.

——— "La mise en nourrice des enfants madrilènes au XVII siècle." *Revue d'Histoire Moderne et Contemporaine* 32 (1985): 125–44.

Lida de Malkiel, María Rosa. "La mujer ante el lenguaje: algunas opiniones de la antigüedad y del renacimiento." *Boletín de la Academia Argentina de Letras* 5 (1937): 237–248.

Reher, David-Sven. *Town and Country in Pre-Industrial Spain: Cuenca, 1550–1870*. Cambridge University Press, 1990.

Roig, Jaume. *Espill o llibre de les dones*. ed. Marina Gustà. Barcelona: Edicions 62 i "La Caixa," 1978.

——— *Espejo*. trans. Ramón Miquel i Planas. Madrid/Barcelona: Alianza/Enciclopedia Catalana, 1987.

Rojo Vega, Anastasio. *El siglo de oro: Inventario de una época*. Junta de Castilla y León: Consejería de Educación y Cultura, 1996.

Saignes, Thierry, and Thérèse Bouysse-Cassagne. "La interrelación creative del quechua y del español en la literatura peruana de lengua española." *500 años de mestizaje en los Andes*. Hiroyasu Tomoeda and Luis Millones, eds. Osaka: Museo Nacional de Etnología, 1992: 14–26.

Sarasúa, Carmen. *Criados, nodrizas y amos: El servicio doméstico en la formación del mercado de trabajo madrileño, 1758–1868*. Madrid: Siglo XXI, 1994.

Sherwood, Joan. *Poverty in Eighteenth-Century Spain: The Women and Children of the "Inclusa"*. Toronto: University of Toronto Press, 1988.

Simón Palmer, María del Carmen. *La Cocina de palacio, 1561–1931*. Madrid: Castalia, 1997.

Valdés, Juan de. *Diálogo de la lengua*. Ed. Juan M. Lope Blanch. Madrid: Castalia, 1969.

Vassberg, David E. *The Village and the Outside World in Golden Age Castile: Mobility and Migration in Everyday Rural Life*. Cambridge University Press, 1996.

Vega, Garcilaso Inca de la. *Comentarios reales*. [1609]. 2 vols. Aurelia Miró Quesada, ed. Caracas: Ayacucho, 1985.

Vives, Juan Luis. *Formación de la mujer cristiana*. En *Obras completas*. T. I: 985–1175. Ed. Lorenzo Riber. Madrid: Aguilar, 1947.

——— *Joannis Ludovici Vivis Valentini Opera Omnia*. Gregorio Mayans, ed. [Valencia: Benedicti Montfort, 1783] facs. London: Gregg Press, 1964. T. IV.

——— *Instrucción de la mujer cristiana*. Juan Justiniano, trans., Elizabeth Teresa Howe, ed. Madrid: Fundación Universitaria Española / Universidad Pontificia de Salamanca, 1995 (based on 1528 edition).

Voltes, María José y Pedro. *Madres y niños en la historia de España*. Barcelona: Planeta, 1989.

Wiesner, Merry. *Women and Gender in Early Modern Europe*. Cambridge University Press, 1993.

Zamora, Margarita. *Language, Authority, and Indigenous History in the "Comentarios reales de los incas"*. Cambridge University Press, 1988.

CHAPTER SEVEN

Motherhood and Protestant Polemics: Stillbirth in Hans von Rüte's *Abgötterei* (1531)

Glenn Ehrstine

In the war of pamphlets and theological tracts arising from the German Reformation, the portrayal of women generally centered around two diametrically opposed stereotypes. In polemic literature, Protestant authors defamed the Catholic faith by associating it with disorderly women who violated accepted norms of behavior, be they domestic, sexual, or otherwise. In such works, corrupt monks fornicated with prostitutes, while the pope himself trafficked with the whore of Babylon (the archetypal disorderly woman) or even became her in the guise of legendary Pope Joan.[1] Meanwhile, the re-evaluation of marriage and family life within the new theology led to the propagation of idealized images of the good wife and mother in sermons and other Protestant writings.[2] On stage, these contrasting stereotypes appeared in two respective dramatic genres, one satirical, one solemn. The first, the carnival play, appropriated the license of the carnival celebration to ridicule ecclesiastical corruption and bring about religious change.[3] In the quintessential example of a Reformation *Fastnachtspiel*, *Der Ablaßkrämer* ("The Indulgence Peddler") by the painter-poet Niklaus Manuel of Bern, peasant women, armed with ladels and halberds, accost and ultimately string an indulgence trader up by his hands to force him to return their money and to confess past misdeeds (Fig. 7.1).[4] In biblical dramas such as Paul Rebhun's *Susanna*,[5] however, female protagonists offered chaste, self-sacrificing role models for Protestant wives and mothers. Traditionally, very little mixing of the above stereotypes occured between genres, unless the woman who usurped authority in patriarchal society was biblically based, such as Queen Vashti or Potiphar's wife.[6] Matters of childbirth and motherhood, beyond the sexual act itself, rarely entered the carnivalesque.

A remarkable exception to this tendency exists in the carnival play

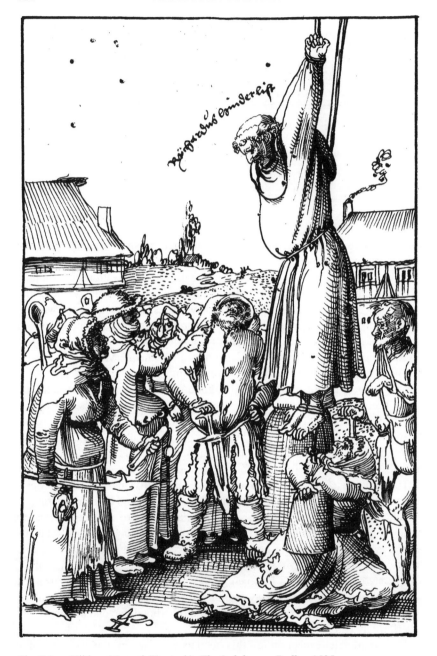

Fig. 7.1   Niklaus Manuel (Deutsch), *The Indulgence Pedler*, 1525

Abgötterei ("Idolatry"; Fig. 7.2), written by Bernese court secretary Hans von Rüte and performed in that town on Laetare Sunday, March 19, 1531.[7] While the play incorporates many licentious elements associated with the topsy-turvy pre-Lenten celebration, it also presents an earnest theological appeal against the veneration of saints and other aspects of the Catholic cult, associating all impious behavior with representatives of the old faith. In particular, Rüte introduces the plight of two would-be mothers, Cordili Syman and Dichtli Schnabelräß, who despite their best efforts have remained childless. Advised by literally demonized clerics to pray to Mary for luck in childbirth, the women make offerings in a stage chapel modeled after the church of Oberbüren, a then Bernese parish near Biel (Bienne) and a place of pilgrimage prior to the Reformation. Their actions, and their ultimate condemnation via association with the play's papal priests, point to the continued survival of the local Catholic cult as well as to the efforts of the newly installed Protestant authorities to combat such "idolatry" with all means at their disposal. To root out the last vestiges of Catholic religious practice, Rüte co-opted the socially sanctioned concerns of childbirth to argue that mothers could best ensure the health and well-being of their newborns by placing their faith in God alone.

The local carnival play tradition had already played a significant role in the dissemination of the new theology or, at the very least, in the denigration of the old. In addition to *Der Ablaßkrämer*, written in 1525,[8] two other works by Niklaus Manuel melded theology and politics in agitating against papal policies perceived as disadvantageous to Bernese interests: *Vom Papst und seiner Priesterschaft* ("On the Pope and His Priests") and *Von Papsts und Christi Gegensatz* ("On the Distinction between the Pope and Christ"), both performed in 1523.[9] The local chronicler Valerius Anshelm recorded that the success of the plays was so extraordinary that "a great mass of people were moved to consider and distinguish Christian freedom and papal servitude."[10] Manuel went on to play a central role in the local Reformation, serving as moderator at the Bernese disputation of January 1528 and, following its resolution in favor of the Protestant participants (including Ulrich Zwingli and a large Zurich delegation), joining the ruling elite of the Small Council, which now assumed control of the local church in addition to overseeing the largest city-state north of the Alps. The residents of the local countryside were, however, not as eager to adopt the new faith as their urban counterparts, and in October 1528 Manuel led a contingent of troops in suppressing unrest in Bern's alpine Oberland territories. Afterwards, in events surrounding the First War of Kappel of June 1529, he became increasingly involved in diplomatic missions to preserve Helvetican unity.[11] He soon began to suffer from ill health, however, and passed away on April 28, 1530. His mantle as local playwright passed to Rüte, who served as court secretary, with a brief intermission, from 1531 to 1555,

Ein Faßnachtſpil den vr

ſprung / haltung / vnd das End beyder/
Heydniſcher / vnd Bäpſtlicher Abgötteryen allenklich verglychende / zů Bern inn öchtland
durch die jungen Burger
gehallten.

Hans von Rüte.

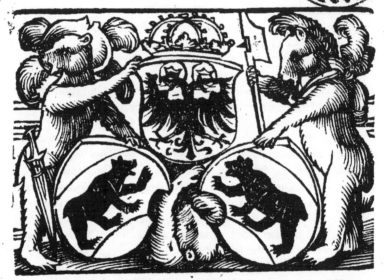

Gedruckt zů Baſel / By Thoman Wolff.

Anno, M. CCCCC, XXXII.

Fig 7.2   Hans von Rüte, *Abgötterei*, 1531

codifying local law in 1539 and occasionally censoring plays to be performed within the Bernese territories.[12] After *Abgötterei*, Rüte continued to propagate the Zwinglian theology of the reformed Bernese church in five biblical plays from 1538 through 1552.

Sixteenth-century Bernese religious drama was thus intimately linked to local government and its support of the new faith, whether countering encroachment from Catholic neighbors such as Lucerne and Unterwalden or, later, from Calvinist Geneva, where the French reformer was initially expelled for refusing to bow to Bernese authority. Moreover, the Oberland uprisings revealed a level of religious dissent that required immediate attention. One of the first matters the council addressed following the local Reformation was the cult of Mary as practiced in Oberbüren. In the final decades of the fifteenth century, reports had spread that the chapel's Marian altar could work miracles.[13] In particular, locals believed that the Virgin could revive a stillborn infant for a few fleeting moments, long enough for a priest to baptize the child. Mothers would place a feather in their infant's mouth and lay the lifeless body near glowing coals and candles; when the warmed air moved the feather, the parents took this as a sign that breath had returned to the child, if only for an instant.[14] Soon, throngs of distraught parents flocked to the chapel, their lifeless children in their arms. Bern afterwards quietly assumed control over the chapel's benefices, which proved to be a source of considerable income. Moreover, the councilors of Bern themselves eagerly demonstrated their devotion. Not only did the council make an official pilgrimage in 1480 to pray for an end to flooding,[15] but several burghers and noblemen of the region were members of the Confraternity of Oberbüren, among them Duke Sigmund of Austria.[16] They no doubt hoped to benefit from their worship of the Virgin as did Hans Stefan, who, sentenced to drown in the river Aare for stealing the sacrament, reportedly prayed to Mary and suffered no harm during an extended period under water.[17] Following this miracle, the council provided Stefan with a letter of recommendation to the pope and otherwise promoted Oberbüren's fame so that it could share in its glory. In 1512, the pope allowed the chapel to dispense episcopal indulgences, greatly increasing the amount of pilgrims. Despite protests from the bishop of Constance concerning the validity of the miracles, the council was intent on protecting such a remunerative operation, advising the chaplains in 1495: "just baptize the children, My Lords wish to protect them from harm."[18]

Following 1528, the new Protestant majority of the Bernese council set about to eradicate this flagrant abuse of naive piety. The reformed view of the Oberbüren miracles appears in an entry in Anshelm's chronicle for 1518:

> And this is also a clear example of the trade of His Papal Holiness …: the great profit of Our Lady of Oberbüren, gained in idolatry through the baptism of dead children and miscarriages, so that this year, under their steward Hans von Erlach,

they erected a new church, steeple and bells and provided two priests and two chaplains with houses and benefices.[19]

When Anshelm subsequently relates the measures of the council to eliminate objectionable images in its territories, he begins with the ceremonious destruction of the Oberbüren altar:

> Thus [the image of] Mary, sought out and venerated far and wide, was hacked and burned by emissaries of the council, not without some trepidation. This transpired, with bells ringing, before a large crowd. Her wonders and workshop, with its idols and service to greed and the mass, were destroyed as well.[20]

The gathered crowd expected divine retribution to be visited upon the councilor who had desecrated the altar, but it waited in vain.[21] Finally, to discourage unwanted pilgrimages, such as those that continued from the Catholic cantons to the supposed cave of Swiss patron St. Beatus near Thun, the council ordered the Oberbüren chapel destroyed in 1530. Similar steps were required in the city itself: as late as 1534, the council required its *Venner* (administrators over each of the city's four quarters) to examine the households in their districts to ensure that all images had been removed.[22]

Such measures, however, addressed mere symptoms, not their causes rooted in centuries of religious habit. For the rural populace to embrace Protestant solafideism, its tenets had to be made readily accessible. While local pastors no doubt regularly preached against the veneration of images, Rüte chose to package the new theology as a popular play, which might appeal to its audience on a more affective level. The similarities between *Abgötterei*'s Dichtli Schnabelräß, Cordili Syman, and the aggrieved mothers who prayed at the Oberbüren chapel for the souls of their children are so striking as to leave no doubt that Rüte had the Oberbüren practices in mind in his criticism of the cult of saints. The women appear among a series of earnest, but naive supplicants ranging from merchants to the emperor, all of whom require aid in various matters. They first approach Roman priests of antiquity, who recommend the help of gods from classical mythology; afterwards, Roman Catholic priests praise the divine intercession of saints. Both women begin by lamenting their difficulties in childbirth; Syman is barren, while Schnabelräß characterizes her experience of stillbirth as follows:

> My friend, although giving birth is hard and a woman would be better off without such pain, nevertheless I would be glad to conceive children and bring them into the world. Indeed, I would take neither money nor possessions in their place if God would only grant that I might let them see the light of the world. But when it comes time for the delivery, even though nothing, neither strap nor belt, is lacking, I cannot give birth. I feel as if I could explode.[23]

The women are first advised to pray to Juno, but then the priest Eusebius Buchsorg ("Book-Worry") makes a more appealing offer:

You shouldn't place too much hope in Juno; Mary can serve you better. ... Her help is great in all matters. She helps those who are infertile that they might conceive the fairest children. ... She is also inclined to aid those whose pain is so overwhelming that they can barely deliver. She helps that it might all take place without suffering, for when she bore her dear child, she had no pain whatsoever.[24]

Buchsorg then instructs the women to enter "the Chapel of Our Lady" ("vnser frouwen Capell"; Ciiij^V), where Schnabelräß, as indicated by one of the play's few explicit stage directions (Dj^r), kneels before an altar:

Mary, my hope, I beseech you, when I suffer heartfelt pain, please do not deny me your succor. In return, I will praise, exalt and glorify you all my days. I also beseech you whom Buchsorg has recommended as special helpers in need, that you help me both morning and evening. I will then sacrifice, celebrate, and fast in your name, donating to your priests so that they may always have nourishment and that poverty may spare their churches.[25]

Though no explicit mention of Oberbüren occurs in these passages, no other Marian altar in the vicinity of Bern was so closely associated with childbirth. Moreover, textual identification would not have been necessary if the stage chapel and altar in some manner resembled the "Chapel of Our Lady" that had been demolished just a year earlier. It is also probable that Rüte omitted explicit topicality to speak to a larger audience. The women's advisers speak only of pain during childbirth – certainly a universal experience among mothers – and Schnabelräß afterwards does not return to the subject of stillbirth, but rather asks to whom she might pray for beautiful children, another common practice of the time.

The portrayal of Syman and Schnabelräß is not unsympathetic. During the sixteenth century, at least one-third of all children died before the age of five, and the likelihood that an infant would die unbaptized before or during birth was indeed great.[26] By the end of the play, however, when demons appear on stage to lead Pope "Starrblind" ("Thoughtlessly/Vapidly Blind") and his followers to hell, it becomes clear that Rüte condemns the women as well, who from a Protestant perspective have endangered their souls through their desire to bear children at any cost. Furthermore, traditional carnivalesque devices mark them as negative examples. In her final lines before the play's review moves on to other gullible victims, Schnabelräß suddenly appears as the stereotypical wife who pilfers what money she can from her husband:

Friend Cordili, we've been told some good saints. I'll now regret no amount of money. Indeed, I intend to give the holy priests everything that I can sneak from my husband.[27]

For the reader of the play, the women are further marked by their satirical last names, a common device in Manuel's works. "Schnabel-räß" means literally "sharp beaked," branding her as a shrew or gossip. Meanwhile, "Sy-man," or "She-Man," refers to either a feminized man or a masculinized woman. The term was most often used for a man who deferred to his wife's wishes in the household, but could also signify a woman who rose first from bed on the feast of Simon and Judas, which implied that she would rule the home for the following year.[28] In either instance, the term indicates a violation of traditional domestic order. The subtext for Rüte's audience was likely that both women would have more success in childbirth if they would tame their tongues and subordinate themselves to the wishes of their husbands. Yet the women are clearly innocent victims; the "blame" for their undecorous behavior lies with the Catholic priests. The implication is that Catholicism, in its supposed perversion of divine order, is ultimately responsible for all types of disorderly women, from shrews to temptresses. Indeed, Rüte equates Catholic theology with feminine unruliness itself in the figure of Frouw Wirrwärr ("Dame Confusion"), a thinly veiled Babylonian Harlot who corrupts Pope Starrblind with bodily pleasures. She, and not the mothers, represents for Rüte the root of all "idolatry" found in the veneration of saints: the corruptibility of the body and above all the fallibility of human reason, which lacking direct biblical guidance ultimately leads Pope Starrblind astray.[29] She thus appears at the top of Rüte's sketch for a title page (Fig. 7.3); all other figures act under her patronage.

Theologically, then, Dame Confusion embodies the play's central thesis, while the mother figures provide a concrete, quotidian example of well-intentioned supplication gone awry. The problem, as would be expected from a Protestant perspective, is not that Syman and Schnabelräß seek assistance for their concerns, but that they do not seek it directly from God, placing trust in human intermediaries instead. Following Buchsorg's initial encouragement to pray to Mary, Syman hesitates, doubting the Virgin's ability to help, since she is far away in heaven and cannot hear her pleas. Though exaggerated for polemic purposes by Rüte, Buchsorg's response reveals the popular conception of the saints' ability to intercede with God:

> So that no one might complain that God and his saints had retreated to a high chamber and were unable to hear people's pleas regardless of what they brought before them, Christ did us much good and left behind a vicar, upon whom he bestowed the Holy Spirit and urged that he show people how they should honor God and the saints. ... This same man has many churches built, which are hewn from precious stone. He consecrates them and places the image of a saint inside who wishes to be venerated there. The saint's grace then finds its way to this place, that he might understand the people's troubles.[30]

Elsewhere in the play, both heathen and Catholic priests portray God as ostensibly passive, distant, and only remotely interested in his creation,[31] a far cry from the universal priesthood of Luther and other reformers. By incorporating such doctrinal issues, Rüte moved beyond the mere criticism of ecclesiastical corruption as found in early anti-Catholic carnival plays to

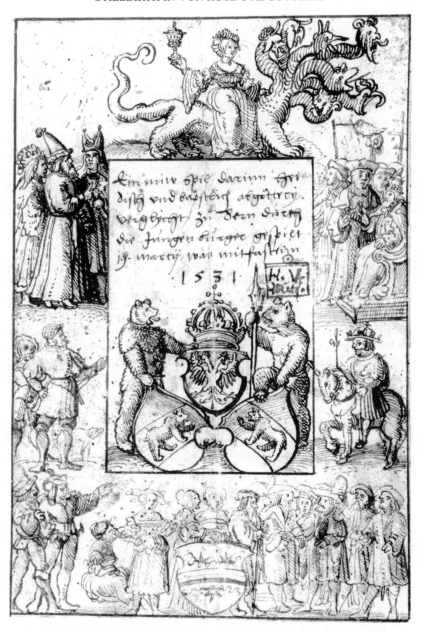

Fig. 7.3   Hans von Rüte, ink drawing for *Abgötterei*

central concerns of the Reformation theological debate. The irony, if Rüte was aware of it, was that, in composing a carnival play against Catholic ritual, he was adapting a literary outgrowth of that very same ritual. The demise of the Bernese carnival play tradition after 1531 is in part an indication of his apparent success: *Abgötterei* was the last of a dying genre whose constitutive licentiousness had become suspect, a transitional work that looked forward to the local biblical plays that were to begin with Rüte's *Joseph* of 1538.

The portrayal of Dichtli Schnabelräß and Cordili Syman lies at the heart of this transitional nature and ultimately reflects, in microcosm, the continuing debate on whether the Reformation expanded or diminished women's role in society. In *Abgötterei*'s carnival context, the mothers are both caregiver and unruly woman. The latter role is linked to plays such as *Der Ablaßkrämer*, in which weapon-wielding, Bible-quoting peasant women, by virtue of an en-gendered license allowing a measure of impunity, bring about true religious change.[32] Rüte's mothers' unruliness, however, is confined to stock carnival motifs and stripped of all political or religious agency. Of the play's parade of supplicants, only two recognize the fallacy of their doing and undergo a conversion on stage: Heiny Kuohorn ("Cowhorn") and his son Cristan, who reads aloud from the New Testament in the final scene before Pope Starrblind's deposition (Lij[r]). The task of nurturing, at least in matters of faith, is thus primarily assigned to fathers; Syman and Schnabelräß do not appear in later scenes and remain passive as regards the new theology. Still, their very appearance among the victims of ecclesiastical impiety acknowledges, within the sanctioned realm of childbearing, the interests of female audience members who were no less active in debating and spreading the new faith as their male counterparts, converting husbands, tutoring children in tenets of faith, and at times even writing God's truth against the Pauline prohibition of women's teaching (1 Timothy 2: 11–15), as done so with pride by Argula von Grumbach.[33] Rüte, then, was no exception to his male contemporaries in confining women's place in sixteenth-century society to the domestic sphere, nor did he portray women on stage as conveyors of Reformation theology. Nevertheless, he clearly recognized that the Protestant project would not succeed without women's active collaboration in embracing the new faith.

Notes

1.   See, for example, Lyndal Roper, "Discipline and Respectability: Prostitution and the Reformation in Augsburg," *History Workshop* 19 (1985): 3–28, a preliminary study for the author's *The Holy Household: Women and Morals in Reformation Augsburg*, Oxford Studies in Social History (Oxford: Clarendon Press, 1989); Barbara Sher Tinsley, "Pope Joan Polemic in Early Modern France: The Use and Disabuse of Myth," *Sixteenth Century Journal* 18 (1987): 381–98; Robert W.

Scribner, *For the Sake of Simple Folk: Popular Propaganda for the German Reformation*, 2nd edn. (Oxford: Clarendon, 1994), 171 ff.

2. See, among others, Thomas Max Safely, "Marriage," in *The Oxford Encyclopedia of the Reformation*, ed. Hans J. Hillerbrand (New York/Oxford: Oxford University Press, 1996), 3:18–23; Merry E. Wiesner, "Studies of Women, the Family, and Gender," in *Reformation Europe: A Guide to Research II*, ed. by William S. Maltby, Reformation Guides to Research 3 (St. Louis: Center for Reformation Research, 1992), 159–87; Steven Ozment, *When Fathers Ruled: Family Life in Reformation Europe* (Cambridge: Harvard University Press, 1983). On sermons specifically, see Susan Karant-Nunn, "'Kinder, Küche, Kirche': Social Ideology in the Sermons of Johannes Mathesius," in *Germania Illustrata. Essays on Early Modern Germany Presented to Gerald Strauss*, eds. Andrew C. Fix and Susan C. Karant-Nunn, Sixteenth Century Essays and Studies 18 (Kirksville, Missouri: Sixteenth Century Journal Publishers, 1992), 121–40.

3. On carnival and Reformation in general, see Robert W. Scribner, "Reformation, Carnival and the World Turned Upside-Down," in *Städtische Gesellschaft und Reformation*, ed. Ingrid Bátori, Spätmittelalter und Frühe Neuzeit 12 (Stuttgart: Klett-Cotta, 1980), 222–52.

4. Niklaus Manuel, *Der Ablaßkrämer*, ed. Paul Zinsli, Altdeutsche Übungstexte 17 (Bern: Francke, 1960). On the author, see Glenn Ehrstine, "Niklaus Manuel (Niklaus Manuel Deutsch)," in *German Writers of the Renaissance and Reformation, 1280–1580*, ed. James Hardin and Max Reinhart, vol. 179, *Dictionary of Literary Biography* (Detroit: Gale Research, 1997), 152–65. On the function of female insurrection in *Der Ablaßkrämer*, see Peter Pfrunder, *Pfaffen, Ketzer, Totenfresser: Fastnachtskultur der Reformationszeit – Die Berner Spiele von Niklaus Manuel* (Zurich: Chronos, 1989), 212 ff.

5. Paul Rebhun, *Ein Geistlich Spiel von der Gotfürchtigen und keuschen Frauen Susannen*, ed. Hans-Gert Roloff (Stuttgart: Reclam, 1980). On the author, see Paul F. Casey, *Paul Rebhun: A Biographical Study* (Stuttgart: Steiner, 1986).

6. On Vashti in Esther dramas, see David Price, "When Women Would Rule: Reversal of Gender Hierarchy in Sixteenth-Century German Drama," *Daphnis* 20 (1991): 158–62. On Potiphar's wife in Joseph plays, see Jean Lebeau, *Salvator Mundi: L'"Exemple" de Joseph dans le théâtre allemand au xvie siècle*, Bibliotheca Humanistica et Reformatica 20 (Nieuwkoop: B. de Graaf, 1977), 1:371 ff.

7. Full title: *Ein Fasnachtspil den vrsprung / haltung / vnd das End beyder / Heydnischer / vnd Bäpstlicher Abgötteryen allenklich verglychende / zuo Bern inn öchtland durch die jungen Burger gehallten* (Basel: Thomas Wolff, 1532). A critical edition of *Abgötterei* and Rüte's five other dramas is nearing publication: Klaus Jaeger, "Zur Edition der Dramen Hans von Rütes," in *Editionsdesiderate zur Frühen Neuzeit. Beiträge zur Tagung der Kommission für die Edition von Texten der Frühen Neuzeit*, ed. Hans-Gert Roloff, Chloe 25 (Amsterdam: Rodopi, 1997), 2:1005–1011.

8. The play survives only in manuscript form, and it is uncertain whether it was ever performed. The manuscript, however, likely circulated among interested parties: In 1529, Manuel asked the Zurich reformer Ulrich Zwingli to return several of his writings, among them "ein aplasz kremmer." *Niklaus Manuel Deutsch. Maler, Dichter, Staatsmann*, ed. Cäsar Menz and Hugo Wagner (Bern: Kunstmuseum Bern, 1979), 512, Nr. 345.

9. All three plays appear in the new critical edition of Manuel's collected works: Niklaus Manuel, *Werke und Briefe*, ed. Paul Zinsli and Thomas Hengartner

(Bern: Stämpfli, 1999), 101–283. Several single editions of *Vom Papst und seiner Priesterschaft* exist, the most recent being "Vom Papst und seiner Priesterschaft," in *Deutsche Spiele und Dramen des 15. und 16. Jahrhunderts*, ed. Hellmut Thomke, Bibliothek deutscher Klassiker 136 (Frankfurt: Deutscher Klassiker Verlag, 1996), 139–209.

10. "Durch dis wunderliche und vor nie, als gotslästerliche, gedachte anschowungen ward ein gross volk bewegt, kristliche friheit und bäbstliche knechtschaft zuo bedenken und ze underscheiden." *Die Berner Chronik des Valerius Anshelm*, ed. Historischer Verein des Kantons Bern (Bern: K.J. Wyss, 1893), 4:475. For Anshelm's complete account with English translation, see Glenn Ehrstine, "From Iconoclasm to Iconography: Reformation Drama in Sixteenth-Century Bern" (Ph.D. dissertation, University of Texas at Austin, 1995), 75.

11. Manuel was instrumental in preserving Swiss unity during the Reformation. See Bruce Gordon, "Toleration in the Early Swiss Reformation: The Art and Politics of Niklaus Manuel of Berne," in *Tolerance and Intolerance in the European Reformation*, ed. Ole Peter Grell and Bob Scribner (Cambridge: Cambridge University Press, 1996), 128–44.

12. "Die Stadtsatzung von 1539," *Stadtrechte*, vol. 1, *Die Rechtsquellen des Kantons Bern*, ed. Friedrich Emil Welti, Sammlung Schweizerischer Rechtsquellen, 2. Abteilung (Aarau: Sauerländer, 1971), 585–683. On Rüte's activities as censor, see Ehrstine, "From Iconoclasm to Iconography," 82.

13. Paul Hofer, "Die Wahlfahrtskapelle zu Oberbüren," in *Neues Berner Taschenbuch auf das Jahr 1904* (Bern: K.J. Wyss, 1903), 103; Richard Feller, *Geschichte Berns* (Bern: Herbert Lang, 1974), 2:95–6. I have been unable to review the most recent research on archeological excavations at the site of the former church: Denise Gaudy, "Die schauderhaften Geschichten um die ehemalige Wallfahrtskapelle 'Chilchmatt': mittelalterliche Ausgrabungen in Büren," *Der Seebutz* 46 (1996): 47–9.

14. Kurt Guggisberg, *Bernische Kirchengeschichte* (Bern: Paul Haupt, 1958), 35.

15. Hofer, 103.

16. Ibid., 117–22.

17. "Uf den 30. Tag Höwmonats hat sich begeben, dass Hans Steffan, von wegen eines kilchendiebstahls, namlich des sacraments mit sinem geväss zuo Bürren gestolen, und hierum daselbs zuo ertränken verurteilt; und als nun der urteil genuog solt sin beschehen, und man in wolt vergraben, erzeigt er lebzeichen und ein grien zwî in siner hand, und als im sin kraft wider kommen was, bekant er, unser frow ze Oberbürren, der er sich in siner not hat ergeben, hätte in also enthalten, dass, diewil er gelegen in der triewen Aren am boden, kein not vom Wasser hät empfunden und alle red des richters und nachrichters gehört, die er ouch erzalt." *Die Berner Chronik des Valerius Anshelm*, 1:279.

18. "Die Kind nur ... taufen, M.H. wellen sie vor Schaden hüten." As quoted in Hofer, 105.

19. "Und das ist ouch ein luter Exempel bäbstlicher heilikeit Gwerbs ... der gros gwin Unser Frowen zuo Oberbürren, alein mit dotner kinden und mispurten touf abgötisch gewunnen, also dass si uber nüw gebuwne kilchen, kilchturn, gros gelüt, zwen pfaffen mit hüser und pfruonden, diss jars under irem vogt, junkher Hansen von Erlach, noch zwen kaplonen mit hüser und pfruonden hat gestiftet und nüw ufgerichtet." *Die Berner Chronik des Valerius Anshelm*, 4:263.

20. "Also ward durch ein rhattsbottschaft zuo Oberbüren mit zuosammengelüteten glogken vor vil volcks nitt ohn grusen zerschytet und verbrennt die lang und wyt gesuochte und vereerete Maria, darzu ire wunder und werckstatt mitt sampt allen

iren götzen, gytts- und mässpfaffendienst zerstört." As quoted in "Die Lücken im Jahrgang 1528 von Anshelms Chronik," Anshelm's missing entries for 1528 discovered at the turn of the century: Theodor de Quervain, *Kirchliche und soziale Zustände in Bern unmittelbar nach der Einführung der Reformation (1528–1536)* (Bern: Grunau, 1906), 249.

21. Guggisberg, 128.

22. Feller, 2:244.

23. "Myn gfatter / wiewol kinden ist gar schwär / Vnd einer frouwen sunst baß wär / Das sy ledig möcht syn des schmertzen / Dennocht wött ich gern von hertzen / Khind machen / vnd bringen an die wellt / Ja / ich näme nit darfür guot noch gelt / Wenn <m>irs nummen Gott wötte gonnen / Das ich sy möcht bringen an dsonnen / Als bald aber khumpt die zyt der purt / Da dann nüt sumpt / wäder band noch gurt / So mag ich die kind nit von mir bringen / Mich dunckt / ich müsß von einandern springen." *Abgötterei*, Ciij^r. The subsequent response by the "heathen" priest Martius Stichfinster summarizes the women's problems: "Eyne macht nit kind / die andre bringt sy todt" ("One conceives no children, the other delivers them lifeless").

24. "Jr sönd nit zuil hoffnung vff Juno setzen / Maria khan üch baß ergetzen .../ Jn allen sachen ist jr hilff gar groß / Sy hilfft denen die vnfruchtbar sindt / Das sy überkhöment die hüpschisten kindt .../ Ouch ist sy gneigt denen zhillff zuokommen / Da der schmertz/ also hat überhand gnommen / Das sy die purt khum mögind bringen an tag / Sy hillfft / das on alles wee beschächen mag / Dann / als sy jr liebes kindt gebar / Hat sy kein schmertzen vmb ein har." *Abgötterei*, Ciiij^r.

25. "Jch bit dich Maria / myn zuouersicht / Wenn mir von hertzen wee beschicht / Wöllest mir dyn hilff nit versagen / So will ich dich inn allen mynen tagen / Rümen / prysen / vnd ouch loben / Jch pitt ouch üch / die herr Buchsorg daoben / Mir zuo bsondern notthellfffern anzöugt hat / Das jr mir helffent fruo vnd spat / So will ich üch opffern / fyren / vnd fasten / Vnd üwern priestern stüren inn casten / Das jnen jr narung nit möge zerrinnen / Vnd jr kilchen mögint der armuot entrinnen." *Abgötterei*, Dj^r–Dj^v.

26. Ozment, 101.

27. "Gfatter Cordily / vns sind guot notthelfferin erzellt / Darumb muosß mich rüwen gar kein gellt / Ja / alles das ich mym man mag verschleicken / Das will ich den heylgen priestern zuo schmeicken." *Abgötterei*, Dij^v.

28. "Simon und Judas," in *Handwörterbuch des deutschen Aberglaubens*, ed. E. Hoffmann-Krayer and Hanns Bächtold-Stäubli (Berlin: de Gruyter, 1936/37), 8, columns 4–5. For other appearances of this name in sixteenth-century German drama, see Price, 156–8.

29. Ehrstine, "From Iconoclasm to Iconography," 186–92, 247–52.

30. "Domit sich niemand möcht erklagen / Wie Gott / vnd syne heylgen überal / Werend gstigen inn ein hochen sal / Das sy die menschen nit hören möchten / Gott gäb / was not sy für sy brechten / So hat vns Christus so vil zguottem thon / Vnd einen Statthalter hinderm glon / Dem hat er geben den heylgen geyst / Vnd das entpfolen aller meyst / Das er den lüten sölle anzöug gäben / Ouch bitten/ wie sy inn jrem läben / Gott / vnd die heylgen Eeren söllend .../ Derselb heißt vil kilchen buwen / Die da syent vß kostlichen steinen ghüwen / Die macht er heylig / vnd stellt darin / Eins heylgen bildnuß / der da will geeret sin / Dohin kumpt dann des heylgen gnad / Do mag er verstan der lüten schad." *Abgötterei*, Ciiij^v.

31. "Dwyl Gott von üch als hoch gescheiden ist" (Aiiij^v); "Sitmals / nun Gott üwer achtet nüt" (Bj^r); "Das gott ein ruowiger gott möcht läben" (Ej^v); "Domit gott ein ruowiger gott möcht sin" (Fj^v).

32. Natalie Davis argues that women could on occasion effect change more easily than men by virtue of their supposed licentiousness: Natalie Zemon Davis, "Women on Top," in *Society and Culture in Early Modern France* (Stanford: Stanford University Press, 1975), 124–51. See also the Lucas Cranach the Elder image "Women Assaulting Clergy" in Merry E. Wiesner, *Women and Gender in Early Modern Europe*, New Approaches to European History 1 (Cambridge: Cambridge University Press, 1993), 187. Wiesner notes that the period during which women most actively participated in the shaping of the Reformation "was the decade or so immediately following an area's decision to break with the Catholic church or while this decision was being made" (p. 186). *Der Ablaßkrämer* appeared at the beginning of this period in Bern, while *Abgötterei* was performed at its waning.

33. "Women were not simply passive recipients of the Reformation message, but left convents, refused to leave convents; preached; prophesied; discussed religion with friends and family; converted their husbands, left their husbands; wrote religious poems, hymns, and polemics; and were martyred on all sides of the religious controversy." Merry E. Wiesner-Hanks, "Women," in *The Oxford Encyclopedia of the Reformation*, 4:290. On the writings of Argula von Grumbach, see *Argula von Grumbach: A Woman's Voice in the Reformation*, ed. Peter Matheson (Edinburgh: Clark, 1995).

The Virgin's Voice:
Representations of Mary in
Seventeenth-Century Italian Song

Claire Fontijn

Just as artists painted vivid depictions of the Madonna and Child and Mary at the Cross, composers evoked the same scenes through music. Seventeenth-century Italy offered up a particularly striking group of works that portray the events of Christ's birth and crucifixion through the voice of Mary herself: lullabies around Christmastime sung by the young nursing mother, and laments for Holy Week and Easter sung by the weeping mother mourning the death of her son on the cross. If the especially strong traditions of Marian devotion in southern Europe no doubt did much to prompt the creation of these songs, so, too, did the growing attention given the solo soprano voice during this period. This study examines eight representative works in which a soprano portraying the Virgin Mary interprets her maternal role through dramatic performance (Table 8.1).[1]

Lullabies

Tarquinio Merula's *canzonetta spirituale* opens with four statements of a semitone ostinato A-B-flat in the bass line, the lullaby or *nanna* (Ex. 8.1). The repeating A-B-flat pair sets a mysterious tone to the work before the soprano sings "hor ch'è tempo di dormire." ("now it is time to go to sleep)." After prompting by the entry of the voice, this ostinato takes on an uneven rocking character that transforms the ensuing music into a soothing cradle song. Now the semitone oscillation can be perceived instead as a comfortably-enclosed space that symbolically connects mother and child. But there is only so much comfort that Mary can provide as she foresees the pain that the outside world will inflict on Jesus; the opening stanzas contrast the safety that she offers

Table 8.1 Marian first-person narratives selected for this study

Composer	Title	Source	Modern Edition
(a) Lullabies			
Tarquinio Merula	Canzonetta Spirituale sopra alla nanna, "Hor ch'è tempo di dormire"	*Curtio precipitato et altri Capricij composti in diversi modi vaghi e leggiadri à voce sola.* Venice: Bartolomeo Magni, 1638.	
Marco Antonio Centorio	Nenia B. Virginis ad X.tum Infantem, "Dormi iam mea vita"	Italy-Vercelli Biblioteca capitolare, sez. musicale-manoscritti, ms. 1302/13 (c. 1615).	
Alessandro Stradella	Cantata per il santissimo Natale, "Ah Troppo è ver"	From two manuscript sources: I-MOe Mus. F. 1145 and I-Tn Giordano 12 (c. 1675).	*Alessandro Stradella, Tre Cantate per voci e strumenti* edited by Carolyn Gianturco. Laaber: Laaber-Verlag, 1997.
Antonia Bembo	Per il Natale, "In braccio di Maria"	*Produzioni armoniche* (F-Pn Rés. Vm[1] 117) (c. 1697–1701).	*Per il Natale,* edited by Clare Fontijn, ClarNan Editions, Fayetteville, AR, 1999.
(b) Laments			
Antonia Bembo	Lamento della Vergine, "D'onnipotente padre"	*Produzioni armoniche* (F-Pn Rés. Vm[1] 117) (c. 1697-1701).	
Claudio Monteverdi	Pianto della Madona à voce sola Sopra il Lamento d'Arianna	*Selva morale e spirituale.* Venice: Bartolomeo Magni, 1641.	
Francesco Capello	"Dic mihi, sacratissima Virgo"	*Sacrorum concertuum.* Venice: Ricciardo Amadino, 1610.	
Luigi Rossi, attr.	Oratorio per la settimana santa	I-Rvat, Barb. lat. 4198–9 (c. 1641–45).	

Ex. 8.1   Merula, "Hor ch'è tempo di dormire," mm. 1–4

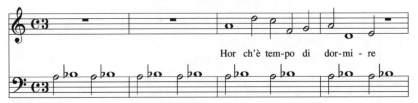

Ex. 8.2   Merula, "Hor ch'è tempo di dormire," mm. 14–16

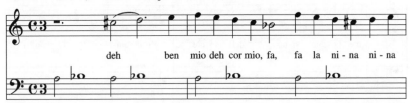

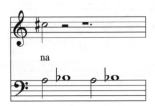

with the dangers that await him (see the entire poem, Text Ex. 1). She rocks the child above the ostinato as if between comfort and warning; she provides equal portions of each as the child goes back and forth between the safety of her protection and her frightening description of his torture. Mary's very realistic lullaby presages the future while celebrating present intimacy, tapering off the initial stanzas with the refrain, "Deh ben mio, deh cor mio, fa, fa la nina nina na" ("Oh my beloved, oh my sweetheart, sleep nina nina na" see Ex. 8.2).

As Mary sings to Jesus she nourishes him with milk from her breasts, which also provide a "soft bed" on which he can rest, in stanzas three and four of the poem. The musical depiction of the nursing Madonna, or *Maria lactans*, parallels those found in visual art.[2] The basso ostinato echoes the meaning of the text: the circular motion of the repeated semitone oscillation depicts the roundness of her breasts, while the two notes symbolize the exchange – the give and take, the soft suck – between two bodies. But the ultimate satisfaction of this meal is disturbed by the image of the food that he will soon eat – not mother's milk but the cruel minister's vinegar and gall – and by the hard cross that will be his final resting place, rather than her soft chest.

Ex. 8.3   Merula, "Hor ch'è tempo di dormire," mm. 79–87

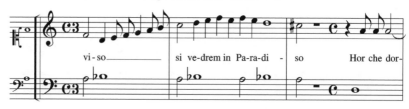

vi - so____   si ve-drem in Pa-ra-di - so   Hor che dor-

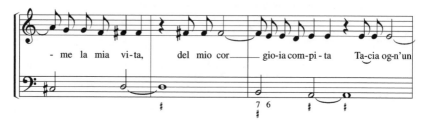

- me la mia vi - ta,   del mio cor____ gio-ia com-pi - ta   Ta-cia og-n'un

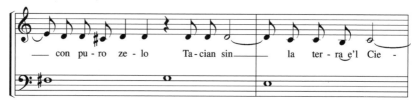

____ con pu - ro ze - lo   Ta - cian sin____   la   ter - ra e'l Cie -

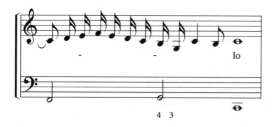

-              -   lo

The ostinato continues for nearly seven minutes, surely the composer's consciously conceived approximation of the real time that it would take for a baby to be sated and fall asleep. At this juncture the ostinato stops; clearly her "nanna" has worked its charm. The lullaby then yields to a freely accompanying basso continuo above which Mary can direct her song to the audience as a way to complete the piece (Ex. 8.3). The effectiveness of Merula's eerily haunting music resides in the power that it has to portray motherhood so vividly and to establish the importance of Mary's omniscience as she nourishes her child's body and mind; the first-person voice invites us to

Ex. 8.4   Centorio, Nenia B. Virginis ad X.tum Infantem, facsimile of the only
surviving part, the "canto"

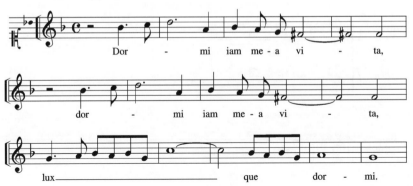

take part in the intimacy between mother and child, bringing us closer to them
than we could come through their customary objective portrayal.

The comfort in repetition is clearly what helps the baby to fall asleep; in a
Latin lullaby, a Latin *nenia*, Marco Antonio Centorio gave Mary a recurring
refrain to lull the child into slumber (Ex. 8.4).[3] She sings the phrase "Sleep here,
my life and light" at the beginning and end of the piece with several repetitions
and transpositions. In the work's central section she elaborates her injunctions
to sleep with a more florid style marked by division work and cadential *trilli*.
Unlike Merula's, the poetry here remains anchored in the present without any
intimation of the future. Little is known of Centorio. Trained in Milan, his
primary activity was in the Piedmontese city of Vercelli; like most of his music,
this piece exists only in manuscript. This *nenia* is a simple song that celebrates
the bond between mother and son.

Although not lullabies in the strict sense, two recently edited Christmas
cantatas by the composers Alessandro Stradella and Antonia Bembo contain
noteworthy Marian narratives that dramatize the role played by the new
mother.[4] Roughly contemporary and with similar titles, the cantatas otherwise
take on wholly different guises. Stradella's cantata employs six characters who
are accompanied by an orchestra in concerto grosso disposition, where two solo
violins add to the ripieno string orchestra. Bembo used an instrumental trio to
accompany one soprano who both narrates the main story and assumes Mary's
role.

In the Stradella cantata, a bass singer and a back-up chorus represent the
forces of evil against which Mary can appear as the gentle heroine who directs
the world toward the good, whether by presenting the Christ child or by
lamenting his loss (Text Ex. 2). Here, after a delightfully bumbling bass
recitative for Lucifer, an angel leads two shepherds to the manger to see the
Christmas miracle. They find Mary there, singing softly to her child

Ex. 8.5   Stradella, Cantata per il Santissimo Natale, opening of Mary's Aria-
           Recitativo

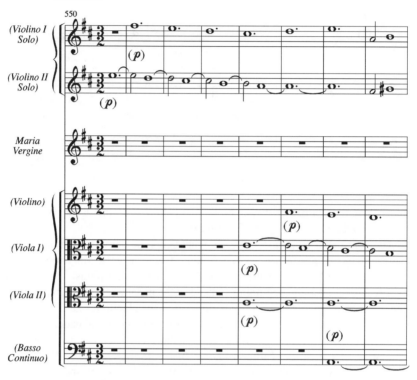

accompanied at first by a pair of violins without the continuo (Ex. 8.5). Even
when the ripieno and bass enter, Stradella took pains to maintain an ethereal
mysterious effect, marking them "sempre pianissimo;" the sensitive handling
of dynamics and textures sets Mary and her music in the sharpest possible
contrast to Lucifer's boastful pyrotechnics.

Bembo's Christmas cantata *Per il Natale* invests Mary with a complex of
characteristic emotions. Her soliloquy shows two sides of a personality
precariously poised between confidence and doubt, wavering between pride in
having borne the Christ child and the fear of appearing to be too arrogant, or
"vainglorious" (Text Ex. 3). At the outset of her soliloquy, in a bright A major
she proclaims her triumph: it is *she* who has brought Christ into the world! The
crowds that adulate her son by association admire her, of whom he is after all a
part (Ex. 8.6). Abruptly, however, she recoils in horror and asks, "What am I
saying?" A shift to the relative minor emphasizes the change that overcomes
her as she catches herself in a vain act. The tonality serves to illustrate the
"supreme mysteries," the powers that are greater than she, which are celebrated

Ex. 8.5 concluded

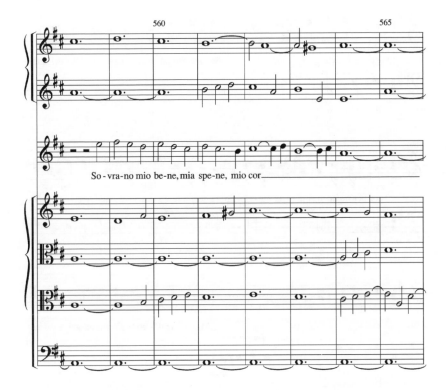

So - vra-no mio be-ne, mia spe-ne, mio cor——

in a tight-knit ensemble aria for the last stanza of her soliloquy (Ex. 8.7). F-sharp minor, the key that had prompted her to avoid pride – to think beyond herself and her own fame – now serves as the vehicle for spiritual meditation.

Laments

The Christmas cantata is followed by a Virgin's Lament in Bembo's manuscript; both *cantate spirituali* feature one singer who can narrate as well as personify Mary (Text Ex. 4). The young mother wavering between pride and shame in the Christmas cantata here becomes an angry and indignant mother who fights as she tries to protect her son and to defend him from death. While the narrator introduces her as sobbing, her opening Aria vivace is anything but, as she lashes out with the questions: "What are you doing? What are you trying to do, tyrannical, evil, dolorous cloud?" while the continuo brazenly moves forward below her (Ex. 8.8).

Ex. 8.6   Bembo, Per il Natale, mm. 47–57

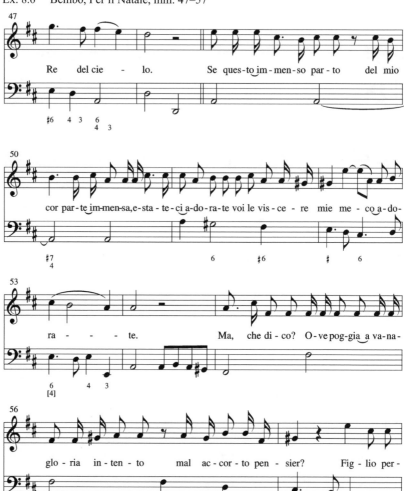

Re   del cie - lo.   Se ques-to im - men-so par - to   del mio

cor par-te im-men-sa,e-sta - te-ci a-do-ra-te voi le vis - ce - re mie me co a-do-

ra - te.   Ma,   che di - co? O - ve pog-gia a va-na-

glo - ria   in - ten - to   mal ac - cor - to pen - sier? Fig - lio per-

Ex. 8.7   Bembo, Per il Natale, mm. 63–78

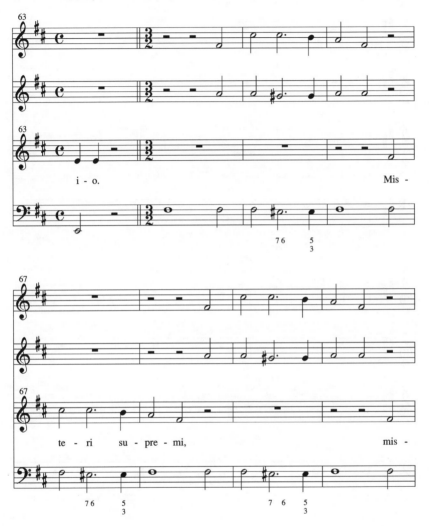

The remaining three laments adhere more closely to the customary image of Mary as the tender weeping mother, one of whose musical models predates the period in question. The *Planctus ante nescia* from the thirteenth-century *Carmina burana* manuscript is a lengthy lament in Mary's active voice. In many societies women are the mourners; one of the strongest images of this practice is that of the *Mater dolorosa*.[5] The enactment and working out of

Ex. 8.7 concluded

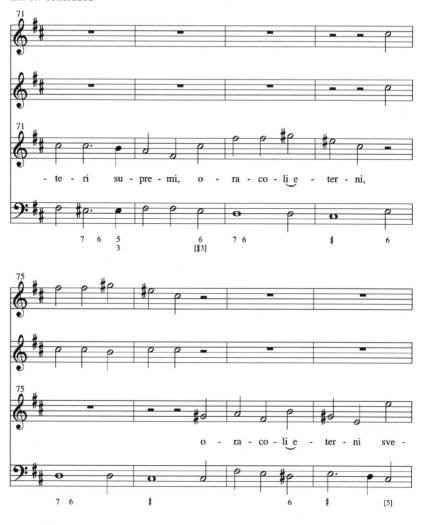

grief occurred in both secular and sacred music at the time and may well have prompted the vast repertory devoted to the lament, whether found at a significant moment in an opera or cultivated as a reflection of grief in the Passion story.

The link between sacred and secular is particularly strong in Monteverdi's *Pianto della Madonna*, a *contrafactum* monody of the *Lamento d'Arianna* from the lost opera, *L'Arianna*.[6] In a study of Monteverdi's religious music, Adelmo

Ex. 8.8   Bembo, Lamento della Vergine, Aria vivace

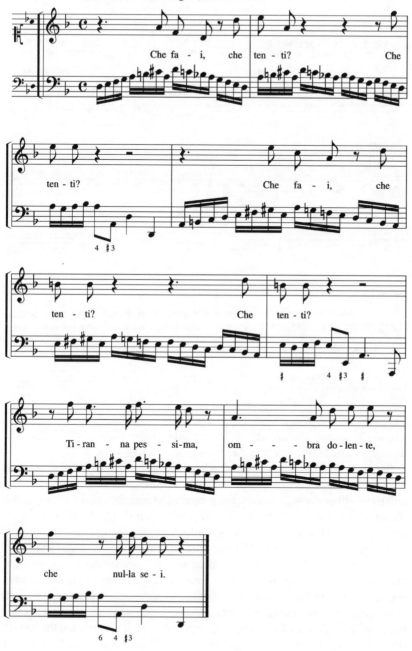

Ex. 8.9   Monteverdi, Pianto della Madona, instances of text painting

Section I

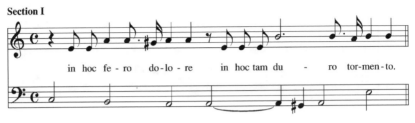

in hoc fe - ro   do - lo - re   in hoc tam du   -   ro tor-men - to.

Section II

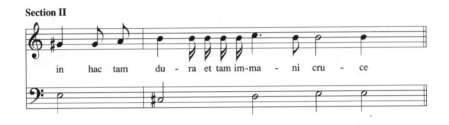

in   hac   tam   du - ra et tam im-ma   -   ni   cru   -   ce

Section III

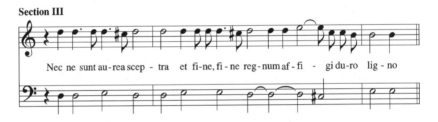

Nec ne sunt au-rea scep - tra   et fi-ne, fi - ne reg-num af - fi   -   gi du-ro lig - no

was to "humanize the divine" as an attempt to unite the duality of God and human; he cited this piece as a good example of the practice.[7]

Set at the foot of the cross, where Mary weeps and speaks to her dying son, Monteverdi's *Pianto* dramatizes the bitter hardships presaged by Merula's lullaby. Particular words convey the pathos of Mary's emotions. Example 8.9 shows successive settings of the adjective "duro" ("hard"); it receives progressively stronger dissonances throughout the lament as it modifies "torment," "cross," and "wood." In the first section the dissonance of a ninth, in the second, a seventh and, at the climax of the piece, the strongest clash of all, a cross relation. The effectiveness of the new text is a credit to the anonymous poet as much as to Monteverdi. The heightened pathos caused by the prolonged dissonance in this setting suggests that he took pains to assure an even more powerful dissonance in the plaint than in the original version of the lament (Ex. 8.10); here the words "fero dolore" strike the dissonant seventh twice (on "fe-ro"), whereas "dura sorte" (on "du-") only strikes it once.

Ex. 8.10   Monteverdi, comparison of dissonance treatment

Pianto della Madona

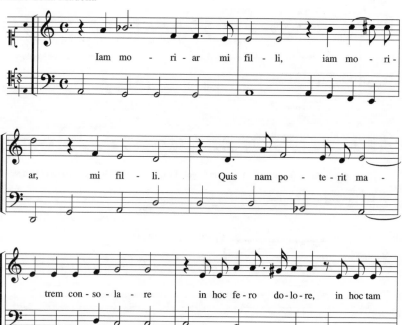

Iam mo — ri - ar mi fil - li, iam mo - ri -

ar,   mi fil - li.   Quis nam po - te - rit ma -

trem con - so - la - re   in hoc fe - ro   do - lo - re,   in hoc tam

Lamento d'Arianna

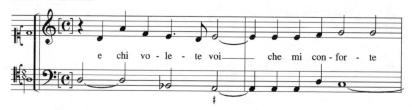

e chi vo - le - te voi___ — che mi con - for - te

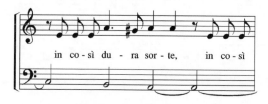

in co - sì du - ra sor - te,   in co - sì

Ex. 8.11   Opening of Capello's "Dic mihi, sacratissima Virgo," reproduced with kind
permission from the editor, Howard Smither

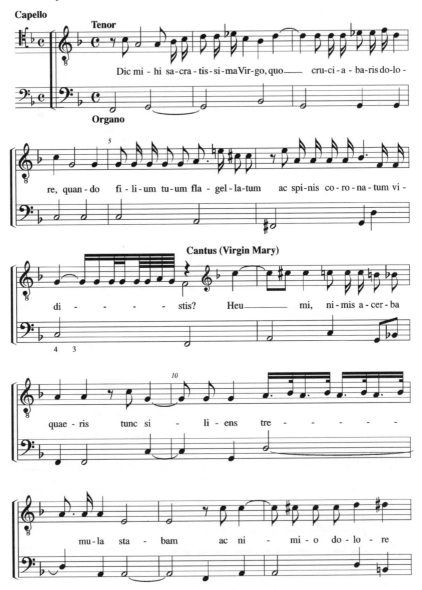

Ex. 8.11 concluded

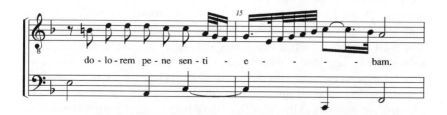

do - lo - rem pe - ne sen - ti - e - - - - bam.

The alternation between statements of first-person narrative ("Here my son dies") and the distance of personal objectivity ("Jesus ... whose breast ... bears such pain, tormenting Mary" – see Text Ex. 5) suggests the ambiguity of Mary's identity through her relation to Christ.[8] He is her son ("mi filli"), but divine ("o Jesu mi, o potens homo, o Deus"), as well as a beloved spouse ("sponse mi, dilecte"). He fulfills the double role of son and incarnation of God the Father, her mystical spouse. That the Virgin sings through the music of *L'Arianna* further conflates eros and filial love, both given extreme feeling through the despair of loss.[9] This most passionate outpouring of the Virgin Mary stands as a tribute to the exquisitely expressive palette of Monteverdi, who gave the character her full share of virtuosity.

The composer Giovanni Francesco Capello set up a brief dialogue between Mary and a tenor, characterized as the soul in a recent recording of the duet "Dic mihi, sacratissima Virgo" (see Text Ex. 6). He poses a series of questions regarding her feelings at the crucifixion, now placed in the temporal past. Each of her answers begins with a sliding ascending semitone, followed by a chromatic descent (Ex. 8.11). The symbolic associations between the sign for the sharp alteration and the cross intensifies the significance of the chromaticism heard in Mary's part. At the conclusion of the dialogue, their alternation gives way to the joining of the two voices in an imitative duet.

The concluding Marian first-person narrative comes from a Roman *Oratorio per la settimana santa* on a libretto by Giulio Cesare Raggioli.[10] This large-scale work has much in common and shares a similar dramatic strategy with the Stradella cantata. A few elements of the piece recall the Stradella cantata: its large scale, the comic foil provided by a bass portraying a demon, and the relatively late appearance of the Virgin's soliloquy. The context emphasizes Mary's redeeming role; her voice seems all the sweeter and her song more tender when encountered side by side with the brusque character of the bass and his attendant demon choruses. Unlike the defiant mother of Bembo's lament, this Mary asks gently for mercy from the start and sings a heartrending lament – based on the descending tetrachord – that stands alongside the best tragic moments in opera. In fact, with many of its passages sounding as dead ringers for scenes from Rossi's *L'Orfeo*, this work suggests the proximity of the opera and oratorio genres. Mary's lament comes in response to the jeering and laughing of those around her, whom Howard Smither has aptly described as "the howling inhabitants of hell."[11] Her tender tune must appease the angry multitudes and convince them to take part in her sadness; in the final phrase of her soliloquy she sings that "one chest alone is too little" to express the grief over the loss of her son (Text Ex. 7). Her beseeching thwarts the demons as all voices join in a final madrigal of mourning. The voice of *Maria mater dolorosa* thus contained the power to affect and transform those around her.

* * *

What might the composers have had in mind as a general vocal concept for the voice of the Virgin Mary? Purity had to be foremost, given that she had been selected as the pure vessel to bear the Christ child, the archetypal mother to whom so many – literate and illiterate alike – could pray in times of need. What does "pure" correspond to in music? Beatless intervals are pure and so are the proportions that determine them; the very notion of purity invokes music's physical nature, prior to the application of the artifice of culture. Linda Austern has recently explored the rich topic of nature and culture in music-making of the early modern period, noting that Mary serves as a nexus between the two realms. In *Parthenia sacra* the seventeenth-century writer Henry Hawkins compared her voice to that of the nightingale, but cleverly stated that her voice exceeds that of the bird, thereby enjoying the gift of pure nature while simultaneously elevated to a divine level; indeed, Austern comments that "Hawkins positions Mary's pure, spiritual voice not only above this little avian's, but far beyond the merely mortal musics of Orpheus, Amphion, Arion, and even the no less legendary Orlando di Lasso and Luca Marenzio."[12]

If the notion of Mary's pure, spiritual voice had some grounding in contemporary European thought, then it would suggest a point of departure for the composers' concept of a naturally beautiful as well as supremely virtuosic instrument. A belief in Mary as the intercessor to Christ for the people could also include one of Mary the singer mediating between nature and culture, between pure physicality and spiritual expression. The humanizing element of the divine, an extension of Mary's long-held associations with the people, prompted the need for the direct quality that the first-person voice provides.

What type of voice might the composers have sought for their portrayal of Mary? A soprano voice in the period could be either male or female. It cannot be ascertained for which gender the pieces were intended, but a consideration of the possibility that several were meant for a woman to sing raises questions about performance venues, about where women's voices could and could not be

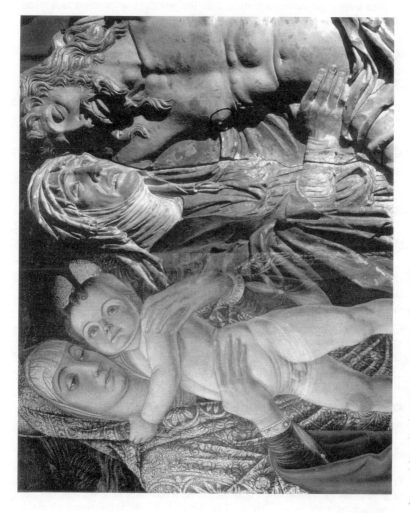

Fig. 8.1   *Mother and Son*, Gardner Museum, 1998

heard. Womens' voices were particularly prized; ducal patronage and the theater in effect prepared the way for them to enter formalized spectacle with solo singing.[13] These voices lent themselves to roles in early opera and in *sacre rappresentazioni* alike. The spawning of first-person Marian narratives may have arisen from a general fascination with the woman's solo voice as well as from the particularly powerful effects obtained through the direct expression of Mary's character. The Church excluded female voices; only in the convents could they participate in sacred musical production, thus requiring boys or *castrati* to represent a female character. The celebrated *Magnificat* and *Stabat Mater dolorosa* settings therefore have stood outside this study; the former generally received a polyphonic setting, while the latter objectifies Mary rather than providing her with an active voice.[14] If a woman was to interpret the role of Mary, however, her voice had by necessity to be heard in an extraliturgical context.[15]

* * *

Through vocal performance of first-person narratives the Blessed Virgin Mary could come to life, whether characterized as *Maria lactans* – the young nursing mother who feels unsure of herself, who feels pride, who enjoys an intimate bond with her child – or as *Mater dolorosa*, the older mother who embodies sadness or indignation (see Fig. 8.1). Each of the foregoing examples brings the listener in close proximity with her formidable character. The newfound appearance of women on stage in this period makes one wonder whether these pieces might have been part of their repertory. The freely-conceived poetry and musical venue for the works neither belonged to church music nor to opera proper, allowing musical performance by sopranos of either gender. Depending on the context, composers found in Mary's subjective depiction the vehicle for highly expressive vocal writing that could link the power of a naturally talented singer with the cultivated *maniere* of the period.

Notes

1. I am grateful to the following people who helped me to formulate the ideas for this essay: Tina Chancey, Michael Collver, Robert Kendrick, Linda Maria Koldau, S. Thomson Moore, Joshua Rifkin, Lea Serafini, Rebecca Soderman, Stefanie Tcharos, Joanna Wulfsberg, and Lucy Yates. It originated as a paper for the Fourth Feminist Theory and Music Conference, University of Virginia, June 1997 and was presented in a substantially revised version at the Eighth Biennial Conference on Baroque Music, University of Exeter, UK, July 1998.
2. See Warren Kirkendale, "*Circulatio*-Tradition, *Maria lactans*, and Josquin as Musical Orator," *Acta musicologica* (January–June 1984), pp. 85–7. For more on this subject, see "The Milk of Paradise," Chapter 13 in Marina Warner, *Alone of*

All Her Sex – The Myth and Cult of the Virgin Mary (New York, Alfred A. Knopf, 1976), pp. 192–205.

3. *Cassell's Compact Latin Dictionary*, s.v. "nenia" ... "nursery ditty, lullaby" (New York: Macmillan, 1963).

4. Gianturco identified another Christmas cantata by Alessandro Scarlatti with a role assigned to *Maria Vergine* in her "'Cantate spirituali e morali', with a Description of the Papal Sacred Cantata Tradition for Christmas 1676–1740," *Music and Letters* (February 1992), p. 17, but only the libretto for the work survives, dated 1695.

5. In an essay examining the power of the image of the Virgin Mary, Julia Kristeva noted that in the Marian cult, "we are entitled only to the ear of the virginal body, the tears and the breast. With the female sexual organ changed into an innocent shell, holder of sound, there arises a possible tendency to eroticize hearing, voice or even understanding. ... under a full blue dress, the maternal, virginal body allowed only the breast to show, while the face, with the stiffness of Byzantine icons gradually softened, was covered with tears. Milk and tears became the privileged signs of the *Mater Dolorosa* ... " "Stabat Mater," pp. 160–86 in *The Kristeva Reader*, ed. Toril Moi (New York: Columbia University Press, 1986), pp. 172–3.

6. See Nella Anfuso and Annibale Gianuario, *Le tre Arianne di Claudio Monteverdi* (Florence: Centro Studi Rinascimento Musicale, 1975). Ulrich Michels clarifies the chronology of the opera monody, the five-voice madrigal setting, and the *Pianto* in "Das 'Lamento d'Arianna' von Claudio Monteverdi," in *Festschrift für Hans Heinrich Eggebrecht zum 65. Geburtstag*, ed. Werner Breig, Reinhold Brinkmann, and Elmar Budde (Stuttgart: Franz Steiner, 1984), pp. 91–109.

7. Adelmo Damerini, "Il senso religioso nelle musiche sacre di Claudio Monteverdi," *Collectanea Historiae Musicae* IV, ed. Mario Fabbri (Florence: Olschki, 1966), pp. 49–50.

8. Michels, op. cit., stated that Monteverdi was very exacting with the texts that he selected to set to music and could even be annoying about it: "Monteverdi war bekanntlich in der Wahl seiner Texte äusserst penibel. Wurden ihm Texte zur Komposition vorgeschlagen, die er nicht selbst ausgesucht hatte, prüfte er sie genau, lehnte sie ab oder machte Verbesserungsvorschläge" (95).

9. The mulitiplicity of their relatedness is treated in music history through such pieces as the sequence *Benedicta es celorum regina* set by Josquin and Willaert. Kristeva pointed out the "threefold metamorphosis of a woman in the tightest parenthood structure ... [she is] *mother* of her son and his *daughter* as well ... and besides his *wife* ... From 1135 on, transposing the Song of Songs, Bernard of Clairvaux glorifies Mary in her role of beloved and wife. But Catherine of Alexandria ... already pictured herself as receiving the wedding ring from Christ, with the Virgin's help, while Catherine of Siena (1347–80) goes through a mystical wedding with him. Is it the impact of Mary's function as Christ's beloved and wife that is responsible for the blossoming out of the Marian cult in the West after Bernard and thanks to the Cistercians?" ("Stabat Mater," p. 169).

10. Howard Smither, liner notes to a recording by Les arts florissants, Harmonia Mundi 901297 (1984–89). While the musical setting has been ascribed to Luigi Rossi, Margaret Murata has called his authorship into question and suggests that the music may actually have been composed by Marc'Antonio Pasqualini. Murata's conjecture about Pasqualini will be explained in her forthcoming *Catalogue of the Barberini Music Manuscripts*, in collaboration with Lowell Lindgren.

11. Howard Smither, *A History of the Oratorio*. Volume I, The Oratorio in the Baroque Era. Italy, Vienna, Paris (Chapel Hill: The University of North Carolina Press, 1977), p. 198.

12. Linda Phyllis Austern, "Nature, Culture, Myth, and the Musician in Early Modern England," *Journal of the American Musicological Society* 51 (Spring 1998), p. 37.

13. During Monteverdi's period of service to the Mantuan court, female *virtuose* were especially treasured and well-rewarded for their singing. The lead singer for *L'Arianna* was to have been Caterina Martinelli, had she not prematurely died before the production. See Edmond Strainchamps, "The Life and Death of Caterina Martinelli: New Light on Monteverdi's '*Arianna*'," pp. 155–86 in *Early Music History* 5 (Cambridge: Cambridge University Press, 1985).

14. See Jerome F. Weber, "Stabat Mater," *Goldberg Early Music Magazine* 3 (1998), pp. 37–45.

15. There were also settings for men to sing. In his preface to an edition of Maurizio Cazzati's *In Calvaria rupe* – a motet for bass voice that contains within it a *Lamento di Maria* – Rudolf Ewerhart noted the preponderance of pieces representing Mary in the basso-continuo period and situated the practice as an extraliturgical one that was based on freely-conceived poetry. See *Cantio Sacra – Geistliche Solokantaten* 19 (Cologne: Verlag Edmund Bieler, n.d.).

Musical Sources

Bembo, Antonia. Lamento della Vergine, "D'onnipotente padre" from *Produzioni armoniche* (France-Paris, Bibliothèque Nationale, Rés. Vm^{1}117, c. 1697–1701), pp. 64–73.

———— Per il Natale, "In braccio di Maria" from *Produzioni armoniche*, pp. 46–63. Edition by Claire Fontijn. Fayetteville, AR: Clar-Nan, 1999.

Capello, Giovanni Francesco. "Dic mihi, sacratissima virgo," from *Sacrorum concentuum unica, & duabus vocibus cum Litanijs B. Virginis Mariae, opus primum.* Venice: Ricciardo Amadino, 1610.

Centorio, Marco Antonio. Nenia B. Virginis ad X[Chris]tum Infantem, "Dormi iam mea vita." Italy-Vercelli, Biblioteca capitolare, sez. musicale-manoscritti: Centorio, ms. 1302/13.

Merula, Tarquinio. Canzonetta Spirituale sopra alla nanna, "Hor ch'è tempo di dormire," pp. 35–9 in *Curtio precipitato et altri Capricij composti in diversi modi vaghi e leggiadri à voce sola*. Venice: Bartolomeo Magni, 1638.

Monteverdi, Claudio. *Lamento d'Arianna*. Venice: Gardano, 1643.

———— "Pianto della Madona à voce sola Sopra il Lamento d'Arianna," pp. 81–9 in *Selva morale e spirituale*. Venice: Bartolomeo Magni, 1641.

Rossi, Luigi, attr. *Oratorio per la settimana santa*. Libretto by Giulio Cesare Raggioli (Italy-Rome, Biblioteca Apostolica Vaticana, Barb. lat. 4198–9, c. 1641–45).

Stradella, Alessandro. Cantata per il santissimo Natale, "Ah Troppo è ver," c. 1675. From two manuscript sources: Italy-Modena, Biblioteca Estense, Mus. F. 1145 and Italy-Turin, Biblioteca nazionale universitaria, Giordano 12; neither autograph but by a scribe commonly associated with Stradella. Edited by Carolyn Gianturco in *Alessandro Stradella, Tre Cantate per voci e strumenti*. Laaber: Laaber-Verlag, 1997.

TEXTS AND TRANSLATIONS

Text Ex. 1. Merula, "Hor ch'è tempo di dormire"

Hor ch'è tempo di dormire
Dormi figlio e non vagire
Perche il tempo ancor verrà
Che vagir bisognerà
Deh ben mio, deh cor mio
Fa la nina nina na.

Now it is time to sleep,
Sleep, my son, and do not cry,
Because the time will come
When crying will be necessary
Oh my beloved, oh my sweetheart,
Sleep nina nina na.

Chiudi quei lumi divini
Come fan gl'altri bambini
Perche tosto oscuro velo
Priverà di lume il cielo
Deh ben mio, deh cor mio
Fa la nina nina na.

Close those heavenly eyes
As other children do,
For before long a dark veil
Will deprive the sky of light,
Oh my beloved, oh my sweetheart,
Sleep nina nina na.

Over prendi questo latte
Dalle mie mammelle intatte
Perche ministro crudele
Ti prepara aceto e fiele
Deh ben mio, deh cor mio
Fa la nina nina na.

Now have this milk
From my virginal breasts,
For the cruel minister
Is preparing vinegar and gall for you.
Oh my beloved, oh my sweetheart,
Sleep nina nina na.

Amor mio sia questo petto
Hor per te morbido letto
Pria che rendi ad alta voce
L'alma al Padre sù la croce
Deh ben mio, deh cor mio
Fa la nina nina na.

My love, let this chest
Be a soft bed for you,
Before aloud commending your soul
To your Father up on the cross.
Oh my beloved, oh my sweetheart,
Sleep nina nina na.

Posa or queste membra belle
Vezzosette e tenerelle
Perche puoi ferri e catene
Gli daran acerbe pene
Deh ben mio, deh cor mio
Fa la nina nina na.

Now rest these beautiful,
Pretty little, tender soft limbs,
Because you will have irons and chains
That will give them bitter pain.
Oh my beloved, oh my sweetheart,
Sleep nina nina na.

Queste mani e questi piedi
Ch'hor con gusto e gaudio vedi
Ahime com'in varij modi
Passeran a cuti chiodi
Questa facia gratiosa
Rubiconda hor più che Rosa
Sputi e schiaffi sporcheranno
Con tormento e grand'affanno

These hands and these feet
That you now see with joy and pleasure
Alas, will be pierced with sharp nails
In a variety of ways.
This graceful face
That is now ruddier than a rose
Will be sullied by spit and insults,
With torment and great anxiety.

Ah con quanto tuo dolore	Oh, with what pain,
Sola speme del mio core	only hope of my heart,
Questo capo e questi crini	This head and these locks of hair
Passeran acuti spini	Will be poked by sharp thorns,
Ah ch'in questo divin petto	Oh, that in this divine chest,
Amor mio dolce e diletto	My sweet love and delight,
Vi farà piaga mortale	Mortal wounds will be made
Empia lancia e disleale	By treacherous, cruel spears.
Dormi dunque figliol mio	Therefore sleep, my son,
Dormi pur Redentor mio	Sleep then, my Redeemer,
Perche poi con lieto viso	So that then with a happy face
Si vedrem in Paradiso.	We shall see each other in Paradise.
Hor che dorme la mia vita	Now that he who is my life is sleeping,
Del mio cor gioia compita	He who is the complete joy of my heart,
Tacia ogn'un con puro zelo	Let all be hushed with pure devotion
Tacian sin la terra e'l cielo.	Let heaven and earth fall silent.
E fra tanto io che farò	And meanwhile, what shall I do?
Il mio ben contemplerò	I shall contemplate my beloved,
Ne starò col capo chino	Stand here with bowed head,
Sin che dorme il mio Bambino.	As long as my child sleeps.

Text Ex. 2. Stradella, Cantata per il santissimo Natale, "Ah Troppo è ver," Mary's Aria-Recitativo:

Maria Vergine [Aria]	*Virgin Mary*
Sovrano mio bene,	Sovereign my beloved,
mia spene, mio cor:	My hope, my heart:
quest'alma ch'in calma	This soul who in peace
gioisce per te,	Rejoices for you,
dal seno materno	From the maternal breast
l'interno suo amor	The core of her love
con piogge serene	With serene rains
riversa al tuo pie'	Pours down again on your feet
e con dovuto omaggio	And with devoted homage
dell'alba tua beata adora il raggio.	Of your holy dawn adores the ray.
[Recitativo]	[Recitative]
Concedi ai falli umani ampio perdono	Grant ample pardon to human error
e sia il mio priego intercessor del dono.	And that my prayer be the intercessor of the gift.

Text Ex. 3. Bembo, Per il Natale:

In braccio di Maria	In Mary's arms
Co' suoi primi vagiti	With his first whimperings,
Spirava aure di pace	The king of the world breathed
Il re del mondo al mondo	Breezes of peace unto the world.
Ella che dal profondo	She who from the depths of her heart
Del cor fiati d'amore al divo infante	Filled with love to warm the divine child,
A riscaldar traea	With devoted piety,
Con divota pietà cosi dicea:	Said thus:
Santi spiriti	"Blessed spirits,
Menti angeliche,	Angelic minds,
Alme fervide,	Fervent souls,
Regi estranei,	Foreign rulers,
Qui venite,	Come ye here;
Riverite	Revere
In santo zelo	In sacred zeal
Il Re del cielo	The king of heaven.
Se questo immenso parto	If this immense product of my labor
Del mio cor parte immensa,	Is an immense part of my body,
Estateci adorate.	You ecstatically
Voi le viscere mie meco adorate	Adore with me my innermost.
Ma, che dico, ove poggia	But what am I saying? From whence
A vanagloria intento	Comes such an evil thought
Mal accorto pensier?	Intent on vainglory?
Figlio perdona, errai, ma non errai	Son, forgive me, I erred; but I did not err:
Che se fuor di peccato originale	If a god without original sin
Dal seno della madre uscito un dio,	Sprang from the womb of his mother,
Impeccabil son'io.	Then I am without sin.
Misteri Supremi	Supreme mysteries
Oracoli eterni	Eternal oracles,
Svelatevi a me.	Open up to me.
V'honora, v'adora	My ever faithful heart
Il cor tutto fe.	Honors you, adores you."
Dal divino sembiante	On the divine face
Del pargoletto infante	Of the infant baby boy
Apparve all'hora insolito splendore	Now appears extraordinary splendor
Che dal sen di Maria	That banishes fear
Scaccia il timore.	From Mary's breast.
In estasi di gioia	In joyous ecstasy
Gloria gridan gl'astanti	The onlookers cry out "gloria"
E ripiglian le voci i spirti santi.	Repeated by the voices of the holy spirits.
E ad eterna memoria	And into eternal memory, echoes
Eco di gloria intuona e gloria, e gloria.	Of this "gloria" resound: gloria! gloria!

Text Ex. 4. Bembo, Lamento della Vergine:

D'onnipotente padre unico figlio
confitto in duro tronco
sovra il Calvario, essangue,
lacero e anhelante,
quel gran verbo divino
temea la morte, al suo morir vicino.
Atre nube il sol copria,
si ascondeano gli astri ardenti
e piangeano gli elementi
al gran pianto di Maria.

Recitativo
Ella che fra i singhiozzi,
dal profondo dell'alma
angosciosi sospir mesta trahea,
contro morte crudel cosi dicea:

Aria vivace
Che fai?
Che tenti,
Tiranna pessima
ombra dolente
che nulla sei?

Recitativo
Pria ch'il ciel fosse
fu il tuo fator.
Tutt'era vita
e non t'è dato
trar all'Eterno
l'esser di morte,
se vita eterna
è il sommo Dio.

Aria
Staccato dal ramo
di pianta fatale,
il fallo d'Adamo
diè frutto mortale.

Seconda
Con pena infinita
congiò trista sorte,
quell'arbor di vita
in arbor di morte.

Of the omnipotent father the only son
attached to a hard shaft
on the Calvary, bleeding,
cut and panting,
this great divine word
fears death, close to mortality.
A cloud covered the sun,
the burning stars hid themselves,
and the elements cried
at Maria's great weeping.

Recitative
She amidst her sobbing
from the depths of her soul,
anguished, drew a sad sigh
against cruel death, saying thus:

Aria vivace
What are you doing? What are you
        attempting?
tyrannical, evil,
dolorous cloud;
you who are made up of the void?

Recitative
I pray that heaven would be
your creator.
Everything was life
and it was not given to you
to take from the eternal
to be one with death,
if eternal life
is the highest god.

Aria
Removed from the branch
of the fatal plant
Adam's fall
gave mortal fruit.

Second
With infinite pain
I meet my sad fate
this tree of life, [turned into]
a tree of death.

Recitativo
Dunque, se l'huomo diè vita alla morte,
contr'il mortal sfoga il tuo sdegno
    atroce,
mostro spietato e rio,
che non può morte dar la morte a Dio.

Recitative
Therefore, if man gives life to death,
against death your atrocious disdain is
    vented,
pitiless and scornful monster
who cannot die gives death to god.

Aria
Larva dileguati,
fantasma inviolati,
cadi nel baratro,
scendi in obio,
che vincer non può Dio altri che Dio.

Aria
Dissipated shadows,
inviolated fantasms,
you fall into the abyss,
descend into oblivion,
That none other than God can conquer.

Recitativo
Volgeva intanto al Padre
il moribondo ciglio il re del cielo,
e presso a l'ultima hora
così, con flebil voce,
sciolse gli ultimi accenti in su la croce:

Recitative
Meanwhile the king of heaven turned
his moribund brow toward his Father,
and, close to the final hour,
with a weak voice, thus
released his last accents from the cross:

Affetuoso Assai
Padre, deh caro Padre,
perché mi lasci?
Ohimé, l'udi la trista
madre e svenuta cade.
Ma perché trino et un voler superno
cosi dispose ne l'empirea corte,

in dar la morte al suo fatto eterno

tremò, sudò, impallidi la morte.

Affettuoso Assai
Father, oh dear father,
why do you abandon me?
Alas, hear the sad mother,
and then he fainted.
But why the trinity and a supernal wish
disposed of such a one in the empyrean
    court,
to give death to he who was made
    eternal,
I tremble, I toil; he grows pale with
    death.

Text Ex. 5. Monteverdi, Pianto della Madona à voce sola Sopra il Lamento d'Arianna. Text based on the original print, with punctuation added:

Iam moriar mi filli.
Quis nam poterit matrem consolare
In hoc fero dolore
In hoc tam duro tormento
Iam moriar mi filli.

Here my son dies.
Who can console this mother,
So fraught with pain,
In such harsh torment?
Now my son dies.

Mi Jesu, o Jesu mi sponse, sponse mi,
dilecte mi, mea spes, mea vita, me
deseris.
Heu vulnus, cordis mei.

My Jesus, o Jesus my spouse, my spouse,
my delight, my hope, my life, my desire,
you leave me. Ah, the wound to my
heart!

Respice Jesu mi,
Respice Jesu precor, respice matrem,
Matrem respice tuam que gemendo pro te,
Pallidas languet atque in monte funesto,
In hac tam dura et tam immani
Cruce tecum petit affigi.

Mi Jesu o Jesu mi
O potens homo, o Deus
En inspectores heu tanti doloris quo torquetur Maria miserere gementis tecum que extincta sit que per te vixit.

Sed promptus ex hac vita discedes o mi fili & ego hic ploro tu confringes infernum hoste
victo superbo & ego relinquor preda doloris, solitaria et mesta, te Pater alme te que fons amoris suscipiant leti & ego te non videbo O Pater o mi sponse. Hec sunt promissa Arcangeli Gabrielis. Hec illa, excelsa sedes antiqui patris David. Sunt hec regalia septra que tibi cingant crines
nec ne sunt aurea sceptra & fine, fine regnum affigi duro ligno & clavis laniati atque corona.

Ah Iesu, ah Iesu mi. En mihi dulce mori ecce plorando ecce clamando rogat.

Te misera Maria nam tecum mori

Est illi gloria et vita.

Hei Filli non respondes,
Heu surdus es ad flectus atque quarellas

O morso culpa, o inferne esse sponsus meus Mersus in undis velox
O terrae centrum aperite profundum et cum Dilecto meo me quoque absconde.

Quid loquor
Heu quid spero misera
Heu iam quid quero o Jesu,
Non sit, quid volo sed fiat quod tibi placet vivat mestum cor meo pleno dolore pascere fili mi matris Amore

Look at me, my Jesus,
Look at me, Jesus, I implore you,
Look at the mother, your mother who,

Pale with weeping for you, languishes and seeks to suffer with you in terrible Death on that harsh and savage cross.

My Jesus, o my Jesus,
powerful man, o God! Lo, you who look on such great sorrow by which Mary is tormented, have mercy on my weeping, that I may die with you, who have lived through you.

But soon you leave this life, o my son, and I weep here. You break the power of Hell, the proud enemy conquered and I am left alone and sad in sorrow. May the kind Father and the Fount of love receive you in joy;
yet I shall not see you, o Father, o my spouse!
Are these the promises of the Archangel Gabriel? Is this the royal crown that encircles your hair? This is not the golden scepter and the end of your kingdom to suffer on the hard wooden cross and your crown to be pierced by nails!

O Jesus, o my Jesus. Lo death is sweet to me!
Lo, with weeping and crying Mary calls on you in wretchedness: for to die with you
Is glory and life for her!

Alas, Son, do you not answer?
Alas, are you deaf to my tears and complaints?
O death, o sin, o hell: lo, my bridegroom is Drowned in the waves!
O quickly open the deep center of the earth and Hide me too with my beloved!

What do I say? Alas, what hope have I, in my wretchedness? Alas now what do I seek?
O Jesus, my Jesus! Let there be nothing that I want that is not pleasing to you! Let my heart live, sad and full of pain! My Son, take nourishment from your mother's love!

Text Ex. 6. Capello, "Dic mihi, sacratissima Virgo." Text and adapted translation from *The Heritage of Monteverdi* (II), *Per la settimana santa*, La Fenice, Ricercar CD, 1995.

Animus	*The Soul*
Dic mihi, sacratissima Virgo,	Tell me, most Holy Virgin,
Quo cruciabaris dolore,	What pain crucified you
Quando filium tuum flagellatum	When you saw your Son whipped
Ac spinis coronatum vidistis?	And crowned with thorns?
Maria Virgo	*Virgin Mary*
Heumi, nimis acerba quaeris.	Alas, I remained silent
Tunc siliens tremula stabam	And trembling;
Ac nimio dolore dolorem pene sentiebam.	I felt the most sorrowful pain within me.
Animus	*The Soul*
Quid filius tuus tibi merenti dixit?	What did your Son say to you as you suffered?
Maria Virgo	*Virgin Mary*
En, dulcis mater, en filium tuum,	O sweet Mother, of what cruel death is
En quam crudelem mortem patior.	your Son dying?
Animus	*The Soul*
Et tu, quid illi morienti dixisti,	And you, what did you say to your dying
O maestissima mulier?	Son, o most majestic of women?
Maria Virgo	*Virgin Mary*
Mi fili, fili mi, solus moreris?	My Son, my Son, shalt thou die alone?
Morior et ipsa tecum.	I also shall die, and die with You.
Animus	*The Soul*
Morior et ipse tecum.	And with you I die.

Text Ex. 7. Rossi, attr. *Oratorio per la settimana santa*. c. 1640s. Translation adapted from Derek Yeld on the liner notes to the recording by Les arts florissants, Harmonia Mundi CD, 1989. Excerpt from Part 2 of the oratorio:

Vergine	*Virgin*
Cieli, stelle, pietà!	Heavens, stars, have mercy!
Demoni	*Demons [chorus]*
Chi si fè prole divina,	He who elevated himself to the progeny of divinity,
Chi di noi gl'oltraggi ordí	Who brought disgrace upon us,
Già nel suol la fronte inchina,	Already inclines hi brow upon the earth,
Già per lui s'eclissa il dí.	Already for him the day darkens.
L'inimico Nazzareno,	The Nazarene foe,
Die viventi la beltà,	The beauty of the living,

Sovra un legno venne meno,
catenato a un tronco stà
chi da regi adorato un tempo fù.

Vergine
Tormenti non piú!
Misera, e quale io sento,
trionfator contento,
con urli e con sibili,
con gridi orribili,
con voci di scherno,
rider gl'abissi e festeggiar l'inferno
e degli orrendi chiostri

dell'estinta beltà pregiarsi i mostri?
Che d'insano livore alto trofeo!
Ogni beltà cadeo
con l'adorato mio figlio Gesú.
Tormenti non piú!

Cieli, stelle, pietà
d'una madre dogliosa, lagrimosa,
ch'a soffrire tanto martire
già perduto il suo cor, piú cor non ha.

Cieli, stelle, pietà!
Maria si more:
S'a me fu tolto il core,

se del fonte di vita io resto priva,
com'esser può ch'io viva?
Fate ch'io mora almeno non senza core in
    seno,
e sia poi di quest'alma alma il dolore.
Rendetemi il mio core!
…

Vergine
Ecco l'ancilla tua pronta a tua voglia:

S'a te piace il mio pianto, occhi piangete;

Se t'aggrada il mio duolo,
È poco un petto solo.

Upon a cross is failing,
Bound to a tree is he
Who once was worshiped by kings.

Virgin
Torments, no more!
But, poor wretch, do I hear,
In happy triumph,
With howls and hisses,
With hideous shrieks,
With jeering voices,
The abyss laughing and hell rejoicing,
And the monsters of the horrendous
    cloisters
Delighting in the extinquished beauty?
What a lofty triumph of insane hatred!
All beauty falls
with my beloved son, Jesus.
Torments, no more!

Heavens, stars, have mercy
On a pain-racked, mourning mother,
Who in suffering so many torments, has
    already lost her heart, and no longer
    has a heart.
Heavens, stars, have mercy!
Mary dies:
If my heart has been torn from me, If I
    am
deprived of the fount of life,
How can it be that I shall live?
Let me at least not die without a heart in
    my breast And let the pain be the soul
    of this soul.
Give me back my heart!
…

Virgin
Behold your handmaid, ready to do your
    bidding:
If my tears please you, then weep, my
    eyes;
If my pain is agreeable to you,
One chest alone is too little.

CHAPTER NINE

"His open side our book":
Meditation and Education in
Elizabeth Grymeston's *Miscelanea*
Meditations Memoratives

Edith Snook

Miscelanea Meditations Memoratives (1604) is a fascinating collection of meditations, penitential psalms, and proverbs written and compiled by Elizabeth Grymeston for the guidance of her son Bernye after her death. Published posthumously, the book also includes a "madrigall" by Bernye, in which he responds to his mother's writing.[1] Like the maternal advice books of Dorothy Leigh (1616), Elizabeth Joceline (1624), and M.R., the author of *The Mother's Counsell* (1623), Grymeston's work offers guidance in conduct and religion. As scholars such as Elaine Beilin, Wendy Wall, and Valerie Wayne have argued, writing about faith and proffering advice to children were common forms in which women could transgress prohibitions against publication.[2] Grymeston's work is also different from later Protestant advice books, however; she was Catholic, and while the collection of proverbs and the prefatory address to Bernye are explicitly directive, the meditations are contemplative, requiring the involvement of the imagination rather than obedience.[3] In this essay, I want to explore the results of these differences. I shall argue that even as Grymeston's work conforms with a conventional view of what is acceptable for a woman author, the conjunction of affective meditation with maternal instruction also challenges customary distinctions establishing gender difference in discourses of religion and education.

Because Grymeston presents her meditations as a work of instruction for Bernye, I first will explore briefly some of the issues related to early modern representations of mothers as educators of their sons. Mothers were considered to be a formative source of moral instruction, especially within the "spiritualized household" – the ideology of the domestic sphere, prominent in seventeenth-century English culture and influenced by earlier humanist writings, that made the family the primary unit of religious education.[4] Juan Luis Vives, for one, attests to the powerful sway that mothers had with their children. He writes in *Instruction of a Christian Woman* that because children love and imitate their mothers, "it lyeth more in the mother, than men ween, to make the conditions of the chyldren. For she may make them whether she wyll, very good, or very badde."[5] Within the privacy of the family that was, as Margo Todd says, the "seminary of church and commonwealth," the mother's daily care for her children gave her an influential role as a teacher of religion and morality.[6]

There were, however, chronological and topical limitations on this guidance. Contingent upon the belief that "the soul both affects and is affected by the body," as Erasmus says in his colloquy "Puerpera"(1526), the mother was thought to best contribute to the development of her son, not by teaching him his letters, which was his father's responsibility, but by nursing him and thereby giving him a healthy body and a virtuous soul.[7] Even though literate women commonly did catechize their children and teach them to read, suggesting that in practice motherhood was not an exclusively physical influence, they still did not often teach their sons to be scholars. Maternal instruction of upper-class boys did not extend past the age of seven, when boys began to be educated by tutors and schoolmasters, and it did not include scholarly topics like Latin and Greek.[8] If the home could be compared to a seminary, it could not be likened to a grammar school or university; moral instruction was not scholarly education. While mothers made a compelling contribution to the former, especially through their material care, they were usually excluded from the latter.

This circumscription on the mother–son relationship can be attributed to restrictions on female education that made mothers simply unable to offer literate instruction and, more fundamentally, to cultural anxieties about gender difference.[9] The mother's exceptional capacity to form a child's character made her a potential threat both to the development of gender difference in her son and to the patriarchal authority of her husband. William Gouge, for example, attests to the effectiveness of a mother's love and daily care at instilling morality in young children – and to her ability to undermine the father's spiritual leadership – when he observes that "if father and mother be of divers religions, most of the children will follow the mother."[10] The compulsion that makes a boy follow his mother in religion could also ensure that he will fail to become a scholar. Humanists, such as Erasmus, Elyot, Vives, and Ascham, express fears that mothers and their love will turn boys from the rigours, reason, and discipline that they associate with scholarship and masculinity toward the life of delicacy, flattery, and foolishness that they attribute to women.[11] Vives, in particular, connects his own ability to become a scholar to his mother's disinclination to reveal her love for him – to a concealing of her influence – and he reports on another scholar's gratitude for his mother's death. If she had not died, this other man is to have said, he would have remained at home "among dicing, drabbes, delicates, and pleasures, as I begonne."[12] Symbolized by the ceremony of breeching, the rejection of qualities and influences deemed feminine and the commencement of a scholarly education indicate the beginnings of a boy's difference from his mother.[13]

Humanist educational discourses demarcate this difference, in part, by laying the boundaries of learnedness over those of gender. Patricia Parker has noted the presence of anxieties about impotence and effeminization in humanist representations of the scholar, tracing them to the abandonment of traditional militaristic signs of masculinity; having relocated manliness in the more feminine world of words, knowledge of Latin ensures that the scholar will be sufficiently unlike women.[14] The foolish is feminine, while the scholarly is what men know – as Erasmus suggests when he urges the Christian Prince to shun the stories of Arthur and Lancelot because they are "utterly illiterate, foolish, and on the level of old wives' tales."[15] The inconsistent representation of the male scholar's mother as both the source of seductive laxity and of moral good perpetuates the exclusion of women from the category of knowledge most associated with power, that of humanist scholarship. Mothers are simply the other against which the scholar constructed his identity as vigorous, manly, and learned. By inscribing gendered domains of knowledge and negative or conflicted definitions of femininity, education discourses manufacture a definition of the masculine scholar, a definition in process without the status of being a stable monolith.

Writing to educate fashions subjectivities – of the author/tutor presenting him or herself as one who knows what should be taught and of the pupil whose character will result from the instruction. Grymeston, I will argue, does two interrelated things to such constructions of gender through education. She creates a version of masculinity for her son that is not dependent upon her absence or the expurgation of femininity, and she writes a positive intellectual, spiritual, and social identity for herself as author, mother, and woman; demonstrating how she can be like men in knowledge and how Bernye ought to know God through feminine terms, Grymeston resists oppositional definitions of their respective genders. She does this first by presenting herself as an educated woman who can address verbal advice of a particularly literary quality to Bernye, a young man old enough to require counsel about marriage and scholarly enough to write a poem in response.[16] In her preface, she gives him practical guidance in moral living and marriage, telling him to marry a woman of the same rank, of moderate beauty, at an appropriate time (A3v,A4). She does not usually speak so directly, however. While claiming that there is no better way for a mother to "manifest hir affection, than in advising hir children out of hir owne experience" (A3), she expresses this experience primarily in the words of other writers and informs Bernye that "thou maiest happily thinke that if every Philosopher fetched his sentence, these leaves would be left without lines" (A3v). Grymeston defers to the philosophers to accrue more authority to her advice, and in so doing inscribes her own words as more humble in origin. Yet, with her citations of an array of classical texts, secular and religious contemporary poetry, and the Bible and other religious works, she also demonstrates that the scholarly category of education that the philosophers represent is integral to her experience.[17] She writes as a well-learned reader to prove that such knowledge is not exclusively for men. Education is important – for she tells Bernye "without learning man is but as an immortall beast" (A3v) – and it is also for mothers. Rather than separating religion from learning, as was typical in descriptions of women's piety, Grymeston integrates them in a way more characteristic of upper-class male education, for whom theology was, according to Deborah Shuger, a "disciplinary matrix" of learned discourses.[18]

While conduct books presented women's religious reading, not as a ground for scholarly exploration but as a method of behavioural control, Grymeston writes of faith as if it were indeed a matrix; from the seeds of various sources she generates a book and an authorial identity. She makes the secular poetry of Virgil and Pindarus, among others, applicable in a sacred context, revealing her ability to judge what is good for herself, without the "wyse and sad men" who Vives would have guiding women's reading to keep them chaste.[19] She also demonstrates her creative engagement with what she has read by altering the texts that she cites. With the exception of those men she mentions by name – Chrystostome (C2v), Pindarus, from whom she quotes in Greek (C3), and Ambrose (C3v) – Grymeston detaches the citations from their authors, as her primary source *Englands Parnassus* (1600) had not done.[20] Furthermore, if the "philosophers" and poets did come to fetch their sentences, they might not recognize them: Rowlands' psalms are in reversed order; Southwell's poem has been broken up and placed in the midst of prose passages; individual words have been changed, as Beilin and Hughey and Hereford have noted; and all the poetry has been placed in different contexts. The citations do the work Grymeston wants of them, not that which they did in their original poems.[21] So, although she writes within the culturally prescribed paradigm of motherhood as a moral influence, she uses its opportunities for authority to place herself within literary and educated culture. She speaks as an active and accomplished reader, an intellectual agent, and one who knows Latin and Greek. As a scholar herself, she can directly contribute to making one of her son, ensuring that he will not define himself in opposition to her or require her silence and absence.

Grymeston also writes a positive social and moral identity for herself by inserting her maternal love into Bernye's education. Grymeston, very much like those writers I discussed earlier, describes a mother's love as a critical impetus in creating the moral character of her child. She tells Bernye:

My dearest sonne, there is nothing so strong as the force of love; there is no love so forcible as the love of an affectionate mother to hir naturall childe: there is no mother can either more affectionately shew hir nature, or more naturally manifest hir affection, than in advising hir children out of hir owne experience, to eschue evill, and encline them to do that which is good. (A3)

Even though Grymeston is not writing for a public audience – unlike Elizabeth Joceline and Dorothy Leigh, she does not self-consciously defend the publication of her work – maternal love does provide a reason for writing. Yet, so does her imminent death, and as Wendy Wall has argued, her absence may be the premise upon which the publication of her work is acceptable.[22] Because maternal love was attended by anxieties that it would become coddling and impede a boy's maturation into masculinity, love could also necessitate a mother's absence. As Mary Beth Rose writes: "Since the mother would remove one from what is conceived as the world of action – the public, socialized world – the best mother is an absent or a dead mother."[23] Maternal love was not invariably a justification for a mother's influence.

Key to Grymeston's assertion of her presence in her son's life is her adamant and particular definition of her love for him. Conceding no benefit to her absence, she instead depicts love as a catalyst, rather than a hindrance, to her son's social development. Her love is an instrument of discipline to which Bernye, described as a brash and reckless youth with a "violent spirit," should submit in order to learn deliberation and to be "seasoned with these precepts." She tells him:

And because that it is incident to quicke spirits to commit rash attempts: as ever the love of a mother may challenge the performance of her demand of a dutifull childe; be a bridle to thy self, to restraine thee from doing that which indeed thou maiest doe: that thou maiest the better forbeare that which in trueth thou oughtest not to doe. (A4v–B)

The bridle was a commonly image of self-government, as in Plato's *Phaedrus*, but it was also an image with particular gender connotations.[24] The early modern gentlemen, like the charioteer in Plato's fable, had to possess self-discipline, for without it the required displays of strength and action could become the excess of violence and rashness.[25] Women, however, were more akin to Plato's vicious horse, associated with appetite and body. Like the horse, too wild to control itself, a woman needed ever-present moral direction. The scold's bridle threatened literal, physical control, while conduct books and education treatises asserted that husbands, fathers, and tutors would guide girls and women; whatever their age, they lacked the capacity to make independent moral judgements.[26] By comparing her love to a bridle, Grymeston can demonstrate her own maturity and her ability to be the self-controlling guide. Even so, her writing about maternal love is not outside of early modern anxieties about parental affection; as the historian Ralph Houlbrooke suggests of familial tenderness: "it was for a long time held undesirable to allow it untrammelled expression."[27] Grymeston, too, values restraint, but she insists upon an important difference. Her love will be expressed. Her love is like that of God, a physician who will lance a wound to heal it and who "if he see thou be softened by the world thy naturall nurse,... can annoint her teate with the bitterness of discontent to weane thee from hir" (Dv). Softness and delicacy, terms associated with femininity, are still morally dangerous, but these are not all that mothers have to offer. Grymeston, like God, has a moral rationale for her love. By redefining maternal love in a way that dissolves the dichotomy between the expression of maternal emotion and the development of masculine discipline, she can make her love, and therefore herself, necessary to, rather than necessarily excised from, the education of an adolescent male.

That Grymeston writes religious meditations for her son also functions within dominant ideologies of maternal moral education and virtuous female speech. But just as her moral instruction reveals her participation in a domain of knowledge from which women tended to be excluded, she makes the faith that she teaches Bernye include attributes of femininity and mothers. In discussions of motherhood, the maternal body was an important source of spiritual influence, and Grymeston, similarly, relates motherhood and spirituality to the corporeal; her meditations connect divine activities to those of mothers through metaphor and attend to the suffering of Christ, transforming the silent corporeal maternal influence into a devotional experience conceptually-related to motherhood through language. Twice Grymeston makes a woman's contemplation of death before childbirth an exemplary way to live. She suggests that one ought to be like the pregnant woman who muses on her delivery and think about life as a way to death, so as to face it without fear (C2v). When life is such a study in preparation for death, it can be endured, like the pains in childbirth, because the result is a new birth: "he feares not his cold sweats, nor forgoing gripes, but taketh them as throwes in childe-bed, by which our soule is brought out of a lothsome body into eternall felicitie" (D2v). These comparisons establish a hierarchy of soul over body, of spiritual over material, but they also create an imaginative sympathy between the "he" who lives and the women who suffer pain in labor. Instead of regarding the female body, with its ability to give birth, as the origin of weak reason, Grymeston writes it as a way of knowing and understanding the abstract concept of redemption.[28] Even in disparaging the body as loathsome, the metaphor is affective and embodying, creating a bond of sympathy between the meditator and mothers.

Grymeston also relates motherhood to faith in a description of Christ. Chapter XI, "Morning Meditation, with sixteene sobs of a sorrowfull spirit," interpolates prose passages based on Psalms 6 and 103 with poetry from Southwell's "St. Peter's Complaint," from which she quotes:

> Christ health of fever'd soule, heaven of the mind,
> Force of the feeble, nurse of infant loves,
> Guide to the wandring foot, light to the blind,
> Whom weeping winnes, repentant sorow moves,
> Father in care, mother in tender hart,
> Revive and save me slaine with sinfull dart. (E3)[29]

As an instrument of God's mercy, an androgynous Christ tenderly nurtures and nurses the weak like a mother and cares like a father. Figuring Christ as partially maternal runs counter to the general trend of the Reformation which was, according to Patricia Crawford, to make all aspects of the Trinity exclusively masculine.[30] Grymeston's citation recalls an earlier tradition, noted by Caroline Walker Bynum in *Jesus as Mother*. Bynum argues that the medieval Cistercian writers she studies use idealized images of motherhood to emphasize the emotion and humanity of Christ in an affective form of spirituality or to figure their authority as affectionate, nurturing, and accessible.[31] The latter practice continues in the early modern period with the Puritans who, according to David Leverenz, represent the nurturing work of ministers as maternal and figure the good church as the mother – and the church of Rome as the whore.[32] The Jesuit Southwell, similarly, describes the church as a mother, but with a different polemical intent: "He cannot have God for his father that refuseth to profess the Catholic Church for his mother."[33] The figure of Christ as mother, to which Grymeston refers, is more exceptional in the early modern period. Using it allows Grymeston to ascribe worth to her work as a mother, for she can connect her care to that of Christ. When metaphors of gender describe the invisible to make it known – more typically in speaking of God as Father – the comparison offers a way of extending the power relations of the family into the cosmos, and consequently for justifying those relations on earth.[34] Grymeston, however, writes a way of knowing God that relates the ideal to mothering, nurturing, and suffering which, in turn, must assert and renew the importance of these values in society. If God is also the ultimate sign of authority, the comparison gives mothering divine authorization and makes divinity more like women, not an exclusively masculine power over them.

Grymeston's gendering of the spiritual through language also affects how Bernye could be a Christian man. She compares the soul to women, again in a way that requires his imaginative sympathy with them. The soul, she tells Bernye, is like a widow (B3), Noah's innocent female dove (B3v), and a beautiful woman: "Thou hast a silly, poore, yet powerfull soule, a soule of noble substance, of exceeding beautie, inspired by God the Father; redeemed by God the Sonne; sanctified by God the holy Ghost: this is the careful charge committed to thy charge to keepe hir" (B3). The representation of the soul as feminine can be explained, as Joan M. Ferrante argues, partly by the gender of the noun, *anima*, and partly by the traditional qualities ascribed to it.[35] Like the good woman, the soul is gentle and simple and possesses a beauty that must be protected. Grymeston reiterates inherited gender metaphors to make the abstract and invisible known, but she also does not undermine the representation of femininity as a positive value by referring to corresponding anti-feminist traditions; just as fallen angels, Adam, and Judas – rather than the more typical Eve – provide the concrete examples of sinners, no masculine *spiritus*, or higher rational soul, appears to rule the soul. When Grymeston tells her son of his feminine soul, she is implicitly suggesting a fundamental way in which he is like her. Ben Jonson's depiction of his recently-deceased son provides a pointed contrast, for he also makes his son's soul like him. This young soul appears, not as feminine, but in "manlie shape" which, as Ronald Huebert suggests, indicates that for Jonson "the shape of the immortal soul is the perfection of manliness."[36] Bernye Grymeston is not being told to attain a moral good that is masculine or to fashion himself upon the rejection of femininity. Rather, he must learn to care for what has been explicitly declared to be a good and feminine part of himself. The message is a contentious one, for that a son could become like his mother is the possibility education is supposed to preclude.

Grymeston's words, because they are addressed to her son and because they are religious meditations, challenge the relationships among maternity, spirituality, and education. The silent communication of morality through material care was contrasted with and surpassed by the textual instruction of male humanist tutors. In her meditations, however, Grymeston speaks that maternal corporeal influence, writing it into words that make motherhood a literate, as well as physical and emotional, value. The idea of Christ as God-incarnate and as logos rests upon an analogous crux of body and language. In Chapter IX, "That Affliction is the coate of a Christian," Grymeston makes the crucifixion central to education by turning the event, and particularly the body, into a lesson:

> [L]et the Mount Calvarie be our schoole, the crosse our pulpit, the crucifixe our meditation, his wounds our letters, his lashes our commaes, his nailes our full-points, his open side our booke, and *Scire Christum crucifixum*, our whole lesson. (D3)[37]

As the body becomes word, the wounds transfigure into letters and the open side to a book, other texts – the literal letters and books – are abandoned. But the metaphors that transform the body into word do not desert the material for the abstract. The text of Christ's body also remains corporeal in order to supersede all texts that are merely language. This makes reading an experience of the body, at once material and spiritual, literal and figurative, present and beyond. The viscerality of a mother's spiritual instruction finds an analogy in Christ because he, too, instructs through his body. Rather than presenting corporeal maternal virtue as a silent ground upon which the scholarly education of a son will be articulated, which requires an opposition between physical and textual,

Grymeston makes the body of Christ, as the mother's body had been, the whole lesson; the corporeal is still a tutorial, but now the mother is speaking it.

Grymeston's meditations also require the involvement of the reader's own body, especially his senses. Grymeston mentions the commonplace that meditation is "the eye wherewith we see God" (B2), and in chapters two and three, expressed respectively "in the person of Heraclitus, who alwaies wept" and "the person of Dives in the torments of hell" (B2v,B4), dramatic speakers ask for particular emotional and sensual responses. The devil of the third chapter, for example, recounts the effects of hell on his senses as a cautionary example: his eyes are afflicted with the fearful sights of "griesely divels," his ears with the "hideous noise of damned spirits," his nose with the stink of "filth," and his taste with "want" (B4v). According to Louis Martz, this technique of meditation through the senses and "imagining the place" is characteristic of Ignatius Loyola's *Spiritual Exercises*, composed 1521–1541 and widely influential in the late sixteenth century and early seventeenth century. Indeed, Ignatius' work seems to provide the model for Grymeston's. His meditator, too, should see hell in his imagination and then ask for an interior sense of the pain suffered by the damned, to see the fires of hell, hear their cries, smell the sulphur and rot, taste hell's bitterness, and touch the flames.[38] Understanding theological concepts by affective meditation, according to Martz, does not preclude reason, but it also does not emphasize exigetical analysis.[39]

The use of the senses in meditation in this way, as well as attention to the body and suffering, can be related to, but not reduced to, the images and methods that Grymeston's Catholicism makes available to her. Barbara Lewalski and others have argued that these properties distinguish Catholic from Protestant meditation.[40] Diane Willen, differentiating Elizabeth Grymeston from the Protestant writers of mother's advice books, also attributes what she sees as Grymeston's lack of emphasis on literacy and Scriptures to her Catholicism.[41] While it is true that Grymeston does not become an advocate for Bible-reading as Dorothy Leigh does, I do not quite agree that Grymeston is unconcerned with literacy; her extensive citations encorporate both the literate and the literary. Further, Grymeston's focus on the senses, emotions, and the material, which makes her representation of faith, education, and motherhood different from her contemporaries, also allows her to use language for a distinct maternal purpose. The affective potential in religious language, which can create emotional bonds among the speaker, the reader, and the object of meditation, facilitates a relationship between Elizabeth and Bernye. She tells him:

> I leave thee this portable *veni mecum* for thy Counseller, in which thou maiest see
> the true portrature of thy mothers minde, and finde something either to resolve
> thee in thy doubts, or comfort thee in thy distresse; hoping, that being my last

speeches, they will be better kept in the conservance of thy memorie; which I desire thou wilt make a Register of heavenly meditations. (A3v)

The meditations are a "*veni mecum*," a portable motherly presence, and her words perpetuate her love and influence. Bernye responds in kind, writing in his "madrigall" of receiving "deadly wounds" from her meditations, as well as being healed. He tells her: "how oft the strokes of sounding keyes hath slaine, / As oft the looks of your kind eies restores my life againe" (E4v). Bernye's poem affirms the value of his mother's writing through describing the effect she has had upon his senses. The sounds that he has heard, the touches that have wounded him, and the looks that she has imparted, judge and then restore him.

That Grymeston did not write an "original" work, but instead composed through citations, may provide an explanation for the relative dearth of scholarly attention to her book. Interest in "women's experience" has been the impetus for the recovery of early modern women's writing, and while it should never be an unproblematic category, Grymeston explicitly resists writing self-referentially about that experience . Because we have used originality to ascribe value to writing, *Miscelanea Meditations Memoratives* also does not fall into the category of literature that would be included in Norton anthologies. Yet, she has her own anthologizing impulse, similarly affixed to declarations of cultural value and suggesting a strategy by which an early modern woman could write authoritatively to her son. While participating in conventional ideas of motherhood by deferring to other writers, offering religious advice, and justifying her counsel by the efficacy of maternal love, Grymeston does not reiterate negative constructions of femininity. Even as she indicates the privileged position of the writing of the "philosophers," she occupies their authority for herself. Grymeston contravenes the frequent exclusion of women from scholarly culture by citing extensively and in Latin and Greek and by demonstrating her ability to make judgments about what she reads. Bernye, for his part, should be a man who esteems feminine attributes, in Christ and in his own soul. Because Grymeston makes her knowledge indispensable to Bernye's development, her affection imperative to his discipline, and her materiality essential to his understanding of God, Bernye will not mark his development in the rejection of his mother. Grymeston will be a mother who remains present, articulate, and necessary, even in death.

Notes

1. All references are to *Miscelanea Meditations Memoratives* (1604; Norwood, NJ: Walter J. Johnson, 1979). The work was also published in 1605/6, [1608?] and 1618 with several additional chapters. See Ruth Hughey and Philip Hereford, "Elizabeth Grymeston and her *Miscelanea*," *The Library* 15 (1935): 61–91 for

a bibliographical study. The added chapters are more argumentative, taking on such topics as oath-taking, treason, and martyrs. I discuss them further in my PhD dissertation from the University of Western Ontario (forthcoming).

2. Elaine Beilin, *Redeeming Eve: Women Writers of the English Renaissance* (Princeton: Princeton University Press, 1987), 266–71; Wendy Wall, *The Imprint of Gender* (Ithaca: Cornell University Press, 1993), 286–7; Valerie Wayne, "Advice for Women from Mothers and Patriarchs," in *Women and Literature in Britain, 1500–1700*, ed. Helen Wilcox (Cambridge: Cambridge University Press, 1996), 65–6. Betty S. Travitsky also briefly discusses Grymeston in "The New Mother of the English Renaissance: Her Writings on Motherhood," in *The Lost Tradition: Mothers and Daughters in Literature*, ed. Cathy N. Davidson and E.M. Broner (New York: Ungar, 1980), 38–9.

3. Hughey and Hereford offer evidence of Grymeston's Catholic connections. Helen C. White also distinguishes between the more common moralistic, aphoristic meditations and "true" meditation which requires "the sustained immediate application of the mind and the imagination and the feelings to one subject." Grymeston's work has affinities with the latter. *English Devotional Literature [Prose] 1600–1640* (New York: Haskell House, 1966), 160.

4. Margo Todd, "Humanists, Puritans and the Spiritualized Household," *Church History* 49 (1980): 18–34. Todd disputes Christopher Hill's earlier thesis that the spiritualized household was a Puritan phenomenon, arguing that English Anglicans and Catholics followed similar theories of household education. Christopher Hill, *Society and Puritanism in Pre-Revolutionary England* (London: Secker and Warburg, 1964): 443–81.

5. Juan Luis Vives, *Instruction of a Christen Woman*, trans. Richard Hyrde (London, 1541), 112v.

6. Todd, 23.

7. Erasmus, "The New Mother" in *The Colloquies of Erasmus*, trans. Craig R. Thompson (Chicago: University of Chicago Press, 1965), 268–85. For more on the transmission of moral characteristics through milk, see Valerie Fildes, *Breasts, Bottles and Babies: A History of Infant Feeding* (Edinburgh: Ediburgh University Press, 1986), 112.

8. Patricia Crawford, "The Construction and Experience of Maternity" in *Women as Mothers in Pre-Industrial Education*, ed. Valerie Fildes (London: Routledge, 1990), 12. Kenneth Charlton, in "Mothers as Educative Agents in Pre-industrial England," *History of Education* 23 (1994): 129–56, notes only two examples of mothers who instructed their sons in Latin, Lady Mary Coke and Lady Brilliana Harley. See also Diane Willen, "Women and Religion in Early Modern England," in *Women in Reformation and Counter-Reformation Europe: Public and Private Worlds*, ed. Sherrin Marshall (Bloomington: Indiana State University Press, 1989), 149–50; Ralph A. Houlbroke, *The English Family 1450–1700* (London: Longman, 1984), 148.

9. For further discussion of female education, see Rosemary O'Day, *Education and Society 1500–1800: The Social Foundations of Education in Early Modern Britain* (London: Longman, 1982) and Hilda L. Smith, "Humanist Education and the Renaissance Concept of Woman," in *Women and Literature in Britain 1500–1700*, ed. Helen Wilcox (Cambridge: Cambridge University Press, 1996), 9–29.

10. William Gouge, *Of Domesticall Duties* (1622; Norwood, NJ: Walter J. Johnson, 1976), 546.

11. Roger Ascham, *The Scholemaster*, ed. John E.B. Mayor (New York: AMS Press, 1967), 21–3; Thomas Elyot, *A Critical Edition of Sir Thomas Elyot's "The Boke*

Named the Governour", ed. Donald W. Rude (New York: Garland, 1992), 33; Erasmus, *The Education of a Christian Prince*, trans. Neil M. Cheshire and Michael J. Heath, ed. Lisa Jardine (Cambridge: Cambridge University Press, 1997), 55.

12. Vives, 116, 116v.
13. For a discussion of breeching, see Anthony Fletcher, *Gender, Sex and Subordination in England 1500–1800* (New Haven: Yale University Press, 1995), 297, 340.
14. Patricia Parker, "Gender Ideology, Gender Change: The Case of Marie Germain," *Critical Inquiry* 19 (1993): 337–64.
15. Erasmus, *Christian Prince*, 61.
16. Though we do not know how old Bernye was in 1604 when the work was first published, Grymeston's advice about marriage and the published response by Bernye, "A Madrigall made by Berny Grymeston upon the conceit of his mothers play to the former ditties," suggest that he is an adolescent rather than a child. Although there is no indication that he was the eldest child, if he were he probably would not have been more than twenty because in 1604 Elizabeth Grymeston would have been married for twenty years.
17. I have been able to identify the following citations, and correlate them between Grymeston's text (1604) and *England's Parnassus* (*EP*): Spenser (B2v:*EP* 282; B4:*EP* 45; C2v:*EP* 167; C3:*EP* 321) Lodge (B3:*EP* 320; C:*EP* 168) Sir John Davies (B3:*EP* 276; Dv: "Nosce Teipsum") Drayton (B3v:*EP* 273; C:*EP* 230; D3v: *EP* 272) Sackville (B4v: *EP* 133) Harington, trans. (Cv:*EP* 121); Daniel (Cv; C2v:*EP* 50) Henry Howard, Earl of Surrey (C2v:*EP* 50) Sylvester (D:*EP* 206). She also quotes from Sylvester's translation of Du Bartas *La Semaine* (A4v), Richard [Rowlands] Versteegan's *Odes in Imitation of the Seven Penitential Psalmes* (1601), Robert Southwell's "St. Peter's Complaint," and works by Gregory, Jerome, Augustine, Seneca, and Terence. See Hughey and Hereford for a further discussion.
18. For descriptions of women's religious reading see Vives, 12–12v; Richard Mulcaster, *Positions* (1581; London: Longmans, 1888), 176, 177; Richard Braithwait, *The English Gentlewoman* (1631; Norwood, NJ: Walter J. Johnson, 1970), G. Debora K. Shuger, *The Renaissance Bible: Scholarship, Sacrifice, and Subjectivity* (Berkeley: University of California Press, 1994), 4.
19. Vives ,12v.
20. Hughey and Hereford, 84, identify *Englands Parnassus* as Grymeston's source.
21. Beilin, 269, 270; Hughey and Hereford, 85–9.
22. Wall, 286, 287.
23. "Where are the Mothers in Shakespeare? Options for Gender Representation in the English Renaissance," *Shakespeare Quarterly* 42 (1991): 301.
24. Plato, *Phaedrus*, trans. Walter Hamilton (London: Penguin, 1973), 256.
25. On connections between masculinity and self-discipline, see Lyndal Roper, *Oedipus and the Devil: Witchcraft, Sexuality and Religion in Early Modern Europe* (New York: Routledge, 1994) and Coppélia Kahn, *Man's Estate: Masculine Identity in Shakespeare* (Berkeley: University of California Press, 1981).
26. Lynda E. Boose, "Scolding Brides and Bridling Scolds: Taming the Woman's Unruly Member," *Shakespeare Quarterly* 42 (1991): 179–213.
27. Houlbrooke, 140; Fletcher, 340 makes a similar point. In *Forgotten Children: Parent–Child Relations from 1500–1900* (Cambridge: Cambridge University Press, 1983), 1–67, Linda A. Pollock offers a useful outline of the argument made by Lawrence Stone, Phillipe Ariès and others that families lacked affection and

that parents and schools treated children harshly. Pollock rigorously disputes these ideas but does not distinguish between fathers and mothers as parents.

28. For discussions of the relationship between the female body and the mind, see Thomas Laqueur, *Making Sex: Body and Gender from the Greeks to Freud* (Cambridge, Mass: Harvard University Press, 1990) and Ian Maclean, *The Renaissance Notion of Woman* (Cambridge: Cambridge University Press, 1980).

29. From Robert Southwell, "St. Peter's Complaint," *The Poems of Robert Southwell, S.J.*, James H. McDonald and Nancy Pollard Brown (Oxford: Clarendon Press, 1967), lines 751–7.

30. Patricia Crawford, *Women and Religion in England 1500–1720* (London: Routledge, 1993), 10–17.

31. Caroline Walker Bynum, *Jesus as Mother: Studies in the Spirituality of the High Middle Ages* (Los Angeles: University of California Press, 1982), 110–69.

32. David Leverenz, *The Language of Puritan Feeling: An Exploration in Literature, Psychology, and Social History* (New Brunswick: Rutgers University Press, 1980), 138–48.

33. Robert Southwell, "Epistle unto his Father," *Two Letters and Short Rules of a Good Life*, ed. Nancy Pollard Brown (Charlottesville: University Press of Virginia, 1973), 18.

34. This conclusion is influenced by Gordon Teskey's discussion of allegory in "Allegory, Materialism, Violence," in *The Production of English Renaissance Culture*, ed. David Lee Miller, Sharon O'Dair, and Harold Weber (Ithaca: Cornell University Press, 1994),293–318.

35. Joan M. Ferrante, *Woman as Image in Medieval Literature From the Twelfth Century to Dante* (New York: Columbia University Press, 1975), 37.

36. Ronald Huebert, "A Shrew Yet Honest: Manliness in Jonson," *Renaissance Drama* 15 (1984):31.

37. The comparison between Christ and the book can also be found in earlier works such as *Meditation on the Life and Passion of Christ* and *The Charter of Christ*. See Richard Firth Green, *Literature and Law in Ricardian England: A Crisis of Truth* (Philadelphia: University of Pennsylvania Press, 1999), 257–63. Grymeston's use of this image is more precisely paralleled in "The Holy Rood or Christes Crosse," by John Davies, although this poem was not published until 1609. It can be found in Volume 1 of *The Complete Works of John Davies of Hereford* (1878), 20. For a discussion of a similar metaphor in Katherine Parr's *Lamentation of a Sinner*, see Janel Mueller, "Complications of Intertextuality: John Fisher, Katherine Parr, and 'The Book of the Crucifix,'" in *Representing Women in Renaissance England*, ed. Claude J. Summers and Ted-Larry Pebworth (Columbia and London: University of Missouri Press, 1997): 24–41.

38. Ignatius of Loyola. *The Spiritual Exercise of Saint Ignatius of Loyola*, trans W.H. Longridge (London: Mowbray, 1919), 66–9.

39. Louis Martz, *The Poetry of Meditation: A Study in English Religious Literature of the Seventeenth Century* (New Haven: Yale University Press, 1962), 27–32, 71–5.

40. Barbara Lewalski, *Protestant Poetics and the Seventeenth-Century Religious Lyric* (Princeton: Princeton University Press, 1979); Marie B. Rowlands, "Recusant Women 1560–1640," in *Women in English Society 1500–1800*, ed. Mary Prior (London: Methuen, 1985), 163, 164; Crawford, *Women and Religion*, 93.

41. Willen, 155.

PART III

DOMESTIC PRODUCTION

Negativizing Nurture and Demonizing Domesticity: The Witch Construct in Early Modern Germany

Nancy Hayes

The construct of the witch as it appears in the illustrations of late fifteenth and early sixteenth century Upper Rhine and southern German treatise, sermon and satire literature as well as in diverse written sources from sixteenth century German-speaking regions perverts the ideal role of the mother as provider of food and comfort to her children.[1] In the context of this volume on caregivers in the early modern era, the German witch figure constitutes the negative maternal, the depriver of her children's food and comfort, the Other to the Mother. The centrality of the maternal role in feeding her child, in ensuring its physical survival, is countered by the centrality of the alleged witch's role in accomplishing just the opposite. While there are a few depictions of the early modern German witch in the act of stealing milk and some accounts of poisoning and contamination of wine and cheese,[2] the most frequent witch portrayals are of weather-makers, the hags who tossed tempests in order to destroy crops, fruit and livestock. When the images are compared to the patterns of witch persecution registered in legal documents from the late fifteenth and again in the later sixteenth century, they can be seen to reflect remarkably accurately what we presume to have taken place in the social history of the period. Of specific allegations of harmful magic found by Richard Kieckhefer in his study of European witch trials from 1300 to 1500, thirty charges for weather magic were documented, as compared to the twelve for child murder and five for milk theft, the other two most frequently cited accusations of *maleficia*, all of which occurred in the late fifteenth century in the Upper Rhine territories.[3]

Perhaps the earliest printed illustration of a witch prototype, for she is not literally called a witch in the accompanying text, is that found in the guise of a milk thief in Tirolian Hans Vintler's 1486 tract concerning virtuous behavior,

Des nachtes auff die schlauffende leút
Das es in hepmliche ding bedeút
Vnd vil zauberp vndapn
Die sebent an dem schulter papn
Was dem menschen sol beschehen
Vnd etlich die geben
Es sep nit gút das man
Den lincken schúch leg an
Vor de gerechten des morgens frú
Und vil die iehen man stoß der kú
Die milch auß der wammen
So sepnd etlich der ammen

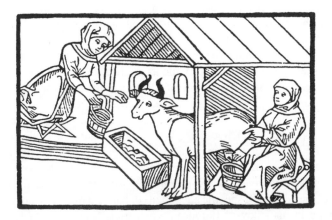

Fig. 10.1   *Milk Magic*, woodcut from Hans Vintler's *Phümen der Tugent*, Augsburg, 1486

Pluemen der Tugent or *Tugendspiegel* (Flowers of Virtue or Mirror for Virtue), published in Augsburg (Fig. 10.1). Illustrating the verse above it which is critical of the many persons (*etliche*) who are superstitious enough to believe such things as the ability of one to "spray" (*stob*) the milk out of the cow's lower belly (*wammen*), the figure of a village woman kneeling on a hexagram hovers near a barn with a bucket of milk in her right hand. Under the roof sits another village woman on a bench evidently trying in vain to milk her cow, as she points to the cow's teat and her empty pail. Similarly clad, both women appear to be going about their domestic tasks nonchalantly enough, and only the position of the one suspended on a traditional hex symbol suggests she is doing something out of the ordinary. Through rhyme but not necessarily syntax, *wammen* is linked to *ammen* (wet nurses) in the following verse, and it is possible that wet nurses may also have been accused of stealing milk from cows when their own supply faltered, although the text is not clear about this. Nevertheless, anxiety about the availability of milk in general, not specifically for infants, and the role of witches (Sigrid Schade provides a caption for this woodcut: *Milchzauber* [milk magic] in her treatment of harmful magic[4]) is registered in the text and image. While Vintler intended to belittle the silly beliefs of the common people, the artist's illustration may have actually planted such notions more visibly in the popular imagination. The same year the Vintler book appeared, Heinrich Kramer and Jakob Sprenger published the notorious witch tract, *Malleus Maleficarum* (The Hammer of Witches), with its anti-feminist bias and multiple citing of examples of witchcraft wrought by village women in the Upper Rhine and southern German areas. Vintler's skeptical, slightly patronizing viewpoint was evidently overshadowed by the violent rhetoric with which the Dominican monks promulgated their conviction of the real harm done by hags and the necessity of persecuting them. According to their own accounts, and affirmed to a degree by Richard Kieckhefer in his account of the trial material, village women were accused and executed on a large scale for deeds including milk theft and more frequently, weather magic.

A generation later, a woodcut illustration for the Strassburg Cathedral preacher Johann Geiler von Kaisersberg's sermon collection, *Die Emeis* (The Ant), alludes to the Vintler image of milk theft (Fig. 10.2), but without skepticism, and adds the *maleficium* of weather-making to the scene. Published in Strassburg in 1517, the book contains sermons against witchcraft that were delivered in the Lenten season of 1508. In this illustration, the artist has borrowed compositional elements from the Vintler version; the kneeling milk-stealing figure is found on the left side of the picture and a wooden pillar supports a roof just right of center. With her knees on the ground instead of on a hexagram and her shoes visible, the milk thief in this image has an earthier dimension. Her facial features are delineated to appear older than those of the women in the earlier woodcut. Across the way under a stable roof similar to the one in the Vintler scene stands the cow, whose milk is supposedly being siphoned away. Contrary to the earlier text, Geiler's does not dispute the actuality of the *maleficium*, but insists, like most of the witch treatises of the time and region, that the witches do not possess the power to execute the alleged deeds, but foolishly believe they do. Demons are responsible for the misfortune, although they are nowhere represented in this depiction.[5]

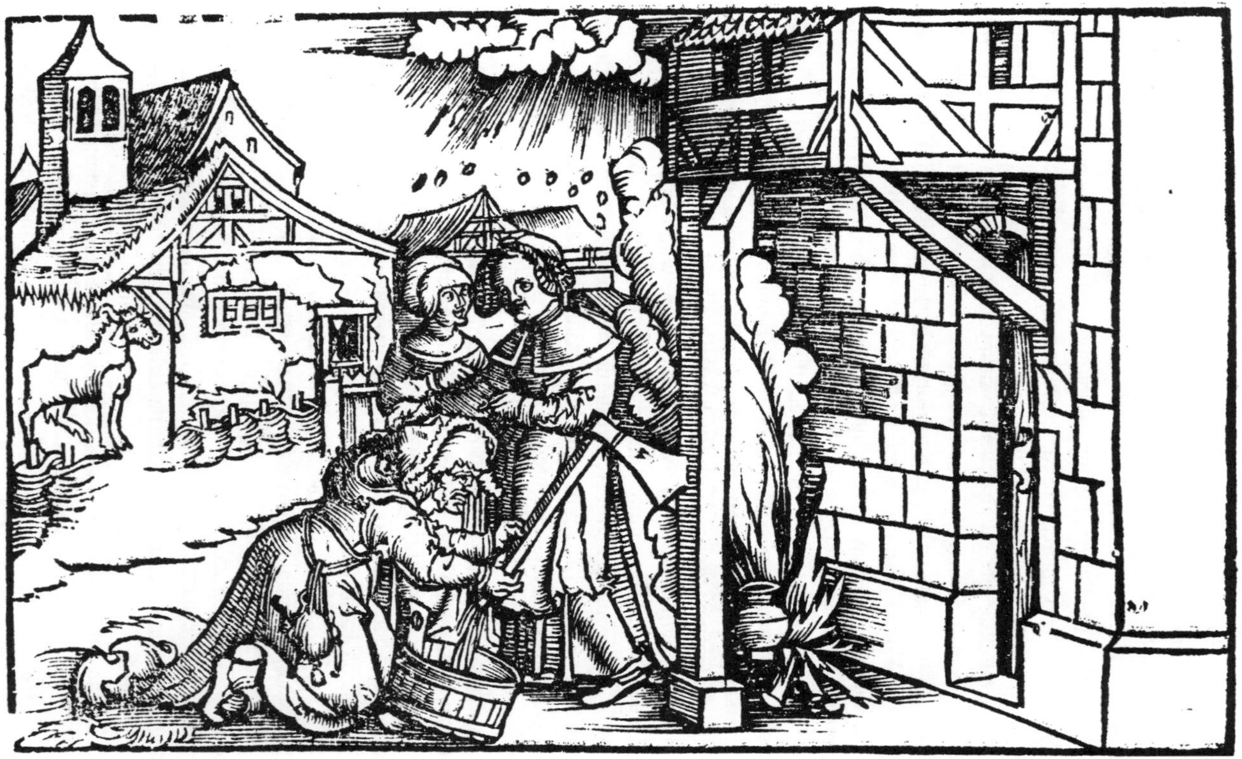

Fig. 10.2   How Witches Get Milk out of an Axe Handle, woodcut from Johann Geiler von Kaiser's *Die Emeis*, Strassburg, 1517

Contributing to the threatening character of the hag in this woodcut is the untended pot to the right under the roof of an overhanging second floor of the house. Ominously close to the wooden pillar, the boiling pot emits billows of smoke that in their upward streaming appear to produce the effects of a hailstorm over the heads of the villagers and rooftops in the village. The vessel serves a literally anti-domestic purpose, cooking up a storm rather than a stew, out on the street rather than on the hearth inside the house, and producing a fire hazard for the house instead of warming it cozily. The connection between these two deeds of harmful magic is that both deprive villagers of food, the one more directly and limited to dairy products and the other more general and widespread involving crops, fruit and livestock in the fields; if the damage were not immediate to the farm animals, the lack of fodder would ruin them eventually. To a rural community completely dependent on successful harvests and healthy livestock for existence, storms were grave threats to survival indeed. Included in Sönke Lorenz and Dieter Bauer's essay collection, *Hexenverfolgung: Beiträge zur Forschung* (Witch Persecution: Contributions to Research), Wolfgang Behringer's article focuses on the link between agrarian crises and witch persecutions.[6] He identifies a recurring pattern of a downward spiral starting with severe weather and dropping through bad harvests, inflation – especially of bread prices, famine to disease and death, and finds that it coincided with the strongest incidences of witch persecutions.

While providing the most documentation for the witch hunts starting in 1560, Behringer, like Kieckhefer, also refers to the bad weather and trials a century earlier. In the years 1481 and 1482 according to a chronicle from the southwest German town of Memmingen, Behringer reports that the area suffered a severe increase in the price of goods.[7] He cites a passage from the *Malleus Maleficarum* about a devastating hailstorm the year of 1481 some thirty miles east of Ravensburg in the diocese of Constance (in the vicinity of Memmingen) which "destroyed all fruit, crops and vineyards in a belt one mile wide, so that the vines hardly bore fruit for three years." Kramer and Sprenger's text further indicates that fifteen days after the storm, two women were taken into custody, and after questioning which included torture, admitted to having carried a little water into the field where each met a devil independently from the other who asked them to dig a little hole and pour the water into it. After each woman stirred the water with her finger, the devil allegedly took the water up into the air, gave the women time to get home and then caused the hailstorm.[8] Three days later both were burned. Kieckhefer also looks to the work of historical climatologists which showed a worsening of the weather with longer, colder winters and wetter, shorter summers beginning in 1300, and continuing through the fifteenth century. In response to a general lack of food and deterioration of physical health across the north European board and the fact that explanation for the natural calamities was sought in supernatural quarters, Kieckhefer is surprised that charges of weather magic do not emerge in the records more frequently than they do.[9] The experiences of destructive storms and crop failures such as the one mentioned above must have convinced Pope Innocent VIII to publish his Bull in 1484 empowering inquisitors to search out and punish men and women who have, among other charges, "slain infants yet in the mother's womb, as also the offspring of cattle, have blasted the produce of the earth, the grapes of the vine, the fruits of the trees, nay men and women, beasts of burthen, herd-beasts, as well as animals of other kinds, vineyards, orchards, meadows, pastureland, corn, wheat, and all other cereals,"[10] the formal charge which gave rise to the publication of the *Malleus*, most likely in 1486. The witches were reportedly engaged not only in destroying human lives, infant and adult, but in attacking the sources of food on which the general population subsisted. The means, weather magic, must have been so obvious that Innocent did not need to name it.

Like milk theft, weather magic was an act that negativized maternal nurture. It operated on a much larger scale that threatened to undermine the domestic entity entirely. The symbolic withdrawal of life-sustaining milk from the household would have raised anxiety levels, even if one had not been personally affected by such a real loss (by whatever means), but the broader loss of the community's complete harvest terrified on a different order. Thus it is no surprise that the most preeminent and most frequent image of the witch to be found in witchcraft treatise illustration depicts the weather witch. An indication that of the many crimes witches were accused of, weather-making was considered most significant, can be found in the early printed visualizations of witches. The very first illustration of witch treatise material, in fact, concerns itself with weather witches. The majority of the title page of the Austrian Archduke Sigismund's attorney Ulrich Molitor's 1489 *De laniis et phitonicis mulieribus* (Concerning witches and soothsayers, being women) is taken up with the image of two older women feeding a flaming cauldron with a snake and a rooster and thereby seeding a severe storm which appears to be emptying its hailstones or huge drops directly onto their own heads (Fig. 10.3). The witches at issue in this tract are solely female, as the inclusion of *mulieribus* in the title infers, and they are not monstrous in appearance but have the features of ordinary village women. The choice itself of *laniis* in the title rather than the more conventional *lamia* for "witch" suggests a certain intensity in Molitor's relatively aggressive conception of the village witch, however, as he has chosen to derive his version of the word for witch idiosyncratically from the Latin verb *laniare*, which means "to tear limb from limb." *Lanius* refers to the masculine term for "butcher" and therefore the addition of "being women" was necessary; the unusual word for "witches" conjured up the image of "female butchers." The word used in other tracts was *lamia*, a term derived

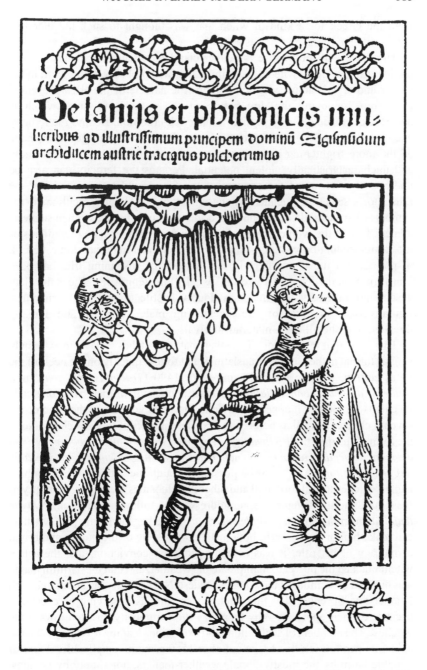

Fig. 10.3 Title page. Woodcut from Ulrich Molitor's De Laniis et phitonicis mulieribus, Cologne, 1489

from the Greek for a kind of witch that was thought to suck the blood of children. *Lanii* threatened adults as well.

The subject of the treatise is neither classical witches nor fantastic ones, but identifiable "real" witches in clothing that was probably being worn in the author and artist's actual vicinity. Perhaps the naiveté of the artist prevented him from conveying the dire nature of the author's mission, which is nevertheless made clear by Molitor's maverick erudition. Behind the ferocity encoded in the spelling must have stood a very basic fear of savage attack, made all the more frightening because of the female gender with its unexpectedly and uncharacteristically violent potential. Perhaps the ferocity can also be understood in terms of the concept of the female witch portrayed, for the illustrator's selection (dictated by the author himself?) of masculine sexual symbols of snake and cock to be tossed into the kettle by the women suggests a latent fear of the women's power over the male gender. The ingredients of the storm-seeding brew suggest that the conventional maternal domestic task of preparing a meal, normally in the interests of sustaining life, has been transformed into a demonic as well as sexually threatening one. The malevolent gesture portrayed by this image is doubly hostile toward vital principles, figuratively destructive of life-engendering male sexuality and literally threatening to the village's material survival.

This particular incarnation of weather-making witches appears in extremely similar format in the German translations that follow quickly on the heels of the Latin edition, starting the following year, 1490 (*Tractatus von den bosen weibern, die man nennet die hexen*, Tract about evil women, who one calls witches). Sometimes it appeared twice in the same volume, at the head of the seventh chapter as well as before the first. The subject of the first chapter took the form of the question, "*Ob mueglich sey auss der uebung der boesen weiben die man nennet die Hexen hagel rueffen und ander ungestömikeit zu verletzung des ertricks zu machen*" (If it be possible through the actions of evil women named witches to call forth hail and other impetuosities leading to the injury of the earth), and the seventh chapter addressed the following question: "*Ob die teufel kuenden hagel oder donder machen*" (whether the devils [not witches] can make hail or thunder). In both instances, in spite of the quirky and brutal etymology of his title, it was actually Molitor's conviction, that the actual witches lacked the power to manipulate the weather, and that the harmful magic was enacted by demons at the witches' behest. Nevertheless, he concurred with Kramer and Sprenger that the witches were just as deserving of execution because of their apostasy. Why then was such animosity directed toward the witches? The numbers of accusations and executions leading up to 1500 and the epidemic persecution that broke out after 1560 remain inexplicable, if fear of tangible harm by the mostly female weather-makers, not simply by demons, were not a factor. If the old women who thought they could harness the winds and call forth the hail were simply fools, as they were purported to be in the satire literature of the early sixteenth century, for example that by the Strassburg humanist clerics, Sebastian Brant and Thomas Murner, and in the sermons of Johannes Geiler von Kaisersberg, evident desire for their violent eradication (on the part of Murner in particular) would not have been so strong. I think personal as well as collective psychological forces are at work and have left their prints on some of the literary and legal, as well as visual, documents of the period.

To illustrate, and I am sure there are many other examples to be discovered, a passage from Thomas Murner's *Narrenbeschwörung* (Exorcism of Fools), printed in Strassburg, 1512, seems overdetermined, weighted down with what may be seen as the man's personal emotional history. The text appears at the beginning of a section entitled "*Ein hagel sieden*" (seeding hail):

> *O Gott / o gott / erhöre myn bit!*
> *Warumb verschluckts das erdtrych nit,*
> *So sy doch dich verleugnet handt*
> *Und zu dem bösen tüfel standt,*
> *Dem sy geben sel und lyb?*
> *O du böses altes wyb,*
> *Verflucht die mutter sy im grundt*
> *Und ouch die selbig ellendt stundt,*
> *Die du uff erdtrych kummen bist!*
> *Kenstu nit des tüfels lisst,*
> *Der all zyt ein lugner ist?*
> *Wie bist du so blindt in disen sachen,*
> *Das du wenst, du kynnest machen*
> *Wetter / hagel / oder schne,*
> *Kinder lemen / darzu me,*
> *Off gesalbten stecken faren!*
> *Wir wolens dir nit lenger sparen!*
> *Nun ins feuer und angezindt!*
> *Und ob man schon kein henker findt,*
> *EE das ich dich wolt lassen gan,*
> *Ich wolts ee selber zinden an.*

> O God / O God / hear my request!
> Why does the earth not swallow them up,
> As they have disowned you
> And have gone to stand with the evil devil,
> To whom they have given their soul and body?
> O you evil old woman,
> May your mother be cursed in the ground
> And also the same miserable hour
> That you arrived on this earth!
> Don't you realize the devil's cunning,
> The devil who is ever a liar?
> How blind you are in these things,
> That you think you can make

Weather / hail / or snow,
Lame children / and more than that,
Ride on anointed staves!
We would no longer spare you!
Now into the fire and let it be lit!
And if no one is able to find an executioner,
Before I would let you go,
I would (before that) light it myself!

Murner's verse moves from prayer to accusation, his rhetoric from supplication to denunciation. He seems to take on the task himself that he originally asks God to perform, that of punishing the old female witch. Although the prayer for vindication appears to be personal at first (*erhöre myn bit!* Hear *my* request!), he speaks for many when he declaims: *Wir wolens dir nit lenger sparen! We would no longer spare you!* Augmented by the plural form, his request gathers steam and exudes authority.

At the end of the passage, however, Murner has returned to the first person singular, and practically screams out a personal vendetta. Murner himself was lame. His mother had explained to him when he was a child that the lameness was due to the work of an old witch. Given such background, one reads the detail of the accusation "*du wenst, du kynnest ... Kinder lehmen*" as a personal, and as such, emotively charged utterance. The examples of misfortunes the witch "thinks" she can wreak are stacked up like faggots at a stake, beginning with the most popularly believed and feared, weather-making, and building up to the most fantastic, the riding on "anointed" staves. Thus the pyre has been prepared, and needs only to be lit. The spark needed to kindle it leaps out of Murner's own deep resentment. The repetition of the little word "ee" ("before") raises the emotional ante, adding to the aural excitement rather than semantic significance. His mother had evidently been unable to save her son from the evil old woman's harmful magic, and perhaps the son had stored up a kind of archaic hatred for such a bad mother, possibly in order to exculpate his own "good" one. The elaborate cursing of the witch's mother, as well as of the witch herself, at the outset of the passage underscores the notion that an anti-maternal subtext informs Murner's mission to burn the evil old woman.

In the 1518 edition of Murner's *Narrenbeschwörung*, the woodcut of a single weather witch appearing at the head of the section quoted from above captures in visual terms the emotional intensity of the passage (Fig. 10.4). The woman moves toward the kettle at a precipitous angle, and only her grip on the spoon seems to keep her from tumbling into her own brew. Angles define the composition as they point toward the pot, angles of the ties from her headgear and her shawl, angles of lightning bolts charging from the upper right corner, the angles of her arms and the long handle of the spoon. The lines of drapery at her feet aim diagonally upward toward the boiling vessel, impelling the figure's movement in that direction. The resulting effect is one of the brew's potency, as

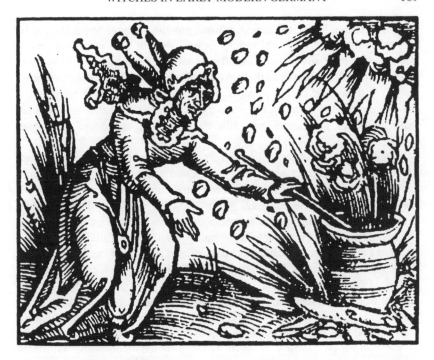

Fig. 10.4 *Weather witch*. Woodcut from Thomas Hurner's *Narrenbeschwörung*, Strassburg, 1518

it appears to emit a force capable of sending her loose head and shoulder cloths flying straight out in the opposite direction, especially because there is no fire under the kettle, which would explain the bubbling naturally. Even though the bells at the end of the bonnet ties should indicate her foolish status, the gale that she has seemingly single-handedly generated (no demons are pictured) appears to be a mighty one. The gigantic size of the hailstones gives credence to the impression that this woman is a powerful weather-maker, a supernatural cook. What kind of satire has Murner in mind here? A bitter and serious one, one that smacks of vindictiveness and speaks of fear.

The visual liveliness of this scene – the lines of steam streaming out of the pot and the huge puffs of smoke that are as large as the storm clouds above crash into and cut across the jagged lines of lightning streaking down – suggests that the artist was impelled by strong emotion and enables us to see the woodcut as an expressionistic work. I imagine the artist read Murner's text carefully, and allowed its emotional dynamism to infuse the illustration of it. The visual violence of the scene bespeaks fear as well as ridicule, just as Murner's shifting between public and private rhetoric and the incendiary impetus of the passage's style and content betray the author's strong emotional engagement even as he tries to outdo Brant's original satire, *Narrenschiff*. In both word and image, intensely negative affect swirls like flames around the subject of the weather witch, who is being bound to the stake by Murner's verse and is left awaiting the torch at the end of the passage. The knowledge that there were actual enactments of this scene in the memory of both writer, artist and original readers imbues the documents with cultural significance and emotional presence.

When weather conditions worsened dramatically around 1562, the construct of the powerful older female weather witch was apparently firmly in place in the popular imagination, as well as in the minds of the more literate levels of society. Historical meteorological research indicates an actual drop of two degrees in general temperatures for northern western Europe beginning in 1560 and lasting through the seventeenth century. Called the "Little Ice Age" by Hartmut Lehman, the drop in temperature caused a series of long, cold winters and short, wet summers like that reported by Kieckhefer for the preceding century. Perhaps the temporal and geographical epicenter for the ensuing temblor of witch persecutions can be situated at the occurrence of a devastating hailstorm on August 3, 1562 in a large region of Swabia including the towns of Stuttgart and Esslingen and extending south and east into the hilly countryside. In his collection of early modern German witch documents, Wolfgang Behringer includes an eyewitness account of the storm found in a personal letter (author unknown):

> *Auff den dritten tag Augusti zwischen 11. vnd 12. vhr zu mittag / Ist ein solch grausame erschrecklich wetter / verfinstert als wann es nacht wer gewest … weren wir zu theil verdorben unn zu grund gangen / Ist also boess genugt / Gleich darauff ein solches grausambs haglen / mit vilen stralen augenblicklich / das menigklich darob erschrocken / und nit gewust was man thun oder lasen solt / vnd sich der Hagel dermasen erzeigt / vnd gewerd biss auff zwelff uhr / ist es alles viruber / vnd der schad geschehen ….*

> On the third day of August between 11 and 12 o'clock noon was such a horrible, frightening weather / [it] darkened as if it were night … [as if] we were to be spoiled and perish / it was bad enough / right after that [there was] such a horrible hail with many bolts [of lightning] at that moment that many were frightened and didn't know what one should do or not do and the hail showed itself and persisted to such a great extent until 12 o'clock / it was all over and the damage was done ….[11]

The letter writer went on to claim that such destruction had not occurred in the Neckar and Rems Valleys in a hundred years, and that many thought Judgment Day had come. As a result the feudal lord even moved away because he could no longer bear the peasants' complaints. The farmers would not be able to pay their debts or have resources enough to plant the next year's crop. The author does not blame witches for the catastrophe, however, but considers it divine punishment of a sinful people. According to the passage, the author and the people – he uses "we" – responded to the sudden intense darkening of the noonday sky with apocalyptic fear, and many responded to the terrific hail and lightning with panic, as the overwrought but idiomatic phrase "*nit gewust was man thun oder lasen solt*" reveals – they didn't know what to do or what to leave off doing.

In the town of Esslingen and the village of Wiesensteig thirty miles to the southeast, citizens did decide what to do and what not to do. The much larger community of Esslingen with its town council and sophisticated judicial body in place, did not act as impetuously or decisively, even though the anti-witch rhetoric of the popular preacher, Thomas Kirchmair, might have riled up the populace to do so. Three women were accused immediately of raising the hailstorm, but none confessed and no witnesses were found, and all were released by December 16 of that year. According to Gisela Vöhringer-Rubröder, however, the social pressure which had not been able to find release may have played a part in the swift trial of January 1563, which resulted in the burning of the so-called Wagenbarbel, although she was not accused of weather-making.[12] In the small village of Wiesensteig in the remoter hill country, Count Ulrich of Helfenstein, the lord of Wiesensteig, had already executed six suspected female weather witches by about August 18 (only about two weeks after the storm), and by the end of the year, sixty-three more had been sent to the stake. In the year following the executions, an anti-witch pamphlet entitled *Hexenzeitung* was published in Wiesensteig, which charged the witches with the general aim of nothing less than the extermination of the human race:

> *Zum andern haben sy nit allain sich gottes verzigen / sondern ihn des Sathans alls des Erbfeinds / Christenliches Names gehorsam und dienstbarkayt ergeben und verpflicht sich ihn allem das zu aussreyttung und verderbung Menschliches Geschlechts geraichen moechte.*

> On the other hand they [the witches] have not only renounced God, but have given their obedience and service to Satan, the arch-enemy of the name of Christ, And have pledged him everything that might benefit the extermination and destruction of the human race.[13]

In the vein of Molitor's title, *laniis … mulieribus*, the pamphlet also accuses the witches of the crime of butchery, of cutting babies out of their mothers' wombs to secure unbaptized infants for their unholy purposes including boiling them into a mush or burning them into a powder:

> *Vnnunder obermelten Kündern haben sy vil / sonderlich aber die ungetaufften widerum aussgraben die vnmenschlicher Jemmerlicher weyss / zu ainem Muess versotten / und zum tayl auch zu ainem Buluer verbrent / Darauss sy ain vergiffte schedliche zauerey Salb gemacht vunv volgende Teuflische / vngepürliche Stuck darein gepraucht haben.*

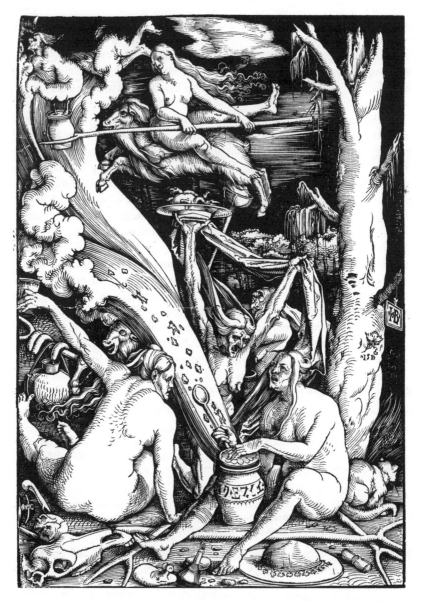

Fig. 10.5   *Preparation for the Sabbath*. Single sheet woodcut by Hans Baldung, 1510

> Of the aforementioned children, they boiled many to a mush, but especially the unbaptized who had been dug out of their graves in an inhuman and pitiful way and in part they were burned to a powder. Out of this they made a poisonous noxious magical salve and used it for the following devilish, improper things.

In the popular imagination, the witches held responsible for the terrific storm had been stirring up more than water in a hole in the ground. They had been hard at some heavy-duty culinary tasks, cooking up concoctions of different textures in order to produce an ointment capable of doing vast harm. While there are other instances recorded of women receiving powders, etc. from the devil, in this pamphlet the women are clearly the cooks behind the broth.

The writer looks back on the devastating storm which "*dem Menschen sein Nahrung, zuentzihen gemacht / Haegel / Regn / Wind / Reiffen / und Newel*" (took away nourishment from the people [by means of] hail, rain, wind, frost and fog). Again, a maternal subtext is worth noting here. Not without reason were the inhabitants fearful for their survival. The crops, fruits and livestock which were destroyed were the villagers' sole means of sustenance; the loss of income would prohibit the purchase of food stuff. For a society completely dependent on local agriculture, such a major disruption of Mother Earth's beneficence did leave *her* children in a state of abjection. The connection between terrible weather and negative maternal constructs – the older female witches who were characterized as perverted cooks and nurses bent on destroying babies to use as ingredients in concoctions that could ruin all of Nature – apparently provided an explanation for such a cataclysm. While clerics might blame the *Volk* themselves for what they considered God's just punishment, the *Volk* blamed the catastrophe on those they considered the bad mothers of their community.

The most famous visual image of the bad mothers was created by the well-known apprentice of Albrecht Dürer, the Swabian-born Strassburg artist Hans Baldung, at the beginning of the century. His single sheet woodcut, "Preparation for the Sabbath," was printed in 1510 for a limited circle of friends, and therefore falls into a very different category from tract illustration (Fig. 10.5). For our purposes in this essay, it is significant for its portrayal of the witch as an assiduous cook, although the lack of any form of apron distinguishes these figures from the weather-making witches that were very popular at the same time. Baldung evidently viewed the work as an aesthetic exercise, both in the sense of practicing the female nude in various positions and ages and in the sense of sharing a smirk as well as a voyeuristic titillation with his educated acquaintances at the expense of the poor village women who were being burned at stakes in his vicinity as he carved. The title is apt, as the accouterments of the kitchen have been carted outside the *domus* to prepare for a kind of feast not intended to satisfy the tongue or fortify the body. Cutlery, pots, plates and oven forks aid the "witches" in their tasks of producing magical substances to enable them to fly to the Sabbath. As we saw in the other illustrations, no fire is necessary to get the vessels to steam and rather than following familiar recipes, the women chant strange incantations. The phallic sausages draped on an ovenfork at the left, the toads in the smoke, and the reptilian pieces on the plate held high by the hag in the center represent a perverse domesticity, food preparation out of body parts that does not transform them into appetizing or remotely edible substances. Ovenforks are endowed with magical powers, set in threes on the ground under the qualming jar and its seated attendant, and are used to carry the flight-inducing vessel on the way to the Sabbath. The purpose of cooking in this night kitchen is the production of harmful magical means to accomplish the damage to crops, fruit, livestock, humans and their shelters, etc., in short, civilization, charged by Innocent VIII and the author of the *Malleus*.

Most of Baldung's witches from 1510 until 1523 are voluptuous, and expressive of the *Malleus* authors' fixation with the lascivious construct of the female witch as she is reported to agitate so vigorously against the male sexual member. Yet in the center of this woodcut, Baldung has imbedded a frightening hag figure who poses a threat of a different sort. In her gesture of lifting a plate of reptiles, seemingly still alive, ceremoniously with a cloth held up between her outstretched arms to form a kind of mysterious triangle complementing that of the ovenforks below her, the hag is quintessentially anti-domestic and anti-maternal. As the formal focus of the composition, and as a leader, a veteran hostess figure sharing her expertise, the hag concentrates the company's effort into a presentation of food calculated by the artist to sicken the viewer, while providing a fulcrum for the other witches' machinations. Her shriveled dug and elongated teat represent the opposite of maternal fullness and generosity; instead of a source of life, her breast signifies barrenness and death. She runs an alternative household whose goal is the ruin of the family and community. While the other witches in Baldung's scene may have entertained their original viewers, the central hag more likely coalesced their fears of hostile maternal power.[14]

Fears of the "antimother," as Diane Purkiss calls the witch in her chapter, "The house, the body, the child,"[15] erupted into violence frequently during the second half of the sixteenth century, beginning with the epidemic reaction to the alleged weather makers of Wiesensteig in 1562. As a final "illustration" of the appearance of the witch figure as a negative maternal and negative domestic construct, I turn to the Bavarian records examined by legal historian Michael Kunze concerning a notorious case from 1600, known as the Pappenheimer trial. Twelve people including members of a vagrant family, the Pappen-heimers, their associates and a miller's family were accused of causing an immense amount of harm by means of witchcraft, and all but the miller who died in prison before, were burned. The most sensational accusations against them involved infanticides (the collective crimes of the Pappenheimers and associates for the first round of executions included four hundred and one infant murders!), but the miller's wife's execution in the second round hinged on her confession of weather-making, a belated confession made under considerable torture:

> If she desired to concoct a weather spell, the Devil would give her certain ingredients or substances, but she did not know exactly what; then she would take ointments, and powder from infants, item toad's eyes she had gouged out, and adders' tails she had chopped off; she would put it all together in a pot, add water, set it on a fire made of hazelwood, let it boil a quarter or half an hour, stirring it with a child's hand or rod of hazelwood until it thickened into a paste ... And then, when she wanted to brew up a storm, she took about half a salt-cellar full of the substance, put it into an earthenware pot, and carried it out into a field, placing it on a stone, or something, and saying: Look, Devil, make a tempest from this. At once the substance began to bubble, seethe, and hiss, rising up into the air in a cloud, causing thunder and lightning ....[16]

In the Wiesensteig pamphlet, weather magic and infanticide were two separate deeds of harmful magic. Here, infanticide occurs in the service of weather magic, making the crime more frightening, and providing a clue to explain the intensity of the fear and anger that led to the kind of persecution which took place in Wiesensteig. A weather-maker has power over growing things – grains, fruits, and livestock – as a mother has power over her infant, who is absolutely dependent on her beneficence. The concocting of damaging weather by stirring a pot containing powders of infant bones with a child's hand for a spoon speaks of a power too horrifying to discount as foolish superstition. The fearful "children" of the age and culture must have felt such a fear as can only be described as the horror of finding oneself at the mercy of a hostile and omnipotent mother, a mother who not only *could* hurt one, but *would* and allegedly *did*!

Incriminating the miller's wife specifically, the only pieces of hard evidence gathered for the entire trial were put forth: a little pot of some sort of paste and some hazel twigs which were discovered in a supposedly secret hearth behind a staircase in the miller's house when the authorities searched the premises. The miller's wife explained that she had had her husband build a second hearth below the stairs for warming milk out of the reach of the cats, who kept on knocking over pots on the main hearth, and had him make a closet around it to keep them out. Such was the lore, Kunze explains, that the witches had to prepare separate hearths to brew their ointments, because predominantly good spirits ordinarily inhabited the hearth, and that hazelwood was used for all kinds of magic.[17] A daunting example of demonized domesticity, the kitchen discovered beneath the stairs was believed to be an evil embodiment of the good hearth, and concomitantly the mother or housewife using it was believed to be the evil cook, i.e., the witch. While the miller's wife maintained that she had only concerned herself with the innocent and positively maternal task of preparing milk, the authorities were convinced that the paste proved otherwise. Torture eventually forced her to corroborate their suspicions.

The other maternal figure among the accused, Anna Pappenheimer, who was put on trial with her husband and three sons, was also condemned as a perverted and perverting mother and housewife. Her accusation was read in Marienplatz in front of the Town Hall in Munich on the morning of July 19, 1600:

> Anna Gämperl [Pappenheimer was the family nickname], being sixty years of age, has assailed over one hundred infants and nineteen old people with her spells, crippling and killing them in godless fashion; she has entered cellars on eight occasions, has committed one murder by her own hand, set fire twice to the homes of others, has caused four gales and hailstorms, and has poisoned meadows and afflicted cattle so often that she herself cannot tell the number."[18]

Each accusation inverts the traditional positive role of the early modern German *Hausmutter*: crippling and killing helpless and dependent young and old rather than nourishing and protecting them, and in the case of small children, helping their legs to grow straight by swaddling them; stealing wine and stores from cellars rather than filling them up with provisions for the family; burning down houses rather than keeping them secure; poisoning crops and livestock instead of raising them to healthy use. The ever-present charge of weather-making ratchets up the offense from a domestic to a cosmic level. Recognizing the kind of demonic caregiving Anna was accused of, it is perhaps not such a total shock to hear what specific torment she was sentenced to in front of the town hall in Marienplatz that July morning. In the words of Christopher Neuchinger, Executive Justice to the Duke of Bavaria,

> ... the aforementioned six culprits' lives are forfeit, they have incurred sentence of death by torment, namely that all six be placed publicly upon two carts, drawn in procession before their deaths to the place of execution, the body of each to be torn six times with red-hot pincers, the mother to have her breasts cut off, the condemned males to have their limbs broken on the wheel, and Paulus Gämperle thereafter to be impaled upon a stake, all six persons then to be put to death by fire.[19]

Anna is not called a witch, but rather a "mother." Accounts of the actual torture before execution survive in pamphlet, chronicle and diary form and include a gruesome detail which was apparently not part of the official sentence. After Anna's breasts were sliced off, they were rubbed around her mouth and those of her two sons (a third, younger son was forced to watch – he was executed less than four months later along with the miller's wife, her daughter and two other men).[20] Betokening the negativizing maternal capacity with which she had evidently suckled demonic children, her severed breasts served some model of popular justice, one motivated perhaps by a collective psychological dread of witches constructed as evil mothers. Kunze attempts some explanation of the torment chosen for the male witches, but leaves the matter of Anna's gender and role specific punishment uninterpreted.

Lyndal Roper's study of trial material from mid-seventeenth century Augsburg confirms the understanding I have garnered of the fear-provoking negative maternal aspects of the witch figure in early modern German regions. Her findings emerged against an expectation of a lascivious witch type such as Kramer and Sprenger promulgated and Baldung cultivated.[21] She had anticipated "a culmination of the sexual antagonism which [she] had discerned in sixteenth and seventeenth century culture. The idea of flight astride a broomstick or pitchfork, the notions of a pact with the Devil sealed by intercourse," but instead she discovered that the "stuff of the accusations" was based on pre-Oedipal rather than Oedipal content, "turning on the relationship to the breast and to the mother in the period before the infant has a sense of sexual identity."[22] The Augsburg witchcraft cases involved women accused by women for crimes concerning delivery, nursing and feeding the new mother, her newborn and other children. The lying-in maids, usually post-menopausal poor women, bore the brunt of the suspicion in cases where the new mother and child fared ill, and several were executed as witches. The old women were accused of reversing the nurturing process, of literally drying out the infants, and of poisoning the mothers instead of preparing a hearty soup for them.

Charges of weather-making, poisoning, milk and cellar theft, and infanticide most commonly constructed the early modern German witch, identifying her as a terrifyingly powerful and aggressive depriver of nutrition and more fundamentally, of life itself. She is cast in the role of a demonic mother who challenges God's natural beneficence. From the cultural documents examined in this essay, it is evident that the witches' anti-maternal nature threatened early modern German communities with the most archaic fear imaginable.[23] In an attempt to articulate such a primary fear which is beyond discursive expression by definition, I turn to the image of horror which Lady Macbeth's fictive "sucking child" might have experienced at her breast, had he been able to decipher her words: "I would, while it was smiling in my face, / Have plucked my nipple from his boneless gums, / And dashed the brains out" (*Macbeth* I, vii, 56–8). The common villager or townsperson in early modern Germany was terrified of an older hostile female who supposedly had not only the power to dash out his or her brains, as well as those of their children and neighbors, and therefore those of future generations, but the *will* to do it! In the form of witch persecutions against predominantly older women, individuals took violent collective measures against the objects which most effectively embodied that demonic maternal threat.

Notes

1. Notions of an ideal maternal construct intent upon promoting the health of her baby in the womb and after birth, and throughout early childhood can be garnered from concerns about maternal and infant health addressed in handbooks such as Eucharius Rösslein's *Rosengarten* (1513), the first printed manual for midwives. In *When Fathers Ruled: Family Life in Reformation Europe*, Harvard, 1983, Steven Ozment discusses advice given to midwives for expectant mothers, and more importantly for our subject here, advice for new mothers concerning feeding and general care such as bathing and swaddling. Rösslein's implicit construction of ideal maternal conduct includes the mother's nursing of her own child, for her own milk is most suited to the baby, being "consistent with the nourishment it had received in the womb" (119). Choice of wet nurse, if necessary, would depend on what would most benefit the physical and spiritual growth of the child (120). Remedies are provided for thirty-five common infant distresses, many associated with the alimentary tract but also that of sleeplessness. Clearly, parents and particularly maternal caregivers who were more intimately involved in the lives of the youngest children, were profoundly interested in contributing to their off- springs' health. According to Patricia Crawford in her article, "'The sucking child': Adult attitudes to child care in the first year of life in seventeenth century England" (*Continuity and Change* I, 1986), "the mainstream of advice to mothers was to satisfy their babies" (31), and not withhold the breast. Swaddling clothes needed to be changed regularly to ensure relative cleanliness and dryness, and aiding the infant in falling to sleep with lullabies as well as placing it in a warm, safe sleeping place were subjects of general discussion (38). It was the mission of motherhood to provide her infant with food and rest, to secure her baby's general physical comfort in the interest of preserving its life.

2. Charles Zika mentions both instances in his essay "The Devil's Hoodwink: Seeing and Believing in the World of Sixteenth-Century Witchcraft" in *No gods except me: Orthodoxy and Religious Practice in Europe 1200–1600* (Melbourne, 1991) about the 1583 witchcraft treatise of Swabian Paulus Frisius. In his concern to address the harm being done by witches, Frisius refers to "recent cases of those tried in Geneva for poisoning, and the attempts made by them to poison preachers, in particular Calvin" (161–2). A preacher himself, Frisius also treats the claims of witches that they have defecated in wine casks and cheese containers (164). Throughout his article, Zika's emphasis is on the relationship between the preach- ers and acts of witchcraft, on the "theologisation" of popular culture as evidenced by demonological writings, rather than on the relationship between the afflicted populace and the witches which I have attempted to study by analysing visual and verbal evidence left by artists and writers.

3. Richard Kieckhefer. *European Witch Trials: Their Foundations in Popular and Learned Culture, 1300–1500*. Berkeley, 1976.

4. Sigrid Schade. *Schadenzauber und die Magie des Körpers: Hexenbilder der frühen Neuzeit*. Worms, 1983.

5. Zika focuses on the same issue in his discussion of Paulus Frisius' argument that the witches' claims of destructive power are evidence of their folly: "Their conviction that they do is simply a result of confusion and blinding ('Verblendung') on the part of the devil." Otherwise, argues Frisius, he too would be also able to use these instruments and techniques: "putting a hatchet into a post in order to milk it, mixing water and verbenum together to produce hail-storms,

beating the dew with a willow rod in the morning to produce frost, blowing under someone's eyes to produce blindness, breaking a backbone by stroking it with one's hand, sticking a knife through a waxen image to commit murder, measuring an enemy with a wax wick and then lighting it in order to destroy him" ("Hoodwink" 162).

6. Wolfgang Behringer. "Sozialgeschichte und Hexenverfolgung. Überlegungen auf der Grundlage einer quantifizierenden Regionalstudie." *Hexenverfolgungen: Beiträge zur Forschung.* Würzburg, 1995.

7. Behringer, 337.

8. Heinrich Kramer and James Sprenger. *Malleus Maleficarum.* Translated by Montague Summers. London, 1996 (originally published 1928). 148–9.

9. Kieckhefer, 61.

10. Kramer, xix.

11. Wolfgang Behringer. *Hexen und Hexenprozesse in Deutschland.* München, 1988. 136–7.

12. Gisela Völker-Rubröder. "Reichstadt Esslingen." *Hexen und Hexenverfolgung im deutschen Südwesten.* Austellungskatalog. Karlsruhe, 1994.

13. Erik Midelfort devotes a section of *Witch Hunting in Southwestern Germany 1562–1684* (Stanford, 1972) to the Wiesensteig trials, which constituted the first massive witch hunt in the German Southwest. 88–9.

14. The year before he died, after a hiatus of twenty years, Baldung produced one last image of a witch. The extremely popular single sheet woodcut (the block is very worn), *Bewitched Stable Groom*, 1544, contains a witch of the hag type discussed above, whose single hanging dug recalls the earlier image and suggests the artist's lingering preoccupation with the figure. Such an image evidently had power over Baldung, as it appears in this, one of his final works, to threaten the unconscious, prone figure of a man who has been thought by many scholars to represent the artist himself. She is depicted in the act of bringing a flaming torch into a straw-strewn stable, a threat to the "household" in its extended sense, if there ever were one.

15. Diane Purkiss. *The Witch in History: Early and Twentieth Century Representations.* Routledge, 1996. This chapter on witchcraft as "a threat to the domestic sphere" draws mostly from English accounts and serves as a rich complement to my study.

16. Michael Kunze. *Highroad to the Stake: A Tale of Witchcraft.* Chicago, 1987. 254. Kunze's dissertation, *Der Pappenheimer Prozess*, 1981, gave rise to this book.

17. Kunze, 245–6.

18. Kunze, 399.

19. Kunze, 404.

20. Kunze, 404–14.

21. In another essay about Paulus Frisius by Charles Zika in which he reworks much of the earlier material of "The Devil's Hoodwink" around the focus of the appropriation of folklore, the author discusses the titlepage woodcut depicting three witches gathered around a steaming cauldron which harks back to Baldung's 1510 "Preparation for the Sabbath" and more directly to a woodcut illustration in Geiler's *Die Emeis* of 1516. His emphasis, following that of Frisius' own, is on the lascivious nature of the witches rather than on their anti-maternal hostility, although he does mention that part of Frisius' subtitle, "The whole business of witchcraft," "is clearly represented as both destructive of human society and intimately related to women's uncontrolled sexuality" ("Appropriating Folklore in Sixteenth-Century Witchcraft Literature" in *Problems in the Historical Anthro-*

pology of Early Modern Europe, Volume 78 of *Wolfenbütteler Forschungen*, 197).
Like Roper, I have discovered more evidence of the first category of "business,"
the fundamental destructiveness of witches and their general threat to survival, in
my documents.

22. Lyndal Roper. "Witchcraft and fantasy in early modern Germany." *Witchcraft in
     Early Modern Europe: Studies in Culture and Belief*. Jonathon Barry, Marianne
     Hester, Gareth Roberts, editors. Cambridge, 1996. 207–36.

23. My choice of documents is eclectic, and I am sure that there are other images and
     texts which I could have included. In an attempt to cross traditional disciplinary
     lines, my use of visual material has been conducted in the same vein as Robert
     Scribner's in his study of popular pamphlets, *For the Sake of Simple Folk: Popular
     Propaganda for the German Reformation* (Cambridge, 1981). In his final chapter,
     "The rhetoric of the image," Scribner expresses the hope "that this study has
     established the value to the historian of visual evidence" (249). I hope to have
     contributed to that goal.

CHAPTER ELEVEN

The Difficult Birth of the Good Mother: Donneau de Visé's *L'Embarras de Godard, ou l'Accouchée*

Deborah Steinberger

In the fall of 1667, Molière's troupe treated Parisian theatergoers to a novelty: Jean Donneau de Visé's one-act comedy *L'Embarras de Godard, ou l'Accouchée* (*Godard's Predicament, or The New Mother*), the first and only seventeenth-century French play about childbirth to be performed on the official stage. The scene is a bourgeois home where Mme Godard, a middle-aged woman, has just gone into labor. This is her fourth pregnancy, and since she is prone to particularly difficult births, her husband is very nervous. M. Godard frantically but ineffectually attempts to fetch the necessary helpers and supplies; his eldest daughter, Isabelle, interrupts a clandestine meeting with her sweetheart, Cléante, to come to her father's aid. We learn that Godard has been planning to send Isabelle to a convent in order to avoid paying a dowry, and thereby reserve more of the family fortune for the couple's son. Mme Godard, however, is sympathetic to her daughter's desire to wed Cléante, and she is instrumental in getting Godard to agree to the marriage: the husband ultimately grants the request of his suffering wife, and permits Isabelle to wed the man she loves.

Early in the play, the lazy valet Champagne, unhappy about being sent out in the dark to fetch the midwife, insists that it's not time yet: Madame, he jokes, is simply suffering from a bad case of indigestion. Isabelle scolds him: "You're laughing at the expense of a woman who's in no position to beat you" (scene 8).[1] It is literally true that Mme Godard is in no position to punish her servant: invisible throughout the play, she remains confined to the room where she is giving birth. She is "present" only insofar as the servant Paquette reports on her progress and conveys her mistress's agony: "Finally, her pains growing, and three strong pangs / Having brought her practically to death's door, / 'Alas!'

she said, 'I suffer torments / So strong, so vehement, / That all the world's treasures could not induce me / To endure again this terrible pain'" (scene 28).[2]

Why does the mother remain offstage in this play? She is arguably the principal figure in this drama, one who exercises decisive power: her "extreme peril" (scene 15) puts her in a position to demand that her wishes be respected and that Isabelle be married. Childbirth is central to the play's intrigue, and the character of the *accouchée* or new mother is the work's most distinctive feature.[3] The play's subtitle attests to her importance; in fact, the work is noted in Molière's troupe's official records, the *Registre de La Grange*, simply as *L'Accouchée*, and it may well have been known by the public principally or exclusively by that title.

One simple explanation for Mme Godard's invisibility is that propriety did not allow labor and birth to be depicted onstage.[4] This is not surprising for a period when, even in the privacy of their homes, most women labored fully dressed: according to Jacques Gélis, "Semi-nakedness and complete nakedness were indecent, even if there were only women present; it went against the labouring woman's modesty and this might hold up the labour.... [G]enerally the woman was decently clad and the midwife worked away under her petticoats."[5] For political reasons, the Queen gave birth before the court; for most women, however, birth was attended only by a midwife and a select group of family and trusted friends.

Childbirth was also perhaps too banal a subject to be considered stageworthy by most dramatists of the period. Nevertheless, *Godard* proved entertainment fit for a king: the play was presented before Louis XIV, and enjoyed success at Versailles.[6] One reason for this success was surely the court's well-known taste for farce. In fact, in his preface to the play, Donneau de Visé claims that the Court requested the addition of two episodes, the first of which happens to be the play's most vulgar: Champagne dresses a drunken servant in the clothes destined for the new baby, feeds the man some improvised baby food, and admonishes him not to wet his diaper (scenes 22–24). In the other episode the midwife, instead of rushing to Mme Godard's aid, enumerates at exasperating length all the items she will need for the delivery: wine, cloth, scissors, string, salt, saffron (scene 18). The addition of this scene suggests that the theme of childbirth had special appeal for Louis XIV, a king who, as is widely recognized, delighted in his virility and his ability to produce numerous children. According to Christiane Northrup, Louis enjoyed the spectacle of labor, and took pleasure in secretly watching women of his court give birth. In fact, Northrup writes that the supine (lithotomy) position for labor was popularized by Louis XIV, "who wanted to watch the births of women in his court without their knowledge of his presence. In the lithotomy position, with her skirts hiked up, the laboring woman couldn't see who was watching."[7]

L'Embarras de Godard is remarkable not only for its unprecedented treatment of the theme of childbirth, but also for its presentation of a kind of mother new to the comic stage. This new character, "the good mother," is a loving and virtuous woman who puts her children's needs before her own. Even in the throes of labor, Mme Godard works to ensure her daughter's happiness by convincing her husband to consent to the girl's marriage. The maidservant Paquette describes the scene to Isabelle, who has been waiting anxiously for news of her mother's condition, as well as for the outcome of her mother's request: "Madame, who thought she had reached her final hour, / And who loves you tenderly, / Implored Monsieur, in a touching manner, / To give your hand in marriage to Cléante; / She demanded this as a last favor..." (scene 28).[8]

This sentimental portrait of maternal love seems out of place in a play that is largely a farce, complete with clownish valets and scatological humor. In fact, the author admits in his preface that court audiences found a couple of the play's scenes "a bit serious," and that the episodes of the midwife and the drunken servants, mentioned above, were added to brighten the work's overall tone. Perhaps the principal reason we never see Mme Godard onstage is that the pain and suffering of a generous, loving mother would have clashed with the prevailing light comic atmosphere. It is tempting to say that the "good mother" is a character waiting to be born, one not yet ready to make her appearance on the comic stage because she is not sufficiently comic for audience tastes.

Indeed, good mothers are hard to find in seventeenth-century French comedy. Comedy has a long tradition of portraying older female characters as blocking figures who delight in either nagging their husbands or frustrating the romantic projects of their children. When present at all onstage, mothers in seventeenth-century French comedy are generally capricious tyrants or selfish, vain coquettes. In the theater of Molière, they are most commonly blocking figures, female equivalents of the *barbon* or graybeard (comparable to Molière's miser, Harpagon, or his imaginary invalid, Argan). Philaminte, the mother in *Les Femmes savantes* (*The Learned Ladies*), is ready to sacrifice her daughter to her own scholarly ambitions: she insists on marrying Henriette to an unappealing pedant. Béline, the greedy, scheming stepmother in *Le Malade imaginaire* (*The Imaginary Invalid*), pressures her husband to send both of his daughters to a convent. And in *Le Bourgeois Gentilhomme* (*The Would-be Gentleman*), though Mme Jourdain does take her daughter's side against the foolish M. Jourdain, this shrill and domineering wife is hardly presented as an attractive role model. In Molière, in fact, it seems that the only truly "good" mother is a dead mother. In *Tartuffe*, it is the late Mme Orgon, whom the grandmother holds up as a moral example to her son's childless, pleasure-seeking, fashionable second wife, Elmire: "And as for you, child, let me add / That your behavior is extremely bad, / And a poor example for these children, too. / Their dear, dead mother did far better than you" (I, 1).[9] In *L'Avare* (*The Miser*), we learn that Harpagon's late wife once tempered his miserly excesses.

His children complain: "It's true that every day he gives us more reason to regret our mother's death" (I, 2).[10]

Benevolent mothers sympathetic to their children's needs and desires are not comic characters; those who seem to have gotten laughs were mothers clinging vainly to youth, masquerading as young girls. In fact, this sort of character had such comic appeal that in 1666 there were two plays called *La Mère coquette* (*The Flirtatious Mother*), one by Donneau de Visé, the other a rival production by Philippe Quinault. In Donneau de Visé's play, a woman named Lucinde, who believes herself a widow, plans to send her daughter to a convent and steal the girl's suitor. Lucinde gladly abdicates her maternal role, the better to hide her age: she does not permit her daughter to call her "Ma mère," ("Mother") but only "Madame." She admits, "I love [my daughter], but I love myself a little more; / I can't stand her, because she's too beautiful."[11]

The dramatist Dancourt, who produced numerous popular comedies at the turn of the seventeenth century, also favored characters like Lucinde, vain and ridiculous older women who refuse to act their age. In his *La Folle enchère* (*The Mad Auction*) (1691), the widowed Mme Argante attempts to block her son's marriage, while she pursues a man his age. The son's valet explains to his master: "Sir, she wants to be young, in spite of nature: by marrying, you'd make her a grandmother, and the title of grandmother usually ages a woman a full fifteen years."[12] In Dancourt's *Les Trois cousines* (*The three cousins*) (1700), a miller's widow, another selfish mother, is described as "a glutton who wants everything for herself": she is too busy planning her next marriage to worry about finding husbands for her daughters. Working against nature, these anti-mothers promote their own sexuality at the expense of their children's. They seek younger men; in Lucinde's case, this is only to satisfy her vanity, for she no longer wishes to have children. Once remarried, Lucinde declares, she will be careful not to become pregnant: "Children make us old before our time," she complains; "Having them spoils our figure, weakens our charms."[13]

Unlike these *mères coquettes*, Donneau de Visé's Mme Godard is a life-giver, self-sacrificing rather than self-serving. She obeys the dictates of both society and nature: she is loyal to her husband, responsive to his needs and desires, and dedicated to her present and future children. She secures and defends the next generation, both by giving birth herself and by arranging for her daughter to become a wife and not a barren nun. Note that in this play, it is the father who wants to send his daughter to a convent, while the mother resists his harsh sentence. Mme Godard prefigures the compassionate *mères confidentes* (mother-confidantes) of eighteenth-century sentimental comedy, for example the title characters of Marivaux's play *La Mère confidente* (1735) and of Nivelle de la Chaussée's *Mélanide* (1741).

The elaboration of the character of the "good mother" and the simultaneous development of sentimental comedy are part of a larger theatrical trend that I call the "domestication" of French comedy. Starting in the 1660s in France, stage settings are transformed as the scene of comedy shifts from the public space of the city square to the private space of the domestic interior. We can see the beginnings of this process in Molière's *L'Ecole des femmes* (*The School for Wives*) (1662), a play which appears to waver between public and private space. The play is set in a city square which is suddenly "domesticated" when the protagonist, Arnolphe, calls for an armchair to be brought outside in preparation for his famous sermon to his intended bride on the "Maxims of marriage" (III, 2). This odd combination of outdoor space and indoor furniture earned Molière the ridicule of some of his contemporaries and rivals. Modern critics, however, have pointed to this scene as a moment of transition in Molière's dramaturgy.[14] After 1665, Molière would choose the domestic interior setting for all of his five-act comedies. But Molière was not alone in this trend: his contemporaries Philippe Quinault, Thomas Corneille and Donneau de Visé followed suit. *L'Embarras de Godard* is among the first "domesticated" French comedies.

There is ample evidence that this theatrical trend, which can be seen to culminate in the *drame bourgeois* one hundred years later, was driven by social forces as well as by esthetic considerations. The domestication of French comedy can be linked to a transformation of social space in early modern Europe which Philippe Aries's *Histoire de la vie privée* explores in depth. The historian describes "a change in the forms of sociability: from the anonymous social life of the street, castle court, square or village to a more restricted sociability centered on the family or the individual."[15] According to Ariès, Roger Chartier and their collaborators, the seventeenth century saw the emergence of privacy and intimacy as values, with growing distinction between the public and private realms. The family home becomes a privileged, intimate space. Ariès and Chartier link the birth of this new "family feeling" to a number of interrelated developments: the growth of literacy, the Reformation and the emergence of new forms of piety, an increase in private reading, meditation, journal-keeping, the rise of individuality. Architectural innovations of the early eighteenth century offer some of the most convincing evidence of this new taste for privacy. Jean-Louis Flandrin and Fernand Braudel, for example, document the compartmentalization of the home: privacy is enhanced as rooms with specialized functions, often opening onto corridors, replace multipurpose rooms arranged *en enfilade*, opening onto one another.[16]

Edward Shorter writes of the growth of family intimacy and closeness in early modern Europe, and he specifically links this development to evolving social attitudes towards the role and responsibilities of the mother: "We won't be able to fully understand the formation of 'domesticity' – that mesh of privacy and intimacy encircling the family as a whole – without understanding how the new relationship between mother and baby came into being."[17]

Building on Philippe Ariès's *L'Enfant et la vie familiale sous l'Ancien Régime*, a groundbreaking study of the evolution of the status of childhood in traditional and modern European society, Shorter cites new maternal behaviors that greatly enhanced infant welfare. Maternal breastfeeding and the decreased use of wet nurses, along with the decline of the practice of swaddling infants to immobilize them, led to increased physical contact between mothers and children, and improved infant hygiene. These measures permitted mother–infant bonding and helped put an end to "the ghastly slaughter of the innocents that was traditional child-rearing": "When the surge of sentiment shattered this grip, infant mortality plunged, and maternal tenderness became part of the world we know so well."[18] Historical research thus indicates that the development of the newly sentimentalized theatrical character of the good mother corresponds to a new chapter in the history of private life.

The domestication of comedy leads to gradual changes in comedy's cast of characters, plot structures and tone. As one might expect, as comedy moves inside the home, one sees increased domestic realism onstage. Donneau de Visé seemed especially interested in writing plays depicting life passages and featuring realistic detail and social satire. This predilection for everyday matters and contemporary manners is doubtless linked to the author's notable career as a journalist: as the editor of the *Mercure Galant*, one of France's earliest newspapers, Donneau de Visé presided over the birth of journalism in his country. His *La Veuve à la Mode* (*The Fashionable Widow*), presented the same year as *Godard*, takes us inside the home of a woman whose husband has just died. We witness her mad rush to secure the possessions that now rightfully belong to her husband's heir, and her simultaneous efforts to keep up appearances by playing the role of the bereaved wife. Among the homey or authentic details featured in *Godard* are the midwife's list of supplies, and the hero's costume: he appears onstage in his bathrobe and nightcap.

A shift in focus in French comedy to the older generation and to mature couples is another feature of domesticated comedy. Like *La Veuve à la mode*, *L'Embarras de Godard* juxtaposes sentimental, idealized notions of love – in this case, those of the young couple Cléante and Isabelle – with the realities of wedlock. Marriage is not portrayed as a simple happy ending, but as an institution fraught with problems, even danger. The play illustrates what almost inevitably followed marriage, and what it meant to be a wife in seventeenth-century Europe: exposure to frequent pregnancies with their accompanying hazards.[19] Mme de Sévigné's letters to her daughter, Mme de Grignan, urging her to avoid this perilous state by abstaining from sex with her husband, eloquently document the very serious dangers of maternity.[20] In *Godard*, Donneau de Visé accentuates this reality by having courtship take place at the very moment of childbirth: Isabelle's hopes for satisfaction in love are overshadowed by fear of her mother's death. Godard exploits this situation to dissuade Isabelle from marrying: "When one is married, how unhappy one is; / Marriage is such a heavy yoke to bear! / Each time, alas! a woman gives birth, / You see how she nears her final moments. / ... / Could you dare think of marrying, / Knowing the state your mother is in?" (scene 11).[21] Also part of this confrontation of idealized romantic love with reality is a scene where Cléante mistakes Paquette for Isabelle in the dark, and passionately kisses the old woman's hand. Paquette remarks, "In the dark, Paquette and Isabelle are just the same to you" (scene 1).[22]

Traditionally, comedy is oriented towards and ends with the marriage of the young people; in a sense, the younger generation supplants the older. In *Godard*, there is a departure from this established structure: Godard and his wife steal the scene from the young lovers. Godard paints a vivid picture of their everyday life and their conjugal contentment:

> The poor woman, alas! who pampers me:
> Who, when I come home late, waits for me all night;
> Who, when I have the tiniest cut on my finger, cries;
> Who always caresses me, and worries I might die;
> Who orders every week, just to be safe,
> That I be bled ...
> When I am the slightest bit indisposed, she is always fearful:
> She herself watches over me at night,
> And keeps the servants from disturbing me.
> You see her zeal in everything she does;
> She always has love-names for me:
> I am her king, her boy, her darling, her sweetheart.
> How I would suffer if I lost her!
> When from time to time we fight,
> Out of affection for me, she's the first to make up;
> She never holds a grudge, and never fails
> To speak to me in bed, to make peace ... (scene 16)[23]

Passages such as these hold our interest. By contrast, the young lovers' conversation is so insipid that it bores even Paquette, who serves as their chaperone. Between yawns, she asks, "Since your conversation is the same every night, / Why bother staying up so late?" (scene 1).[24]

This is comedy, so there is a happy ending: Isabelle gets to marry Cléante, and Mme Godard gives birth to a healthy baby. According to Paquette, while in labor Mme Godard had sworn that this would be her last child: "'From now on, my husband can beg all he wants,' she said, followed by something else / That I don't wish to say, or rather, I dare not.'"[25] But Paquette reports that once her mistress's ordeal was over, "She judged she'd made a frivolous vow: / 'It looks like you'll keep that promise to your husband,' we joked. / She surprised us with a smile / That showed the opposite was true" (scene 28). But although this is comedy, the play does not shy away from the theme of death: we are constantly reminded that Mme Godard is in great danger. In the play's first scene, her daughter Isabelle declares, "We must fear for her life, / Knowing that she will give birth any minute. / I can't bear the thought of losing her." Christiane Northrup notes that an emphasis on the pain of childbirth, and the characterization of the pregnant woman as weak and sick, are part of our internalized patriarchy: "At some very deep level, we are all awed by pregnant women and their power. But instead of emphasizing a woman's power, in classic patriarchal reversal our culture attends to the fear that that power brings up."[26] The historian Jacques Gélis notes how giving birth empowered women, at least temporarily: "Bereft of self-expression, with little say in community decisions ... women became themselves at birth, grouped round the midwife ... [who] became the symbol of resistance to a kind of morality, a regulation of life, which people were attempting to impose on them from the outside."[27]

As we have seen, in *L'Embarras de Godard* the laboring woman acquires the authority and power to determine her daughter's fate. And for a brief moment, women reign. Isabelle, the daughter of the house, takes charge, organizing the servants and preparing for the new arrival when her father proves too distraught to perform these tasks (scene 7). Paquette orders Champagne about (scenes 14 and 15). The midwife is greeted ceremoniously as a great lady: Champagne cries, "Make way, make way for Madame!" as she enters; Godard embraces her joyfully (scene 17). And the new baby is a feisty girl ("From its cries I thought it was a boy," says Champagne, who had at first reported the wrong sex). But this matriarchal moment fades as quickly as Mme. Godard's resolution to abstain from the pleasures of the marriage bed. We remember that the mother's power stemmed only from her perceived proximity to death; in the end, patriarchal order is restored. The play's last line enjoins us not to celebrate the mother, but to serve the man of the house: "Servez Godard, car sa femme est en couche" ("Serve Godard, for his wife has given birth"). Ephemeral too were the play's fortunes: after its presentation at court, it was performed another fifteen or so times, again by Molière's troupe, at the Palais Royal theater. The play had only one run, and it was never revived. Not until the eighteenth-century vogue of sentimental comedy would French audiences wholeheartedly welcome the sight of the good mother at center stage.

Notes

1.   "Mais tu ris d'une femme qui ne peut à son gré te battre." Jean Donneau de Visé, *L'Embarras de Godard ou l'Accouchée*, in *Les Contemporains de Molière*, ed. Victor Fournel, vol. 3 (Geneva: Slatkine Reprints, 1967), 465. Subsequent references to this play will be followed by scene number. Unless otherwise noted, all translations of French texts are mine.
2.   "Enfin, son mal croissant, et trois douleurs de suite / Jusqu'à l'extremité l'ayant presque réduite, / 'Hélas!,' a-t-elle dit, 'je souffre des tourmens / Qui m'abattent si

fort et sont si véhémens / Que, pour souffrir encore cette peine profonde, / On m'offriroit en vain tous les trésors du monde.'"

3.   This figure is often present in Latin comedy, but these new mothers are invariably teen-age girls, all first-time mothers; the matrons are all past childbearing age. These young mothers are usually one-dimensional characters: about all one hears from them are offstage cries of pain and appeals to Juno, the protectress of women in labor.

4.   This is true for the official French stage. We possess much less information about what happened onstage in the popular, unofficial genres of the time, such as the *théâtre de la foire* (fairground theater). I am grateful to Barry Russell, an expert on this genre, for bringing to my attention two plays which portray childbirth in an allegorical or burlesque manner. Seventeenth-century poetry collections such as the *Recueil de Sercy* and the prose work *Les Caquets de l'accouchée* (1622) treat the subject of childbirth with considerable frankness. For more on the *Caquets*, see Domna Stanton's article, "Recuperating women and the man behind the screen," in James Grantham Turner, ed., *Sexuality and Gender in Early Modern Europe* (Cambridge: Cambridge University Press, 1993), 247–65.

5.   Jacques Gélis, *History of Childirth: Fertility, Pregnancy and Birth in Early Modern Europe*, trans. Rosemary Morris (Cambridge: Polity Press, 1991), 120.

6.   Pierre Mélèse, *Un homme de lettres au temps du Grand Roi: Donneau de Visé* (Paris: Droz, 1936), 74. See also Victor Fournel's introduction to his edition of the play (450), as well as Donneau de Visé's own preface, which Fournel reproduces (452).

7.   Christiane Northrup, *Women's Bodies, Women's Wisdom* (New York: Bantam Books, 1994), 394–5. I have thus far been unable to find confirmation of this fascinating information in any historical work on Louis XIV. If true, this account would lend added resonance to the king's memoirs, where he writes, "All that is most necessary for this work [kingship] is at the same time pleasurable; for it is, in a word, my son, to have our eyes fixed upon the entire land … to be informed of an infinite number of things of which we are supposed to be ignorant; to penetrate that which our subjects hide from us with the greatest care. …" ("Tout ce qui est le plus nécessaire à ce travail est en même temps agréable; car, c'est en un mot, mon fils, avoir les yeux ouverts sur toute la terre … être informé d'un nombre infini de choses qu'on croit que nous ignorons; pénétrer parmi nos sujets ce qu'ils nous cachent avec le plus de soin…"). Louis XIV, *Mémoires*, ed. Jean Longnon (Paris: Librairie Jules Tallandier, 1978), 42.

8.   "Madame, qui croyoit estre à son dernier jour, / Ayant beaucoup pour vous de tendresse et d'amour, / A conjuré monsieur, d'une façon touchante, / De vous donner, dans peu, pour épouse à Cléante, / Et l'exigeant de lui pour dernière faveur. …"

9.   "Ma bru, qu'il ne vous en déplaise, / Votre conduite en tout est tout à fait mauvaise; / Vous devriez leur mettre un bon exemple aux yeux, / Et leur défunte mère en usait beaucoup mieux" (I, 2, 25–8). Jean Baptiste Poquelin de Molière, *Tartuffe*, in *Oeuvres complètes*, vol. 2 (Paris: Flammarion, 1965). The English given in the text is from Richard Wilbur's translation of the play (New York: Harcourt Brace Jovanovich, 1965), 171. It is worth noting here that Elmire escapes the general rule that makes literary stepmothers self-serving tyrants.

10.   "Il est bien vrai que tous les jours il nous donne de plus en plus sujet de regretter la mort de notre mère …." Jean Baptiste Poquelin de Molière, *L'Avare*, in *Oeuvres complètes*, vol. 3 (Paris: Flammarion, 1965).

11.   "Je l'aime, mais je m'aime un peu plus qu'elle. / Je ne la puis souffrir, pource

qu'elle est trop belle" (I, 2). Jean Donneau de Visé, *La Mère coquette* (Paris, 1666). All citations from the play are taken from this original edition.

12. "Monsieur, elle veut estre jeune, en dépit de la nature; en vous mariant vous la feriez grand'mère, et le titre de grand'mère vieillit ordinairement une femme de quinze bonnes années des plus complètes" (scene 2). Florent Carton Dancourt, *La Folle enchère* (Paris, 1691).

13. "Les enfants ... nous font vieillir avant notre temps, / Gâtent souvent la taille, aféblissent les charmes ... (III, 1).

14. See especially Roger Herzel's study, "The Décor of Molière's Stage: The Testimony of Brissart and Chauveau," *PMLA* 93 (1978): 925–54. For more on domestication in Molière, see my own article, "Molière and the Domestication of French Comedy: Public and Private Space in *L'Ecole des femmes*," *Cahiers du Dix-Septième* 6, no. 2 (1996): 131–39.

15. Philippe Ariès and Roger Chartier, eds., *A History of Private Life*, vol. 3 (Cambridge, Massachusetts: Belknap Press, 1989), 9.

16. Jean-Louis Flandrin, *Familles: Parenté, maison, sexualité dans l'ancienne société* (Paris: Seuil, 1984), 92–4; Fernand Braudel, *The Structures of Everyday Life: The Limits of the Possible*, trans. Sian Reynolds (New York: Harper and Row, 1981), 308–309.

17. Edward Shorter, *The Making of the Modern Family* (New York: Basic Books, 1975), 168. Lawrence Stone documents a related phenomenon in England, the birth in the late seventeenth century of "affective individualism": the walling-off of the nuclear family from either interference or support from kin, accompanied by the development of warmer affective relations between husband and wife and between parents and children. See his *The Family, Sex and Marriage in England, 1500–1800* (New York: Harper and Row, 1977).

18. Shorter, 204. Elisabeth Badinter, also inspired by Ariès's work on childhood, argues that mother love is a relatively modern concept; she claims that the "good mother" is born and the myth of maternal instinct engendered during the late eighteenth century, thanks in large part to the writings of Rousseau. See her *Mother Love: Myth and Reality* (New York: Macmillan, 1981), 117; originally published in French as *L'Amour en plus* (Paris: Flammarion, 1980).

19. This was especially true for those women most likely to employ a wet nurse: city dwellers and members of the upper classes. On the relationship between class, fertility, and lactation practices, see Jean-Louis Flandrin, *Familles: Parenté, maison, sexualité dans l'ancienne société* (Paris: Seuil, 1984), 195–7.

20. Of Mme de Grignan's seven pregnancies, only four children were born alive and survived infancy, and Mme de Grignan twice came perilously close to death during labor. See Jacques Gélis, Mireille Laget and Marie-France Morel, *Entrer dans la vie: Naissances et enfances dans la France traditionnelle* (Paris: Gallimard/Julliard, 1978), 70–71.

21. "Quand on est marié, que l'on est malheureux! / Et que le mariage est un joug rigoureux! / Toutes les fois, hélas! qu'une femme est en couche, / A son dernier moment tu vois comme elle touche. / ... / Mais à vous marier oseriez-vous songer, / Sçachant en quel état se trouve votre mère?"

22. "Paquette, la nuit, vaut pour vous Isabelle."

23. "La pauvre femme, hélas! Qui me dorlote tant, / Qui, lorsque je viens tard, toute la nuit m'attend, / Qui, quand au bout du doigt j'ay le moindre mal, pleure; / Qui toujours me caresse et craint que je ne meure, / Qui veut, tous les huit jours, que, par précaution, / Je me fasse saigner. ... / ... / Quand je suis un peu mal, toujours elle appréhende; / Elle-mesme a le soin de me veiller la nuit / Et d'empescher mes

gens de me faire du bruit. / Dans tout ce qu'elle fait on remarque son zèle; / Par des noms caressans toujours elle m'appelle; / Je suis son roy, son fils, son mignon et son coeur. / Ah! Si je la perdois, que j'aurois de douleur! / Quand quelquefois tous deux nous sommes en colère, / Son amitié la fait revenir la première; / Elle tient peu son coeur et ne manque jamais / De me parler au lit, pour refaire la paix. …"

24. "Puisque vostre entretien est tous les soirs de mesme, / Pourquoi veiller si tard?"
25. "'Mon mary désormais aura beau me prier,' / A-t-elle dit encore, avec quelque autre chose / Que je ne veux pas dire, ou plutost que je n'ose'" ; "Jugeant bien qu'elle avoit fait un serment frivole: / 'A vostre époux je crois que vous tiendrez parole,' / A-t-on dit en riant. Elle, par un souris, / A fait voir le contraire et nous a tous surpris."
26. Northrup, 378.
27. Gélis, *History of Childirth*, 110.

CHAPTER TWELVE

"Players in your huswifery, and huswives in your beds": Conflicting Identities of Early Modern English Women

Mary Thomas Crane

In current debate over ideologies of the home and family, few terms are so loaded as "housewife," a word which we generally now use to describe a woman who does not work outside the home and thus devotes all her time to domestic and familial caretaking.[1] This term was perhaps even more problematic and contested in the early modern period, when (along with its alternate form "huswife") it could mean simultaneously *both* "a woman (usually a married woman) ... who manages her household with skill and thrift" and "a light, worthless, or pert woman or girl ... now (as of around 1650) Hussy" (*NED*). In a period when women's domestic roles were changing at all levels of society, the conflicting uses of this term can provide a kind of paradigm of issues at stake as women became increasingly confined to and associated with caregiving within the home and domestic matters. I want to look at an array of uses of the term (largely by male writers – women seem generally to avoid it), in order to trace a pattern of anxiety, first, over working-class women's wage-earning potential within the home (with fears of a concomitant sexual independence) and, later, anxiety over upper-class women's increasing idleness (with fears of concomitant sexual freedom) as they were confined to a domestic sphere where servants did most of the work.

In both cases, anxiety about the role of women seems to center around the unstable boundaries between their potential as "producers," of income, goods, children, and a literally "conservative" sense (emphasizing its etymological connection with "conserve") of their role as caretakers and preservers of money, goods, and offspring produced by the husband. Although prescriptive accounts of women's roles often attempt to separate these two functions, it is, in practice, very difficult to do so, and also very difficult not to imagine production eliding with prodigality and waste. I want to end by looking at two early country house poems, Ben Jonson's "To Penshurst" and Emilia Lanyer's "A Description of Cooke-ham," in order to trace some of the differing ways that a male and female writer negotiate the boundary between production and conservation in their representations of the ideal domestic woman.

An early account of the duties of a good housewife is provided by Thomas Tusser's "The Points of Huswiferie United to the Comforts of Husbandrie" (1570).[2] Tusser attempts to prescribe a daily round of activities for the wife of a small farmer who is to prepare meals, bake bread, brew beer, manage the dairy, mend clothing, supervise servants, and, in general make sure that the money and produce her husband provides is not wasted: "if thrift by that labour be honestlie got: / Then is it good huswiferie, else is it not." Tusser's housewife doesn't earn money, but is instead expected to work day and night to conserve what her husband has earned: "Ill huswiferie othing / or other must crave. / Good huswiferie nothing / but needfull will have" (181); "Il huswiferie bringeth a shilling to naught / Good huswiferie singeth her cofers full fraught" (181). Tusser, a younger son and former courtier/musician who failed as a small farmer seems largely concerned to define the housewife as subordinate to and supportive of her husband's financial interests. In this prescriptive work, the alternate sense "hussy" is carefully suppressed.

In descriptive contexts, however, "huswife" often seems to focus more narrowly on the housewife's archetypal occupation as spinner of yarn. Initially, good huswives (like Tusser's) were to spin their own thread for domestic linens in order to spare the expense of buying such goods: "set some to peele hempe or else rishes to twine, / to spin and to card" (163). Thus, for example, George Herbert in "The Pearl" can describe "what reason hath ... of it self, like a good huswife, spun" (3–4).[3] In addition to production of yarn for domestic consumption, spinning of flax or wool remained in the early seventeenth century a kind of cottage industry in which women could still participate for wages. Tusser, in fact, seems to allow his huswife to have others help with this work, instructing her to "pluck up thy flax, for the maidens to spin, / First see it dried, and timelie got in" (116). Wages for such "spinsters" were, in most cases, too low to provide subsistence, and as a result spinning was largely (in Alice Clark's words) "a tertiary occupation for married women. She who was employed by day in the intervals of household duties with her husband's business or her dairy and garden, could spin through the long winter evenings when the light was too bad for other work".[4] Still, women who were so employed could supplement household income, and it is significant that Tusser does *not* recommend that his huswife undertake anything beyond the gathering and spinning of flax for domestic linens, despite the straightened means of her household.

That he did not probably indicates nervousness about women's ability to earn wages in a domestic sphere which was increasingly separated from commodity production. In this sense, anxieties about women's potential as wage earners within the home seem conflated with worries about their independent sexuality. In *Twelfth Night*, for example, Sir Toby Belch describes Andrew Aguecheek's lank hair hanging "like flax on a distaff; and I hope to see a huswife take thee between her legs, and spin it off" (1.3.103).[5] Here, "huswife" clearly means both domestic spinner and "hussy," with some part of the joke probably dependent upon the position of the spinning wheel between the spinster's legs. In *The Winter's Tale*, Leontes calls Hermione "as rank as any flax-wench that puts to / Before her troth-plight" (1.2.277–8), suggesting a common association between transgressive female sexuality and the spinning of flax. Similar anxiety and play on both senses of the word comes up in *As You Like It*, where Fortune is a huswife because she spins the length of human life, but also because she is as changeable and wanton as a hussy. In this regard, Shakespeare's male characters seem to imagine something like the Wife of Bath; a woman who, because of her success in the textile industry, is able to travel widely and subsidize a voracious sexual appetite. Of course, the small wages available to a seventeenth-century huswife render this improbable, and register the narrowing opportunities available to women in England in the early modern period.

Huswifely spinning, whether for wages or for domestic use, seems also to have been connected to anxiety about sexuality and fertility within as well as outside marriage; thus, attempts to separate the huswife from the hussy prove problematic in this instance as well. George Herbert, records in his *Outlandish Proverbs*, the injunction that "she spins well that breedes her children" (144), perhaps suggesting that a woman would be better occupied in domestic nurturance than in supplementary wage earning. Robert Herrick also suggests a link between huswives, spinning, and female sexuality. In "Connubii flores, or the well-wishes at a Wedding," he depicts choruses of shepherds and matrons urging the bride to earn money by spinning. The shepherds present her with a fleece and suggest that spinning is an occupation for married women: "Nor Faire, must you be loth / Your Finger to apply / To huswiferie. / Then, then begin / To spin: / And (Sweetling) marke you, what a web will come / Into your chests, drawn by your painfull Thumb" (35–41).[6] There is, here, I think, an unspoken analogy between spinning and marital sexuality – both of which seem to begin upon marriage, both of which will be productive, and both of which can be initially "painfull" (here with a primary sense of "careful," but probably also suggesting a Cinderella-like prick of the spindle). Indeed, this section of the poem follows immediately after a chorus of youths who deliver an ambivalent view of sexuality within marriage: "Love is a thing most nice; and must be fed / To such a height; but never surfeited … Go then discreetly to the bed of pleasure; and this remember, *Vertue Keepes the measure*."

A chorus of matrons proceeds explicitly to describe the wage-earning potential of the bride: "Set you to your Wheele and wax / Rich, by the ductile wool and Flax. / Yarne is an income; and the Huswives thread / The Larder fills with meat; the bin with bread." A chorus of old men immediately signals ambivalence about this idea, urging that "wealth come in by comely thrift / And not by any sordid shift," presumably cautioning against improper means of female wage earning, including prostitution. *Othello*, a text similarly concerned with female sexuality in relation to marriage, may provide a gloss on this connection when Iago describes Bianca as "a huswife that by selling her desires / Buys herself bread and clothes (F1 reads "cloath"). Instead of spinning her own cloth, Bianca sells herself in order to buy it. Othello himself similarly links his fear of Desdemona's sexual power over him with the huswife's power within her home (though not in this case connected to spinning) when he vows that whenever "my disports [with Desdemona] corrupt and taint my business / Let housewives make a skillet of my helm" (1.3.271–2). Herrick's wedding poem concludes with a chorus of virgins whose reference to "the blessing of encrease," possibly continues the discussion of the bride's potential to contribute to household income through her huswifery but primarily indicates her role as producer of offspring.

Indeed, a woman's power as producer of offspring was, like her potential to augment family income, a quality both desired and feared. Although fertility in women seems to have been prized even at lower levels of society, its consequence – numerous children – could cause financial distress.[7] Thus, although Herbert's proverbs could reflect that "she spins well who breedes her children," they also note that "he that hath children, all his morsels are not his owne" (423). Tusser, author of the treatise on huswifery cited above, describes just such mixed feelings in his poetic autobiography:

> Behold of truth, with wife in youth,
> For joie at large, what dailie charge,
> Through childrens hap, what opened gap
> To more begun.
> The childe at nurse, to rob the purse.
> The same to wed, to trouble hed.
> For pleasure rare, such endlesse care
> Hath husband wun.

Tusser, however, seems unwilling to have the expense of huswifely fertility in this regard offset by her productivity as a wage earner.

Tusser's instructions on "The good motherlie Nurserie" are, not surprisingly, focused on saving money. He comes out as a clear advocate of maternal breastfeeding, a position that would have been controversial at the time. He seems initially to do so for reasons of health:

> Good huswifes take paine, and doo count it good luck,
> To make their owne breast their owne childe to give suck
> Though wrauling and rocking be noisome so neare,
> Yet lost by ill nursing is woorser to heare (180).

He goes on, however, to point out the financial advantage: "But one thing I warne thee, let huswife be nurse, / least husband doo find thee too franke with his purse" (180). The rest of this brief passage on maternal caregiving is devoted to proper discipline, clearly presented as part of the huswife's conservative role: "Teach childe to aske blessing, serve God, and to church, / Then blesse as a mother, else blesse him with burch." Tusser emphasizes the waste involved in the case of a child who does not receive proper discipline at home, "fit neither for prentise, for plough, nor for schoole" (180).

Significantly, by the second decade of the seventeenth century the term "spinster" no longer designates the employment of a (usually married) woman as a spinner of yarn, but comes to be used as the legal term for an unmarried woman. The *NED* cites its use to denote occupation as late as 1580 in a legal document: "Margaretta Tirrell spinster, alias dicta Margaretta Tirrell uxor Thome Tirrell." By 1617, however, it cites Minseu's dictionary as defining spinster in this way: "a terme, or an addition in our Common Law, onely added in Obligations, Evidences, and Writings unto maids unmarried." It seems possible that a solution to anxieties about huswifely spinning was to confine this occupation primarily to unmarried women, or at least to confine the legal sense of the word "spinster" to a designation of single status.[8]

Another attempted solution to this swirl of uncertainties surrounding women's changing roles in society was to attempt to separate huswives from hussies by confining women within the space of the home. Jean Howard has argued that anti-theatrical tracts from the period, such as Stephen Gosson's *The Schoole of Abuse* (1579), express repeated concerns about the presence of women at performances in public theaters. As Howard notes, "the threat the theater seems to hold for Gosson in regard to ordinary gentlewomen is that in that public space such women have become unanchored from the structures of surveillance and control 'normal' to the culture and useful in securing the boundary between 'good women' and 'whores.'"[9] However, as another anti-theatrical tract reveals, the relatively clear boundary between "good women" and "whores" becomes more difficult to maintain when the word "huswife," with its innate ambiguity, comes into play. The author of *A Second and third blast of retrait from plaies and Theaters* (1580) states that he has heard women swear on their death beds that attendance at theaters, being "mere brothel houses of Bauderie," have "made them of honest women light huswives."[10] Tusser, who uses the term only in its positive sense, urges huswives to stay at home for financial reasons: "As huswives keep home, and be stirrers about, / so speedeth their winnings, the yeere thorow out" (159).

However, the tensions traced so far suggest that it was within the home itself that women, as huswives, proved most threatening. As Iago argues in *Othello*, there seems always to have been a nagging fear that all domestic women were "players in your huswiferie, and huswives in your beds" (2.1.112).

In the case of upper-class women, the term develops somewhat differently, but with an ultimately similar attempt to separate proper huswives from hussies. Indeed, the two words do separate around the middle of the seventeenth century, when "hussy" first appears in English sources as a separate term for a loose woman. Initially, "huswife" seems to designate women of lower gentry status or below, often in rustic situations. Tusser includes women who may have several servants, but the huswife is always described directly in relation to household labor – either as supervisor or as performing the work herself. In the course of the seventeenth century, however, a variety of factors combined to confine upper class women to the domestic sphere even as servants took over most of the work. When country houses were manor houses at the center of a large network of dependent workers, women were often involved not only in conducting business in their husband's absence but also in seeing to the welfare of feudal dependents. Alice Friedman has argued that the "removal of the country house from its agricultural context" served to enforce "a clear separation between public and private life," thus limiting "the sphere in which upper-class women could move." According to Friedman, the creation of the new style country house "helped to place domestic work and family life directly under women's control" even as it physically embodied "the virtual exclusion of women from public life."[11]

By the middle of the seventeenth century, as Alice Clark has suggested, many gentlewomen came to lead lives of "idleness and dependence" (38). Clark cites Pepys' expressions of concern in his diary about his own wife's idleness: "Nov. 13, 1662. Our discontent again and sorely angered my wife, who indeed do live very lonely, but I do perceive that it is want of work that do make her and all other people think of ways of spending their time worse" (297), or, again, August 20, 1664 "I see that she is confirmed in it that all I do is by design, and that my very keeping of the house in dirt, and the doing this and anything else in the house, is but to find her employment to keep her within, and from minding her pleasure, which though I am sorry to see she minds it, is true enough in great degree" (297). Pepys himself, of course, knew a great deal about minding his own pleasure with other men's idle wives, and it is easy to see that there is a short distance between such women and the idle, pleasure loving women of the restoration stage.

Beginning early in the century, however, some men undertook a campaign to keep upper-class women engaged in domestic labor which was a bit subtler than Pepys' "keeping of the house in dirt." These writers attempted to redefine an ideal of "noble" or "high huswifery," urging ladies of means to return to the kinds of work within the house and neighborhood that the mistress of the feudal manor traditionally undertook. Gervase Markham's "The English Hus-wife, conteyning, The inward and outward vertues which ought to be in a compleat woman" (1615), differs from Tusser's earlier treatise in its intended audience of gentlewomen. Markham's book is dedicated to the Countess Dowager of Exeter, although he hastens to assure her that "it can add nothing to your own rare and unparalleled knowledge."[12] It begins with a long section "Of Physical Surgery," providing directions for the treatment of illness ranging from fever, to the plague, to stinking breath, bones broken in the head, worms, sore breasts, and "privy parts burned" (3–5). Although Markham urges the necessity of medical knowlege for treating members of the household, this section must also allude to the tradition that the lady of the manor (or country minister's wife) dispensed medical care to surrounding villagers. The diary of Lady Margaret Hoby, for instance, notes that she "dressed a poor boy's leg that came to me, and then brake my fast with Mr. Hoby. After, I dressed the hand of one of our servants that was very sore cut."[13]

Markham's chapter on cookery includes recipes for fancy banqueting dishes, and his chapters on distillation of perfume and the making of wine (rather than ale or beer) similarly suggest that the book is directed to women of more than modest means. Markham urges that housewives learn "the manner of serving and setting forth of meat for a great feast," since "it is the office of the clerk of the kitchen (which place our housewife must many times supply) to order the meat at the dresser and deliver it unto the sewer, who is to deliver it to the gentlemen and yeomen waiters to bear to the table" (121). Markham emphasizes that even the housewife who has such a panoply of servants under her command must attain to "a perfect skill and knowledge in cookery, together with all the secrets belonging to the same, because it is a duty really belonging to a woman; and she that is utterly ignorant therein may not by the laws of strict justice challenge the freedom of marriage, because indeed she can then but perform half her vow; for she may love and obey, but she cannot serve and keep him with that true duty which is ever expected" (60).

Significantly, Markham's chapter on spinning allows for hiring other women to do that work: "forasmuch as every housewife is not able to spin or tear in her own house, you shall make choice of the best spinners you can hear of, and to them put forth your tear to spin, weighing it before you go, and weighing it after it is spun and dry, allowing weight for weight, or an ounce and a half for waste at the most: as for the prices of spinning, they are according to the natures of the country, the fineness of the tear, and the dearness of provisions: some spinning by the pound, some by the lea, and some by day, as the bargain shall be made" (162). This housewife's thrift is thus confined to making sure that she is not cheated by the lower-class women she hires to do her spinning for her. Nevertheless, Markham would insure that she busy herself with supervision of all domestic labor that she does not carry out herself.

Markham's book does not address the care of children, although a few of his medical receipts are suited for the treatment of children or for child-bearing women. As historians have documented, upper-class women in this period did not usually breastfeed or care for their own young children, sending them out instead to wet nurses. For women of this class, often under pressure to produce an heir, fertility itself could replace caregiving as a maternal imperative.[14] At the same time, emphasis on women's productive capacities, especially when linked directly to their sexuality, can easily lead to the very kinds of anxiety that these treatises are concerned to prevent. In Markham's work, there is a great deal of emphasis on the housewife's occupation as caregiver – as provider of medical care and food – to adult members of her household and surrounding community, a role which stands in for the less socially acceptable nurture within the home of babies and small children and possibly counters the threatening fact of female fertility with a more conservative caretaking role.

Perhaps the most prominent literary treatment of the "noble huswife" is to be found in Ben Jonson's "To Penshurst." Don Wayne has established the role of the poem in what he calls the "preliminary 'mapping' of an ideological domain" where "traditional, feudal notions" are redefined to contribute to the bourgeois ideology of the home.[15] As an important part of Jonson's "mapping," he attempts to define a role for the lady of the house along the lines suggested by Markham. When King James visits the house unexpectedly in the absence of its mistress, she has so well directed domestic matters that everything is in order:

> what praise was heaped,
> On thy good lady then! who therein reaped
> The just reward of her high housewifery:
> To have her linen, plate, and all things nigh
> When she was far; and not a room but dressed
> As if it had expected such a guest![16]

It is important to note that Barbara Gamage Sidney, the lady of the house, does not seem to be present to receive this praise herself. Ironically, she manages to be a good housewife by not staying at home and by effectively delegating domestic work to others – this is evidently "high housewifery," as distinguished from lower versions that involve doing the work oneself. Anxiety about sexuality and fertility nevertheless surface within a few lines, when we learn that Penshurst's lady is "noble, fruitful, chaste withal; / His children thy great lord may call his own, / A fortune in this age but rarely known." Lady Sidney's fertility (she had twelve children) must be immediately qualified by assurances of her chastity, and further qualified by repeated assurance of her marital fidelity, which Jonson acknowledges to be unusual among women of her class.

Intimations of the "hussy" thus creep in, although Jonson tries very hard to exclude them.

Interestingly, parental nurture, in this poem, consists of a disciplinary function very similar to that outlined by Tusser: "They [the Sidney children] are and have been taught religion; thence / Their gentler spirits have sucked innocence. / Each morn and even they are taught to pray / With the whole household" (93–6). In this case, although this training in religion is not specifically attributed to either parent, it seems to stand in for the maternal breastfeeding which women of Barbara Sidney's class rarely undertook; here, their "spirits have sucked innocence" from the religious atmosphere of the home. Jonson thus further manages the potentially threatening nature of Lady Sidney's fertility by describing the careful disciplining of its products in language that associates it, however indirectly, with her role as thrifty caretaker.

A link between Lady Sidney and huswives of a lower class is also implied, as Wayne has suggested, by the repeated image of "fruit" when the "ripe daughters" of Penshurst's feudal dependents bear gifts of fruit to the manor house, hoping to find "husbands" in the process. "Husband," the correlative of "housewife," never develops a pejorative sense equivalent to "hussy." Here, there is a play on its secondary sense as "agricultural worker," with the implication that a husband's role is to cultivate his wife into a pattern of regulated fertility and domestic responsibility. Indeed, it is unclear whether the husband or huswife is truly the person who will "reap" the rewards of high huswifery.

It would be interesting to know what Lady Sidney herself would have to say about the practice of noble huswifery.[17] Amelia Lanyer, author of another early country house poem, "The Description of Cooke-ham," does *not* praise the domestic skills of its mistress Margaret Clifford; instead, housework becomes part of the *sponte sua topos*, a conventional passage in country house poems where nature itself celebrates and serves the lord or lady of the manor:

> Oh how (me thought) against you thither came,
> Each part did seeme some new delight to frame!
> The House receiv'd all ornaments to grace it,
> And would endure no foulenesse to deface it.
> The Walkes put on their summer Liveries,
> And all things else did hold like similies[18]

Similarly, when Clifford is forced to depart, the house participates in the mourning of all nature on the estate and (as houses tend to do) reverts to messiness: "The house cast off each garment that might grace it / Putting on Dust and Cobwebs to deface it" (201–2).

Raymond Williams read the *sponte sua* passage in Jonson's poem as a mystification of the actual means of production – the labor of dependent workers – through a kind of magical depiction of the estate as paradise: "the magical extraction of the curse of labour is in fact achieved by a simple extraction of the existence of labourers."[19] Jonson, however, is at pains to establish the organizational labor of the housewife as necessary to the maintainance of the ideal home. Indeed, Barbara Sidney is the only person at Penshurst who seems to do any work at all. Although Jonson imagines the master of the estate as its moral center, he is able to ensure its order simply by his presence: in a famous Jonsonian formulation, Penshurst's lord "dwells." It is his wife who must actively work to organize its hospitality and discipline the children.

Lanyer, on the other hand, exempts the mistress of the house from labor as well, freeing her to spend her time in meditation. Barbara Lewalski has argued that Lanyer's poem depicts Cookeham as a "female Eden," a "happy garden state in which women lived without mates but found contentment and delight in nature, God, and female companionship."[20] Lanyer emphasizes "pleasure" and "grace" as the organizing virtues of Cookeham, in marked contrast to Jonson's more austere valuing of order, discipline, and chastity. She depicts Margaret and Ann Clifford wandering over the grounds of the estate, taking pleasure in its natural beauty, engaging in "sports" and meditation on Biblical topics. Neither Clifford is imagined as producing or conserving anything, but rather seems free to enjoy what nature has produced for their pleasure. On the other hand, Lanyer suggests that given unlimited leisure time and freedom from domestic duties, women will choose to use it chastely and nobly in religious meditation.

It is the poet herself who must work for a living, and who produces something – her poetry. And it is around the speaker that anxieties about women's roles are clustered in this poem. The poet/speaker announces early on that Cookeham and the Cliffords have been instrumental in enabling her to write. Cookeham is where

> the Muses gave their full consent,
> I should have powre the virtuous to content.
> Where princely Palace will'd me to indite,
> The sacred Storie of the Soules delight. (3–6)

Like domestic labor, poetic work is also, oddly, displaced onto the house itself; it is the Palace, and not its inhabitants, who "will'd" her to write her poems. Lanyer here seems simultaneously to empower a community of women to authorize literary production (the Muses and the Cliffords both seem to contribute to this authorization) but also to stress its conservative nature: her poems are about religious topics and are intended "the virtuous to content" while the masculine "princely Palace" suggests that, as at Penshurst, a male agency ultimately authorizes and controls production. A few lines later Lanyer more directly attributes her productivity to Clifford's patronage, addressing "you (great Lady) Mistress of that Place, / From whose desires did spring this worke of Grace" (11–12). Here Lanyer both glances at the production of children (offspring of the Mistress's "desires") and firmly replaces them with the less threatening "worke of Grace" that she has written. "Worke of Grace" is, itself, paradoxical, since it admits the labor that has produced the poem but also suggests that it has come about through the grace of God, and Margaret Clifford. Lanyer, then, seems simultaneously to assert the dangerous concepts of female leisure, pleasure, and production while also taking pains to represent them as managed and controlled (if indirectly) by religion, and by the estate itself.

It is no surprise, then, that Lanyer, far from advocating traditional housewifely virtues, urges "all vertuous Ladies in generall" (in one of many dedicatory poems directed addressed to influential women which begin her long work, *Salve Deus Rex Judaeorum*) to clothe themselves "as did the beauteous Lilly of the field." The allusion here is to Matthew 6.28–9, where Christ, in the Sermon on the Mount, urges his listeners to "consider the lilies of the field, how they grow; they toil not, neither do they spin. And yet I say unto you, that even Solomon in all his glory was not arrayed like one of these." Lanyer, who seeks in these dedicatory poems to obtain patronage for herself as a writer, calls on Biblical precedent for the avoidance of housewifely thrift. Her avoidance of the term "huswife" itself and all it had come to stand for, in these dedicatory poems and, more importantly, in her depiction of an all-female domestic ideal at Cookeham, suggests that it was possible for a woman in early modern England to at least imagine alternatives to the limited and limiting visions of women's roles offered by male writers. By shifting women's productivity from the sexual and monetary to an intellectual and religious realm, Lanyer may attempt to alleviate the anxieties which caused male writers to insist that women should conserve, not produce. The leisured pleasure and grace afforded the three women at Cookeham is dependant on the exclusion of the "huswife" in both complex senses of that word. Until real houses learn to clean themselves, however, Lanyer's vision of a classless comradeship of women will remain an unattainable ideal.

Notes

1.	See Ann Oakley, *The Sociology of Housework* (London: Martin Robertson, 1974), 29, who uses the following definition of "housewife": "the person, other than a domestic servant, who is responsible for most of the household duties (or for supervising a domestic servant who carries out these duties)." Oakley further notes that "the equation of femaleness with housewifery is basic to the structure of modern society, and to the ideology of gender roles which pervades it."

2.	Thomas Tusser, *Five Hundred Points of Good Husbandry* and *The Points of Huswiferie United to the Comfort of Husbandrie*, ed. Geoffrey Grigson (Oxford: Oxford University Press, 1984).

3.	F. E. Hutchinson, ed., *The Works of George Herbert* (Oxford: Clarendon, 1941; reprint, 1970), ll. 3–4. Further quotations from Herbert are cited from this edition.

4. Alice Clark, *Working Life of Women in the Seventeenth Century* (London: Cass and Co., 1919; reprint, New York: Kelley, 1968), 95.

5. G. Blakemore Evans, ed., *The Riverside Shakespeare* (Boston: Houghton Mifflin, 1974). All quotations from Shakespeare's plays are cited from this edition.

6. L. C. Martin, ed., *The Poetical Works of Robert Herrick* (Oxford: Clarendon, 1956; reprint 1968), ll. 35–41. All further quotations from Herrick are cited from this edition.

7. However, evidence suggests that in the sixteenth century poorer women were more likely to breastfeed their children than were wealthy women and therefore had lower fertility rates. See Dorothy McLaren, "Marital Fertility and Lactation, 1570–1720," in Mary Prior, ed., *Women in English Society 1500–1800* (London: Methuen, 1985), 22–53.

8. However, see Carol Z. Wiener, "Is a Spinster an Unmarried Woman?", *The American Journal Of Legal History* 20 (1976): 27–31, for an argument that in English legal records between 1589 and 1603, the term "spinster" when applied to married women does not designate their occupation but is instead a "legal fiction" used by Justices of the Peace to apportion blame fairly between husband and wife.

9. Jean E. Howard, "Women as Spectators, Spectacles, and Paying Customers," in David Kastan and Peter Stallybrass, eds., *Staging the Renaissance: Reinterpretations of Elizabethan and Jacobean Drama* (New York and London: Routledge, 1991), 71–2.

10. Anthony Munday (?), *A second and third blast of retrait from plaies and Theaters*, excerpted in E. K. Chambers, *The Elizabethan Stage* Vol. 4 (Oxford: Clarendon, 1923), 209.

11. Alice T. Friedman, *House and Household in Elizabethan England: Wollaton Hall and the Willoughby Family* (Chicago: University of Chicago Press, 1989), 48–9.

12. Gervase Markham, *The English Housewife*, ed. Michael R. Best (Kingston and Montreal: McGill-Queen's University Press, 1986), 3.

13. From the diary of Lady Margaret Hoby, January, 1600, excerpted in Ralph Houlbrooke, ed., *English Family Life, 1576–1716: An Anthology from Diaries* (Oxford: Blackwell, 1988), 59.

14. See McLaren, 27, who notes of upper class women that "poets and playwrights eulogized their fertility. Artists painted them caressing their big bellies. Monuments proudly depicted their numerous boys and girls."

15. Don Wayne, *Penshurst: The Semiotics of Place and the Poetics of History* (Madison: University of Wisconsin Press, 1984), 25.

16. Ben Jonson, *Poems*, ed. Ian Donaldson (Oxford: Oxford University Press, 1975), 87–90. All quotations from Jonson's poems will refer to this edition.

17. Barbara Lewalski notes that the over 300 surviving letters from Robert Sidney to his wife "project a portrait of Barbara as highly valued domestic helpmeet, manager of the estate and its hospitality, and devoted mother of his children (she bore twelve in all)." However, Barbara Sidney's letters do not survive, so her thoughts on high huswifery are lost to us. See Barbara Kiefer Lewalski, *Writing Women in Jacobean England* (Cambridge: Harvard University Press, 1993), 399 n. 60, and 235–41 for a valuable comparison of Jonson's and Lanyer's poems.

18. Susanne Woods, ed., *The Poems of Aemilia Lanyer* (Oxford: Oxford University Press, 1993), 130–38.

19. Raymond Williams, *The Country and the City* (New York: Oxford University Press, 1973), 32.

20. Lewalski, 241, 240.

Maternal Textualities

Susan Frye

The domestic, maternal spaces occupied by early modern English women defined and demarked the forms of writing that they produced within those spaces. While many valuable studies have considered women's writing in relation to men's lives and the traditions of male authorship, scholars increasingly have access to information about women's domestic lives that allows us to consider a women's textual tradition. This tradition, while necessarily intertwined with the lives and work of men, stands apart from the male tradition of authorship because women's writing was once thoroughly associated with women's maternalistic roles within their households, those living and work spaces occupied by members of a group of men and women closely connected through their domestic interactions and their work.[1] Although only some of the forms of what I call "household writing" have been actively considered by scholars, women's writing – defined as recording any part of the alphabet worked or drawn in any form – encompassed a number of activities. These activities may be placed on a continuum, from those that provide very little information about their composers to those that provide a great deal of information. The traces of women's textuality in brief notes and messages, alphabets in stitchery or calligraphy, initials, ciphers, and sententiae, tease us with what they suggest about the importance of these less articulate forms of household writing. Account books, art work, receipt or recipe books, letters, diaries, calligraphic manuscripts, and published texts offer more fulsome although sometimes no less mysterious means to consider the textuality of early modern women. This essay concentrates on four such types of trace writings: vestigial notes or messages, initials, a cipher, as well as two diaries in order to demonstrate that the examples available of women's textuality complicate our sense of maternal roles in the early modern household.

Needlework in particular offers small glimpses of English maternal and filial relations because girls and women by the thousands left behind whispers of their historical "selves" in the form of needlework projects. Their work –

produced to add to the well-being and wealth of the household rather than as an indication of leisure – ranges in the sixteenth and seventeenth centuries from the samplers of early girlhood to the bed testers, cushions, and curtains of womanhood, many of them initialed, some signed, and a few carrying additional written information. The earliest dated sampler, a spot sampler registering a variety of patterns for later reference, contains a name and an inscription that makes momentarily visible the relation between an embroidered text and the maternal: "JANE BOSTOCKE 1598 / ALICE LEE WAS BORNE THE 23 OF NOVEMBER : BE / ING TUESDAY IN THE AFTERNOONE: 1596."[2] This message links Jane Bostocke's claim to her identity as a distinct and single subject with her identity as the mother of Alice Lee. Why Jane Bostocke would work this record two years after Alice's birth could almost equally be attributed to the baby's birthday, death, or both, but its existence records a maternal connection painstakingly worked for us to find. Far more ubiquitous are the samplers of daughters, into which they worked their initials, like "MF" on a spot sampler recording two ways to embroider strawberries (829–1902) or "SID" worked as part of a white cut-work sampler dated 1649 (T.124–1992). Occasionally, embroidered names, like Hannah Pittman, Elizabeth Mackett, and Hannah Downs (T.83.1913; 433–1884; T.34–1935), register identity via familial connections. Despite differences of class, wealth, and location, the girls and young women who worked their initials or names used the letters of the alphabet to claim their affiliation with the work of their hands and minds. Their needlework, as Margreta de Grazia, Maureen Quilligan, and Peter Stallybrass point out about material objects in general, "Might constitute [the] subjects who in turn own, use, and transform them,"[3] just as the materials worked by women once defined and were defined by them.

Such fragments of literacy – the initials, the sewn alphabets, the notes left signed and unsigned within worked boxes, many of which were writing boxes – constitute a distinct feminine textual tradition, however difficult it may be to recover. The woman writer's audience is limited to herself and her household, to her sewing circle of kin and neighbors, to her descendants whose care has preserved these objects, and, inadvertently, to people like us interested in material artifacts. Likewise, manuscript receipt books, with recipes for cooking and healing added by family members and friends across generations, become in their aggregate, as Janet Theophano says, "a memoir, a diary – a record of life."[4] Such fragments comprise brief commentaries on sixteenth- and seventeenth-century households and the place of the mother and child within them that in lengthier form became letters and diaries and, still more boldly intellectual and more demanding of a wider audience, translations, calligraphic manuscripts, and printed texts. Even the alphabet worked into countless samplers implies either some literacy or at least a sense of the cultural capital of literacy for girls and women. The sampler, which began as a memory aid of worked stitches, marks the value of knowing the shapes of letters that one worked with the needle or the pen.

The extent to which the needle and the pen both functioned to create women's texts is evident in the epitaph that George Ballard records of Elizabeth Lucar, a London merchant's wife who died in 1537. In its verses, the double play of "wrote" as "wrote" and "wrought" makes Lucar's sewing and writing activities interchangeable: "She wrote all Needle-workes that women exercise / With Pen, Frame, or Stoole, all Pictures artficiall. / Curious Knots, or Trailes, what fancie could devise / … Three manner Hands could she write them faire all." Lucar "wrote" with needle and pen alike her "Curious Knots," or embroidered designs, as well as "Three manner hands," or types of handwriting.[5] Jonathan Goldberg has recently maintained that the phrase "female pen" "sounds like a virtual impossibility" because "pen sounds so much like and is so often analogized with the penis." Indeed, for Goldberg, a woman who wields a pen requires "a revaluation of the sense in which the writer remains female in any cultural sense of the word."[6] Goldberg's use of the word "female" here assumes that the subjects whom this culture classified as "women" were defined entirely within masculinist definitions, as if culture itself were necessarily masculine and "women" who disturb masculine definitions therefore cease to count as women. If we consider, however, that the masculinist attempts to limit and define the feminine served to create a rich interaction that we might call a women's culture, a culture that flourished less visibly but no less actively than men's culture, then we might also consider how generations of women worked to create and re-create what a "female" was and what she did. Any woman who worked a chosen needlework pattern or picture within a group of other women while sitting and talking, or while being read to, participated in an ongoing redefinition of the masculinist equation between women's work and women's silence.

For Lucar and the girls and women literate enough to form letters, if only as needlework patterns, female textuality was an everyday occurrence that grew out of the forms of women's culture that itself simultaneously conformed to and challenged the masculinist, outsider view of their domestic roles. In consequence, I see women's taking up the pen as inseparable from their creating a variety of texts, all of which represent a recontouring of masculinist categories. Lady Grace Mildmay, who worked with the "plummet ['chalk (or possibly lead) pencil or pen'] on paper," makes connections among drawing on paper, designs for embroidery, and her own penned account of the years that she spent as a "daughter" in the home of her in-laws: "Every day I spent some time in works of mine own inventions, without sample of drawing or pattern before me, for carpet or cushion work [i.e., embroidery], and to draw flowers and fruits to their life with my plummet on paper."[7] The fact that Mildmay records this activity in her manuscript autobiography completes the implicit connection between drawing embroidered patterns, performing the needlework, and the activity of writing as related and integral ways to create both visual and written texts within the distinctly female experience.

Although sixteenth and seventeenth century theories of women's education made it clear that girls should be educated only insofar as it would benefit their households and be consonant with their station in life,[8] it would be a mistake to think that all English people regarded the education of women with disinterest or suspicion. We are aware of the privileged educations that many aristocratic women and women of the gentry received during the early modern period, but increasingly in the seventeenth century a limited education for indigent girls that included sewing and some reading was advocated, while education was highly valued in religious households of many classes. Among the merchant classes the efforts of brilliant daughters, hard-working wives, and advice-dispensing mothers were celebrated in sermons and epitaphs like Lucar's. The number of "hands" that a woman acquired was a ready indicator of the extent of a young person's education because they provided the means to negotiate a number of different social, domestic, and intellectual contexts. "Writing" in the sense of what we would call "calligraphy" constituted part of an upscale education for girls and women especially fashionable in the sixteenth century and then emulated in the seventeenth.

To teach girls to form letters themselves and to acquire different hands assumes a need for this knowledge beyond self-display or an association with Protestant humanism. For aristocrats, gentry, and the wealthier classes of merchants who owned land and interests across the country, female letter writers and receivers of letters like the women of the Thynne and Lisle families allowed travelers to keep up with what was going on at home or to report on business abroad, providing a necessary link in communications. Letters frequently passed between women and their children, from Lady Brilliana Harley to her son Ned,[9] for example, or from Margaret Clifford to her daughter Anne, who records in her diary her frequent responses. For these same groups as well as for all classes of merchants, women who could keep inventories and accounts, like Elizabeth Talbot or Katherine Windham,[10] were often crucial to household operations in an era when personal lives and household businesses remained virtually indistinguishable. Less organized but more fragmentary accounts, like those in the margins of the *Madison and Morison Families Receipt Book*, note particularly maternal expenditures in the usual accounting method of listing first pounds, then shillings, then pence: "My Dater Margret August the furst / sent hur to by a petecot – 3-3-0 / fer a yerd and a half of / Bengall for a Aprone 0-4-0 / She had more 0-15-0." Another entry records money given another daughter: "August the furst 1688 what my Dater / that is at home Mary / she had 0-2-0."[11] In writing letters, receipts, or accounts, women's hands fulfilled several household functions, while offering the possibility of recording discreet moments in a life.

In spite of the evidence of a tradition of women's household writing, early modern theories of the separation between the public and the domestic, between who is permitted literacy and who holds the authority to write, have made it difficult to conceptualize the connections among domestic space, maternal roles, and women's writing. The connections go much further than the recognition that women who wrote or produced other texts tended to take their subject matter from their households. In thinking through these connections, social and psycho-analytic theory provides ways of talking about how maternal domestic space and the identity of the women living within that space intersect at the point where space and language produce the individual subject. In exploring the relation among domestic space, the maternal, and the development of language, Julia Kristeva points out in "Women's Time" that

> Studies on the acquisition of the symbolic function by children[,] show that the permanence and quality of maternal love condition the appearance of the first spacial references which induce the child's laugh and then induce the entire range of symbolic manifestations which lead eventually to sign and syntax.[12]

I would argue, that like the child who moves within domestic spaces into the symbolic and the sign and thus into language and text, the women who occupied domestic spaces first as children and then as adults lived the connection between biological and textual reproduction – that is, in occupying the roles of "girl," woman," and "mother," they occupied the linguistic categories that authorized women's (limited) speech in general and the categories of household writing in particular. If we focus attention on maternal domestic space, we make visible women as well as children coming into identity through the same language through which they would later attempt to express that identity. Indeed the linguistic and symbolic aspects of maternal space invite us to address the fact that these interactions between women and children resulted in passing the symbolic from one generation to the next, whether as language, oral and visual traditions, reading, or even writing.

My consideration of the early modern household as a maternal site for texts would not be complete without taking into account the complexity of those households as well as the ways in which that complexity shaped textual production and writerly selves. In describing domestic space as "maternal," I do not assume that all households in this period were composed according to a normative heterosexuality, but rather that the "maternal" can be expanded to include a variety of roles, spaces, and textualities occupied by women. At the same time, in a society in which women were defined culturally by the injunction to marry as the means to reproduce – as the author of *The Lawes Resolutions to Womens Rights* declared, "All of them are understood either married or to bee married"[13] – "maternal" is a category that includes women's reproductive capacity as fulfilled in a variety of roles. We have ample evidence of same-sex households, as well as households with absent fathers, separated or otherwise estranged couples, households that include the childless woman, the single parent, the unmarried aunt, the spinster, and the widow.[14]

Moreover, domestic establishments tended to include a variety of members: farming, trade, and upper class households comprised helpers, apprentices, servants, retainers, young people raised away from their natal homes, as well as assorted kinfolk. The female body existed as maternal in all of these spaces to the degree that its place in the world was determined by its inter-related capacities to reproduce and to produce the goods and services that nourished, clothed, taught, and otherwise managed the household. It is this variable but always central maternal identity that women household writers articulate within the space and time of the early modern English household, where "identity" points to the ever-becoming sense of a stable "self" that individual subjects attempt to generate through their relations to space, time, and discourse. The subjectivity of the women whom I am considering at a temporal and cultural remove of four hundred years is the nexus of that space and the identities fashioned in response to and as the means to define the household. Identity in this sense emerges as agency when expressed through the production of texts, however humble or domestic.

Such a definition of subjectivity opens the door to a consideration not only of the centrality of the maternal role in the household, but also to the fact that the stability of that role is a fiction. The maternal role, like all subject positions, is necessarily unstable, varying both with historical circumstance and the ongoing effort to imagine a "self." The maternal role is also unstable because it was composed of a dialectic between each individual who occupied that role and the domestic spaces to which she had been delegated. Or put another way, instabilities of the maternal are inevitable because women, while valued as reproducers, worked to define the domestic spaces in which they found themselves at the same time that the spaces, their people and activities, defined the women. Because increasingly the definition of "woman" depended on the occupation of certain spaces, it is not enough to assert with Kristeva that women's reproductive capability determined the nature of the spaces they inhabited. Rather, to consider the textuality of women it is important to understand the extent to which they fashioned their own activities and forms of self-expression within the reciprocal concepts of "woman" and "domestic space."

The wrought initials of aristocratic women tell us more within the contexts of their more recoverable lives and homes than the occasional names and initials on samplers. What emerges from upper class women's trace writings is a non-normative view of the maternal role. One exceptional woman, the most successful social climber of the late sixteenth century, displayed her initials prominently enough to shed some light on the significance of the initials and names left behind on material objects by less privileged women. At New Hardwick Hall in Derbyshire, the giant initials ES dominate the skyline. Through her initials, which appear eight times around the cornice of the building that she built after her last husband's death, "Bess of Hardwick," who clearly thought of herself as "Elizabeth [Countess of] Shrewsbury," declares to the countryside that she is the owner of this magnificent home on the hill and the wealth that produced it – a bold declaration and construction of her power. That name, acquired with the last of her four husbands, is also the one represented in the vast majority of her needlework. Elizabeth Talbot, Countess of Shrewsbury, a great needleworker and enterprising mother whose dynastic ambitions produced an heir to the English throne in her granddaughter Arabella Stuart, saw to it that her initials appeared in many of her textile productions, like the large worked hanging of Diana and Actaeon in which arcs of power, represented by colorful, broad lines, extend from Diana's fingers to an Actaeon who, depicted with the head of a stag and the legs of a man, is changing into an animal before our eyes. Shrewsbury even had her initials painted into Elizabeth's motto above the mantlepiece in her magnificent Great Hall by changing the "et" in "Dieu et mon droit" to the unmistakable "Dieu eESt mon droit" as the means to graft her own name, with its attendant dynastic ambitions, onto the supreme expression of royal privilege, "God and mine right."

Still other textile hangings at Hardwick declare a familial, even maternal, identity. Her larger needlework pieces from the 1570s in the series called the "Virtues" dominate the main story of Hardwick Hall, with appliquéd designs composed from medieval priests' copes that she and her helpers cut into new compositions featuring powerful female figures. In Elizabeth of Shrewsbury's case, two of her designs – Temperance and Lucrece – were also the names of two of the daughters that she bore her second husband, William Cavendish. Temperance, her second child born in 1549, and Penelope, her eighth child born in 1557, both died in childhood (Durant, 17, 28). Thus Elizabeth Talbot's choice of female figures connects the wall hangings she designed during her fourth marriage to the Early of Shrewsbury with the memorialization of daughters born into that earlier – and happier – marriage.

Like the Countess of Shrewsbury, Elizabeth Tudor, when a girl whose destiny in life seemed to be a political marriage, also used initials to assert her identity. A half-century before Elizabeth Talbot designed and decorated Hardwick Hall, Elizabeth Tudor at the age of twelve composed a complex cipher using her own initials together with those of her father, Henry VIII, and her stepmother, Katherine Parr, and worked them on the matching covers of two volumes of translations that she presented to them as New Year's Gifts.[15] In fact, the cipher-covered translations presented in 1545 had been preceded by what was probably another matched set of needlework-covered translations (of which only one remains extant) in 1544. For all their display of her abilities in needlework and in writing two different Italic hands, these gifts also demonstrated her intellectual and religious relationships to the court. The three extant volumes contain ambitious translations: in 1544, for her stepmother, Elizabeth translated a section of Calvin's *Institutes*, and for her father, she translated Katherine Parr's prayers into Italian, Latin, and French. In 1545, again for Parr, she translated Marguerite de Navarre's *Glass of the Sinfull Soul*, a Protestant text that John Bales published on the Continent in 1548 – Elizabeth's first publication.

To her stepmother, Katherine Parr, Elizabeth's gifts demonstrated her commitment to an already existing alliance that offered her more intellectual and emotional nurturance than her dynastic ties to her father. Through her gifts to Parr, the Lady Elizabeth articulated her attachment to a woman who had helped to reconnect her father with his children, a woman who took a vital interest in Elizabeth's education. Moreover, Parr was, as Elizabeth's gift to her father of the queen's prayers demonstrates, herself an author in the acceptably pious vein of the 1530s and 40s.[16] In the absence of her father's interest, Elizabeth reached out to Parr through the association of the discourses of protestant humanism and emblematically ciphered needlework. Elizabeth's translations of Protestant texts for Parr asserted the bond between herself and her stepmother through religion, female kinship, and authorship. As Elizabeth wrote in her "Epistle Dedicatory," the work came from her "humble daughter," who "knowing the affectionate will and fervent zeal which your highness hath toward all godly learning as also my duty toward you … hath moved so small a portion as God hath lent me to prove what I could do." In other words, this is a gift that "proves" what the twelve-year-old Elizabeth can do.

Elizabeth's gifts to Parr connect Elizabeth, whom parliament had declared to be a bastard, with the memories and activities of queens who were for the most part motherly or grandmotherly figures: Marguerite de Navarre, Katherine Parr, Anne Boleyn, and even Lady Margaret Beaufort, Henry VII's mother and Elizabeth's great-grandmother. In his edition of the first of Elizabeth's two translations for Parr, *The Glass of the Sinful Soul*, Marc Shell points out that Marguerite de Navarre very likely had presented Elizabeth's mother, Anne Boleyn, with a copy of her Protestant work when they renewed their association in 1534–35.[17] Moreover, Elizabeth's choice of the title, "The Glass of the Sinful Soul," echoes the choice that her great-grandmother made when she translated a work from the French titled "The Mirror of Gold for the Sinful Soul." Elizabeth's gift, covered and even screened by her hand-worked initials or cipher, brings her into association with these women through a composite self-display of needlework, calligraphy, and translation.

Elizabeth Talbot, Countess of Shrewsbury and Elizabeth Tudor, the future

Elizabeth I, emblematize the painstaking effort of women to connect initials with their productions – whether architectural, textile, dynastic, intellectual or artistic. Initials express a sense of identity, but they also reach out to connect women with the names of powerful figures into whose company they might literally work themselves. Initials are thus doubly important, pointing both inward toward a domestic subjectivity and outward toward a public identity. Our awareness of the significance of initials for privileged women allows us to map the significance of initials for those women whose needlework is the only evidence that they once lived. Initials make a different if related kind of announcement than the linked coats of arms or initials of husband and wife, which locate property and territory within the specific context of heterosexual union. Initials locate a moment of self-identification within an object registered as one's own, however precarious locating that "one" among changing female names may be: if we count the initials of her maiden name, Elizabeth, Countess of Shrewsbury went through four different sets of initials before acquiring the exalted "ES." In the effort to continue in memory beyond one's life span, these initials in stone point to the initials worked in the more fragile medium of needlework performed by the classes of women engaged in embroidery, as well as to the textile artifacts – the christening blankets, napkins, and handkerchiefs – that the wills of working class women hand on to their loved ones.

If initials and ciphers represent a momentary identity in relation to the political and familial, diaries present us with far more articulate means to assess the physical spaces in which privileged women lived, as well as the different forms that "maternity" might take. One of the earliest known women's diaries of this period, that of the Lady Margaret Hoby, presents a well-known puzzle. For although Hoby, a childless woman, kept her diary from August, 1599 to July, 1605, her entries provide only brief accounts of the management of her estate, her healing activities, religious reading, needlework, "goodly" conversations, and self-examination, while maintaining a strict emotional distance from her own life. Unlike Anne Clifford's diaries, which leave accounts of the interrelated love she bore her mother, her daughter, and her land, Margaret Hoby's diary says little about her fears, frustrations, desires or joys. Her husband led the busy life of a member of the Council of the North, and, being well-connected as the son of Elizabeth Lady Russell and the cousin of Robert Cecil, frequently conducted his affairs away from home, while during the years of the diary Hoby remained at the Yorkshire estate, Harkness, gained through her first marriage, except for one visit to London. Her entry of Friday, September 7, 1599 is if anything unusually forthcoming:

> After priuat praiers I wrett my notes in my testement, which I geathered out of the Lector the night before: then I did eate my breakfast, then I walked abroad and talked of good thinges, so that I found much Comfort: after I Cam hom I wrett my sermon that was preached the saboth day before, then I went to priuat praier, and

so to dinner: after which I taked a litle with some of my frendes, and exercised my body at bowles a whill, of which I found good: then I Came home and wrought tell 4, then I praied with Mr Rhodes, and after walked abroad: and when I Came hom I praied priuatly, and sonne after went to supper: after which I went to the Lector, and then to bed.[18]

The phrase about playing at bowls, "of which I found good," is one of the most effusive moments in the diary. But entries like these record how integrated writing was in her daily activities: "I wrett my notes in my testement," and "I wrett my sermon," note religious writing that she then records in her diary. Rarely do we glimpse how populated her world actually was, although in this entry she provides the rare notation that she "walked abroad and talked of good thinges" and later talked "a litle with some of my frendes." She also performed needlework nearly every day except on Sunday ("I Came home and wrought til 4") – even heiresses were expected to provide a steady supply of turkey carpets, cushion covers, bed testers, and wall coverings, produced with the help of maids and other serving people, often regardless of sex or class. Elsewhere in the diary she lets slip that she actually performed her needlework in the company of the girls and women she was raising in her house: "I went and wrought with my Maides tell allmost night" (Hoby, p. 170). For the most part, however, we must rely on secondary evidence for information about what her activities in raising the children of others in her household might have been like.[19] The "maids" to whom Hoby refers were doubtless the daughters of friends and local gentry, whom she raised, according to the custom, as she herself had been, in the Puritan household of Catherine, Countess of Huntingdon (Hoby, p.5). Although in 1603 Hoby's chaplain, Richard Rhodes, married a "girl of good family in attendance on Lady Hoby" (Hoby, p. 244 n.180), in her diary itself there is only one specific mention of such a young woman who must have been in the family the entire time Hoby was keeping the diary and whose upbringing Hoby must have overseen: "Euerill Aske went from Hacknes to Mr Robert Stillingtons, wt whom Mr Hoby send 30li (besides hir wages) wch was all the monie that he had receiuied before, in 4 yeares, that was dwe to hir, Lefte hir by hir father, wch Mr Bethell had, by his will, for the bringing hir vp" (pp. 199, 283n.545). This Euerill Aske, then, had come to the Hoby household with a dowry of £30 at her father's behest. When she left to marry Robert Stillington, she took with her the £30 and her wages. Clearly, Aske had lived with Hoby, wrought with her, ate and prayed and walked with her during four years in which she kept her diary – the kind of nurturing relationship readily available to a childless heiress whose husband was so frequently absent. Yet Aske appears in the diary only as a point of honor, an entry certifying that the Hobys had done well by her.

Even as Margaret Hoby fulfills every other role expected of a woman of her class and position, the construction of a mother–daughter relationship so visible in the textiles of Elizabeth Talbot and Elizabeth Tudor and the diary of Anne Clifford is notably absent. Indeed, the diary maintains such an eloquent silence on the subject of motherhood that I must speculate that her inability to have children may have been the principal reason for keeping the diary in the first place. Born Margaret Dakin, Margaret Hoby had been married three times when she began her diary. First, at the comparatively advanced age of twenty, she married Walter Devereux, who was killed in France while following his brother, the Earl of Essex, into action in 1591. At twenty-four she married Thomas Sidney, and at twenty-five in 1596, Sir Thomas Hoby. The diary covers her life from the age of twenty-eight to thirty-four, as she was reaching the end of her child-bearing years and the realization that she would not bear children. As a memorial to her blameless life and the means to examine the moments when "satan" tempted her and was overcome, the diary suggests not only her personal piety, but a deep need to record and puruse it. Certainly in this period the belief was widespread that a childless woman was a sinful woman. As Sara Mendelson and Patricia Crawford point out, "barrenness was seen as an unhappy female condition, perhaps even, as the Bible suggested, a punishment for sin." They cite in particular the diary of one Sarah Savage, who kept "a poignant record of her prayers to the Lord about 'a Particular matter' – her long-desired pregnancy."[20] The determination with which Margaret Hoby sets down the purposefulness and piety of her existence may be read as a response to the unspoken criticism that her childlessness was a judgment of God. Illness she certainly considered to be such a judgment: "After dinner, it pleased, for a Iust punishment to corricte my sinnes, to send me febelnis of stomak and paine of my head, that kept me vpon my bed tell 5: a clock" (Hoby, p. 64). If her health stood in such direct relation to God, why not her infertility? In its repression of her childlessness, the diary of Margaret Hoby actively seeks an alternative to traditional maternity in domestic, highly textual activity.

Women's maternal textualities, whether in the form of diaries, art work, trace writings, initials, or ciphers, formed the tradition which enabled some women to publish their work. From the earliest publications by women in the sixteenth century to those of the seventeenth century, women authors wrote from the subject position of daughter, mother, wife, and widow whether they married or not, had children or not. Their published work forms one end of a continuum of women's textuality that begins with traces of texts and initials and ends in complex forms of public utterance. From Margaret More Roper's authorization from her father to publish *A devout treatise upon the Pater Noster* (1524) and Katherine Parr's filial prayers in *The Lamentation of a Sinner* (1547), Dorothy Leigh's *The Mother's Blessing* (1616) and Elizabeth Clinton, Countess of Lincoln's *Nursery* (1622), to the poems of Anne Bradstreet and Amelia Lanyer's *Salve Deus Rex Judeorum*, the household formed the conceptual space from which so many of women's published texts emanated and whose occurrence in manuscript or print provides the most visible means to assess how women worked within and reworked the place of women. The published work of women that began to proliferate in the seventeenth century stemmed from the tradition of household writing that I have outlined in this essay, but in order to see this relationship we must be willing to see how women's textuality connects to household tasks like needlework, cooking, healing, and raising children. Elizabeth Talbot and Elizabeth Tudor constructed the connections between written and embroidered texts that so many anonymous women also were ready to assert, while Margaret Hoby and Anne Clifford recorded their daily, monthly, and yearly responses to the injunctions to lead virtuous and active lives and to bear children. The maternal textualities of lesser-known women must likewise be treated as variable, unstable, and open to restructure, because these women too continually re-created the patterns and contours of domestic space.

Notes

1. On the structure and meaning of the household, see Lena Cowen Orlin, *Elizabethan Households: An Anthology* (Washington, D.C.: The Folger Shakespeare Library, 1995); Amy Louise Erickson, *Women and Property in Early Modern England* (London: Routledge, 1993); Mary Abbot, *Life Cycles in England 1560–1720* (London: Routledge, 1996); and Sara Mendelson and Patricia Crawford, *Women in Early Modern England* (Oxford: The Clarendon Press, 1998).

2. Textile citations, unless otherwise indicated, refer to items from the Victoria and Albert Textile Collections, whose curators I would like to thank for showing me so many embroidered pieces. The Jane Bostocke sampler is identified as T.190–1960.

3. Margreta de Grazia, Maureen Quilligan, and Peter Stallybrass, *Subject and Object in Renaissance Culture* (Cambridge: Cambridge University Press, 1996), p. 5.

4. Janet Theophano, *Household Words: Women Write from and for the Kitchen: An Exhibition of Materials Selected from the Esther B. Aresty Collection of Rare Books on the Culinary Arts* (Philadelphia: University of Pennsylvania, 1996), p. 7.

5. On handwriting during the early modern period see Jonathan Goldberg, *Writing Matter: From the Hands of the English Renaissance* (Stanford: Stanford University Press, 1990).

6. Jonanthan Goldberg, "The Female Pen: Writing as a Woman," in Jeffrey Masten, Peter Stallybrass, and Nancy Vickers, eds., *Language Machines: Technologies of Literary and Cultural Production* (New York: Routledge, 1997), p. 17.

7. Grace Mildmay, "From *Autobiography*," in Randall Martin, ed., *Women Writers in Renaissance England* (London: Longman, 1997), p. 221.

8. See Juan Vives, *The Instruction of a Christian Woman* (1523); Richard Mulcaster, *Positions* (1581), pp. 132–3, 167–78; John Amos Comenius, *The Great Didactic* (1657), ed. M.W. Keating, 2nd edition (1910), p. 68; see also David Cressy, *Education in Tudor and Stuart England* (New York: St. Martin's Press, 1975) and Erickson, *Women and Property in Early Modern England*, pp. 55–6.

9. Thomas Taylor Lewis, *The Lady Brilliana Harley, Wife of Sir Robert Harley* (London: The Camden Society, 1854), reproduces these letters.

10. Many account books and inventories kept by Elizabeth Talbot, Countess of Shrewsbury ("Bess of Hardwick") are extant. Katherine Windham, who "managed her investments with the help of her father" is mentioned in Mendelson and Crawford, *Women in Early Modern England*, p. 313. Mendelson and Crawford cite her personal account book, kept from 1669 to 1680 as Norfolk RO, WKC 6/12.

11. *Madison and Morison Families Receipt Book*, University of Pennsylvania Library, marginalia on pp. 95 and 98. My thanks to Peter Parolin for making these entries available to me, and for all his invaluable suggestions regarding this essay.

12. Julia Kristeva, "Women's Time," trans. Alice Jardine and Henry Blake, in Nannerl O. Keohane, Michelle Z. Rosaldo, and Barbara C. Gelpi, *Feminist Theory: A Critique of Ideology* (Chicago: University of Chicago Press, 1981), p. 33.

13. *The Lawes Resolutions to Womens Rights* (London: John More, 1632), p. 6.

14. See Erickson, *Women and Property in Early Modern England* and Mendelson and Crawford, *Women in Early Modern England 1550–1720*.

15. See Susan Frye, "Sewing Connections: Elizabeth Tudor, Mary Stuart, Elizabeth Talbot, and Seventeenth-century Anonymous Needleworkers," in Susan Frye and Karen Robertson, *Maids and Mistresses, Cousins and Queens: Women's Alliances in Early Modern England* (New York: Oxford University Press, 1999), pp. 167–9 and 180n.3. Margaret Swain first concluded that the three extant manuscripts point to a fourth missing manuscript. See Swain, "A New Year's Gift from Princess Elizabeth," *The Connoisseur* (August 1973), pp. 258–66.

16. On Katherine Parr's prayers see Janel Mueller, "Devotion as Difference: Intertextuality in Queen Katherine Parr's *Prayers and Meditations (1545)*", in *Huntingdon Library Quarterly* 53(1990), pp. 171–97; Elaine V. Beilin, *Redeeming Eve: Women Writers of the English Renaissance* (Princeton: Princeton University Press, 1987), 72–5; and John N. King, "Patronage and Piety: The Influence of Catherine Parr," in Margaret P. Hannay, ed., *Silent But for the Word: Tudor Women as Patrons, Translators and Writers of Religious Works* (Kent, Ohio: Kent State University Press, 1985), pp. 43–60.

17. Marc Shell, *Elizabeth's Glass* (Lincoln: University of Nebraska Press, 1993), p. 3. But see also Anne Lake Prescott's argument that Elizabeth was working from the Geneva edition of 1539, in "The Pearl of the Valois and Elizabeth I," in Hannay, *Silent but for the Word*, pp. 66–7.

18. Margaret Hoby, *Diary of Lady Margaret Hoby 1599–1605*, ed. Dorothy M. Meads (Boston: Houghton Mifflin, 1930), p. 70.

19. On the ways in which the children of the upper classes circulated among households, see Patricia Fumerton, *Cultural Aesthetics: Renaissance Literature and the Practice of Social Ornament* (Chicago: University of Chicago Press, 1991), pp. 43–4.

20. Mendelson and Crawford, *Women in Early Modern England*, pp. 149–50; The summary of the diary's contents is from Patricia Crawford, "The Construction and Experience of Maternity in Seventeenth-century England," in Valerie Fides, ed., *Women as Mothers in Pre-Industrial England: Essays in Memory of Dorothy McLaren* (London: Routledge, 1990), p. 19.

PART IV

SOCIAL AUTHORITY

CHAPTER FOURTEEN

"My Mother Musicke": Music and Early Modern Fantasies of Embodiment

Linda Phyllis Austern

[T]here are some who conceive in the soul more than in the body, what is proper for souls to conceive and bear. And what is proper? – Wisdom and virtue in general – to this class belong all creative poets, and those artists and craftsmen who are said to be inventive.

Plato, *The Symposium*

[C]raftsmen of Western art reveal better than anyone else the artist's debt to the maternal body and/or motherhood's entry into symbolic existence – that is, translibidinal jouissance, eroticism taken over by the language of art.
Julia Kristeva, *Motherhood According to Giovanni Bellini* (1975)

From the seminal ideas of Plato through feminist psychoanalytic philosophy, the Western mind has considered male creativity in mirror image to female procreation and maternal love. Aristotle and his followers had privileged masculinity and intellect above femaleness and the body, influencing philosophy, medicine, science, and theology for millennia thereafter. Yet metaphors for mental productivity continued to evoke the female bodily processes of conception, gestation, and lactation. Long before the early modern era, metaphysical creation had become signified by the maternal body in a myriad ways, her womb a place of transcendental growth and her breasts a site of nourishment for the spiritual faculties. "The bodies and the souls of all human beings are alike pregnant with their future progeny," proclaims the disembodied voice of Diotima through the lips of Socrates in Plato's *Symposium*, "and when we arrive at a certain age, our nature impels us to bring forth and propagate."[1] It is significant that even here, the woman's living, laboring body is banished in favor of her former pupil's, the descendent of her mind.

The artist in particular has long been considered to sublimate Woman's creative powers, compelled by the image of her body and the desires of his soul.

His quest for eternal beauty mingles eroticism and inventiveness as he seeks the
eternal and himself becomes divine:

> Whosoever, therefore, from his youth feels his soul pregnant with the conception
> of these excellences, is divine; and when due time arrives, desires to bring forth;
> and wandering about, he seeks the beautiful in which he may propagate what he
> has conceived.[2]

Based largely on a tradition of clothing abstract concepts in female flesh and on
the complexities of an ancient and medieval heritage that held the idealized
maternal body as an object of perfection, desire, and inspiration, the liberal
arts, including music, were embodied as nurturing women in literary and visual
depictions throughout early modern Europe. In such flesh, Music stood as
the passive conduit for male creative power, an embodied mother-lover, ever
virgin, ever fertile, the material vehicle for intellectual creativity and the milk
of inspiration. She was at once the untouched maiden "fitte to wedde mens
eares and heartes unto her," and "as pregnant as *Libia*[,] alwaies breeding some
new thing."[3] Daughter of God and Nature, she endowed her sons with the raw
material which their masters could help them form into high artifice.[4] She was
the mother who could never die, her lover-sons as fecund as herself with
intellectual progeny. Under her influence, musical instruments were likened to
hollow vessels awaiting the creative principle of metaphysical life, and music
soothed perturbations of body and soul like a mother's lullaby. In addition,
literate male composers and music theorists presented their creative products
as their children, and attributed to abstract, audible music the powers and
capacities most often ascribed to female caregivers. Like all idealized products
of a fertile imagination, the embodiment of early modern music in the form of a
sweetly nurturing woman bore only a superficial relationship to real women
and their daily struggles. Yet she has much to teach us about her era's
conceptions of nurture and creation.

Music, Maternity, and Nurturance

> The project invented or created, unwonted and new, emanates from a solitary
> head to illuminate and to comprehend. It dissolves into light and converts
> exteriority into idea. Whence we can define power as presence in a world that by
> right resolves itself into my ideas. But the encounter with the Other as feminine is
> required in order that the future of the child come to pass from beyond the
> possible, beyond projects.
>
> Emmanuel Levinas, *Totality and Infinity* (1979)

Early modern thought especially associated music with the female capacities
for creation and nurture for several reasons. Firstly, Christian Europe had
absorbed and expanded the Classical legacy of representing virtues, vices, and

abstract concepts as women. By the seventeenth century, an entire category of womanhood was reserved for such personifications. As the Puritan thinker John Wing explains in his exposition on women and marriage of 1632,

> The Booke of God maketh mention of *Women* of divers kinds, but all of them ... may be reduced to one of these heads, eyther the *Mysticall*, *Naturall*, or *Matrimoniall* Woman. The *Mysticall* Woman, is found in the Scriptures to be the embleme or representation of *good* and *evill*[.][5]

Although there is an essential difference between exegetical and allegorical traditions in the West, both contributed musical personifications which became driving intellectual forces and were treated as real and overlapping.[6] Within the Augustinian tradition, Eve, the mother of humanity, was associated with the invention and practice of the arts, just as knowing, feeling, and experiencing were located in the body; even today, an essential function of music is to reveal itself as hidden, and to entangle performers and auditors in a sensual embrace.[7] Within secular allegory, Musica had been embodied as a woman since antiquity, perhaps because of the Latin gender of the word. Not later than the fourteenth century, the female embodiment of Musica had also become associated with the Augustinian musical tradition. By the Reformation, Music was accounted Queen of Heaven as well as of the arts, and the figure of St. Cecilia came to embody the positive powers of music across sacred and secular contexts.[8]

Such allegories as Music continued to absorb the gendered attributes of their personifications until further concepts were actually produced.[9] As Musica became more feminine, considerations of her art acquired more womanly characteristics parallel to the Virtues and Vices. The negative aspects of music were subsumed within dangerous women; the unnatural predilections of the seductress and monstrous body of the siren especially served as warnings against the lure of auditory pleasure as both were accounted superb musicians.[10] In contrast, the positive, productive attributes of music were rendered yielding and maternal until beneficial music reflected these qualities in its most abstract form. Musical achievement thus joined a wider tradition in which creativity was not simply linked to gestation and birth, or an illuminating and ethereal "encounter with the Other as feminine." On the ultimate bases of Platonic philosophy and Aristotelian-Galenic medicine, it became conceptually linked to the defining materiality which enabled creation within the mother. The very Archetypal Feminine in Western thought has been considered the mysteriously creative vessel which brings forth the male in itself and from out of itself, which nourishes and protects within all bodies.[11] Music especially fits this abstract conceptual scheme, for it is an immaterial art which fills space with living resonance, and space has long been conceived as a woman in the West.[12] The composer, the performer, the theorist imposed form on passive matter as father on mother, seed in womb. Thus could the Swiss music theorist and humanist

Heinrich Glarean (1488–1563) present the poetic image of a lyre's swelling belly that conceals a thousand tones, awaiting the performer's plectrum.[13] In an era of fluid association between gender and sexual characteristics, this principle of action on passive materials of music also enabled the female musician to serve as the (male) agent acting on "empty guts of beasts, and hollow wood" to create music on her lute.[14] Similarly could the Franco–Flemish music theorist and composer Johannes Tinctoris (1446?–1511) explain that his treatise had gestated within him and been brought forth, and the Elizabethan publisher Joseph Barnes refer to a posthumous work as "an Orphan of one of Lady Musickes children."[15] The female element necessary for creation was unresisting, bodily, and contributed gestational space to the final product.

Secondly, and completely related, many of the positive capacities ascribed to music mirrored those of the early modern mother and caretaker of family and children. The powerful, productive aspect of music, that which was embodied as a good and loving woman, assumed and magnified her presumed aptitudes even as it took on her form. The primary duty of the early modern mother was the bearing and nurture of the young.[16] So too on Classical and Biblical authority did music nourish unformed minds and set them on the path toward virtue.[17] These parallel ideas particularly came together in the recognition of the power of lullabies to calm tiny nurslings, a virtue rooted, like motherhood itself, in nature rather than in artifice and special training. In the most famous words of Baldessare Castiglione's influential humanist courtesy manual

> nature hath taught [music] unto nurses for a speciall remedye to the contynuall waylings of sucking babes, which at the soun[d]e of their voice fall into a quiet and sweete sleepe, forgetting the teares that are so proper to them.[18]

Music was considered parent and guardian of morality, and a teacher of godliness. Both of these were duties widely ascribed to the early modern mother. She taught virtue and morality to her young charges in the home, whereas music was the "parent and guardian of public morals."[19] According to numerous early modern thinkers of both genders, a mother's highest duty was the early religious education of her children. Within several intellectual traditions, her gender was accorded an intense, natural propensity for simple devoutness of the sort most easily taught to the young. "And can any man blame a Mother (who indeede brought foorth her Childe with much paine) though she labour again till Christ be formed in them?," asks Dorothy Leigh in her much-reprinted *Mothers Blessing*.[20] Likewise, "No one science draweth neerer to the essence of God, then this of Musicke," the passionately moving art central to public and private Judeo-Christian worship.[21] These parallel ideas are beautifully united in Berny[e] Grymeston's comments on his mother's moral lessons, which he likens to the majesty of an organ's penetrating sound. Yet unlike the awful pipes of that instrument most associated with public worship, her grim keyboard strokes and sounds are softened by "the looks of [her] kind eies."[22]

The early modern woman of the middle classes and higher served as mentor and doctor to the community of her household, in which capacity she prepared cures, maintained supplies of food and medicinal herbs, and watched over the sick.[23] Like the mother and lady of the house, music healed, nourished languishing soul, and served as caretaker to those within its physical reach. For it was an art of secret sympathy with human body and soul, as with all forms of balance and harmony within the universe. Music was thus invoked to cure bodily imbalances, fever, and depressive disorders, to lull the sufferer into healing sleep or drive away his ills "as to entrance his paine, or cure his woe."[24] The powers of music to work between the visible and invisible aspects of the world were greater still. It sounded with the magnetic force of cosmic love, which it inspired in its mortal hearers. "Love is born from Music ... and ... never parts from her," explains Giorgio Vasari in description of an allegorical image.[25] On the ultimate authority of Plato, music was "a science of love matters occupied in harmony and rhythmos," bringing together in magical sympathy all pairs of loving elements.[26] Early modern mothers loved if anything excessively; tract after tract emphasizes their emotional bond with their children, their great affection. "There is nothing as the force of love; there is no love so forcible as the love of an affectionate mother to hir naturall childe," writes Elizabeth Grymeston to the same son who likened her heartfelt instructions to music.[27]

Thirdly, the natural sound and innate sensuousness of the mother's voice was recognized as an extraordinary influence on the development of her children. The female voice in general, with its perceived warmth and high register, exerted endless fascination for medieval and early modern thinkers. In an early seventeenth-century defense of women, the English writer William Austin links "beauty *Corporall* and *Vocall*" until the two merge and the voice "not only sets forth the [bodily] *forme*, but declares the disposition as well as the face." Woman thus becomes her voice. Significantly, voice follows breasts in this treatise as a source of erotic pleasure and nurture, and yields great "*Pleasure* and *Profit*," as if Austin retained an infant's memory of the dual sources of maternal comfort.[28] Where vision has long been associated with masculine privilege, hearing and vocality have been linked to women's interiority and irresistible invitation to comfort or seduction; the female body dissolves and is re-membered in music, or becomes eroticized as an ear.[29] The mouth of an unchaste woman is like an uncovered vagina, from which flows a siren's lubricious song or primal words of evil; it sings of deadly fruit. But the maternal voice still remains a thing of comfort and sweet dreams, an auditory caress of sublime, all-enveloping love and the remembered taste of true nourishment.

Early modern theories of perception emphasized the intimacy between the sounding body and the hearing body, the mutual action and affection between sentient thing and thing sensed.[30] Not only was the early modern woman responsible for setting the habits and patterns of speech in her children by the example of her own voice. They were, in turn, encouraged to make music from infancy, presumably first by her example.[31] Austin explains that, other than birds, women are the most innately musical creatures of the earthly realm, whose voices are gentle, tender, and "angel-like." "[F]rom *their voyce* men learne to frame *their owne*, to be understood of others," he explains,

> For in our infancy, we learne our language from them. Which men (therein not ingratefull) have justly termed our *Mother tongue*: but for the *Profits* and *Commodities* that proceed from *their Body* comitting the *pleasure* that it gives in their beauteous forme they are so great, that *Pliny* is *amazed* to write them, and holds them rather miracles than *effects of nature*[.][32]

Austin's sensuous language, rich with suppressed desire, reminds his readers that both music and the mother–child bond are held to be oceanic experiences, all-encompassing pleasures that close out the rest of the world.[33] His description moves fluidly between her singing and speaking voice, dissolving any difference between them. Developmentally, the child first locates the world through the sonorous envelope of the mother's sound and touch and smell. His or her first utterances imitate the mother's voice, which teaches both communication with, and separation from, the external world. Her voice, and her seemingly fragmented body centered on the breast, becomes the pleasurable milieu which sustains him and first arouses his sexuality.[34]

These forms of musical caregiving are brought together in numerous subtle ways in the era's compositions. Richard Edwardes's (1524–1566) song "Where Gripinge Grefes" (Ex. 14.1), most famously quoted in Act IV, scene v of William Shakespeare's *Romeo and Juliet*, presents an auditory portrait of a female Music who sweetly soothes all ailments of heart and mind with her versatile salve. The music is full of unexpected harmonic shifts, brief phrases, dissonant melodic leaps, and falling motives that suggest an unsettled psyche. But yet it resolves to consonant stability and a melodically higher pitch than its beginning, to demonstrate the efficacy and uplifting effect of Music's medicine. Its limited vocal range, frequent rests, predominantly one-note-per-syllable setting, and simple, imitative melodic structure render it particularly easy for untrained singers to follow, imitate, or anticipate each section. It is the easiest sort of melody to learn by ear, perhaps suggesting early auditory-vocal experience. Francis Pilkington's "Rest, sweet Nymphs" of 1605 (Ex. 14.2) gives the composer/narrator's lute the power to lull not just the title characters to whom the song is addressed, but also the hearer, into peaceful, contented rest. The music enhances the effect of the text by shifting into triple meter right after the soothing "lulla lullaby," and slowing down to elongated note-values to induce "calm contentment." In these ways do two male composers from the same country both represent and usurp the comforting, maternal powers of music.

Ex. 14.1   Richard Edwards's "Where Gripinge Grefes." Edited by Frederick Sternfeld
from *Songs from Shakespeare's Tragedies* © Oxford University Press, 1964.
Reproduced by permission

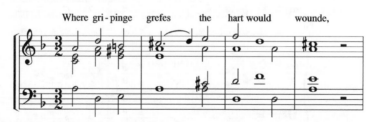

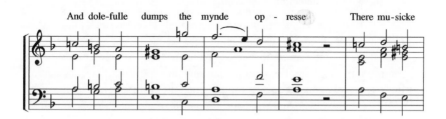

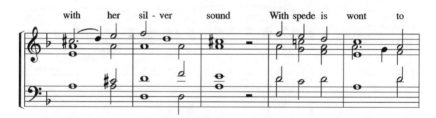

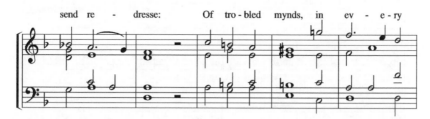

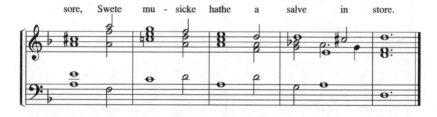

Ex. 14.2   Francis Pilkington's "Rest, sweet Nymphs," © 1922. Stainer and Bell Ltd, London, 1971

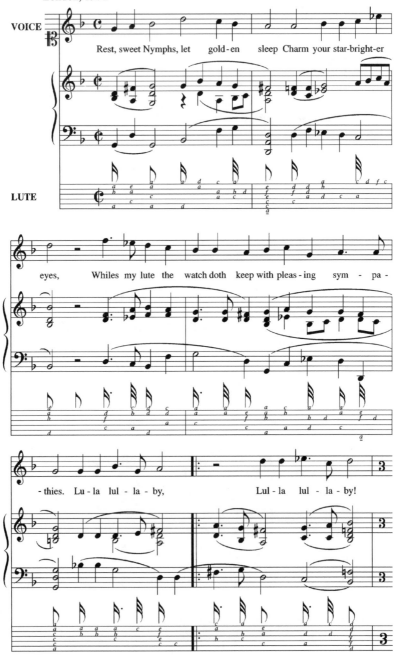

Ex. 14.2 concluded

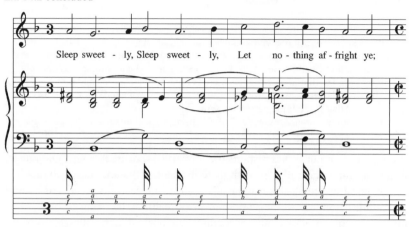

Sleep sweet - ly, Sleep sweet - ly, Let no - thing af - fright ye;

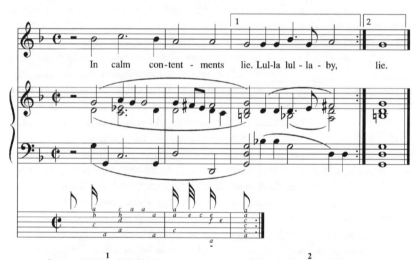

In calm con-tent - ments lie. Lul-la lul - la - by, lie.

1
Rest, sweet nymphs, let golden sleep
Charm your star-brighter eyes,
Whilst my lute the watch doth keep
With pleasing sympathies.
Lulla Lullaby!
Sleep sweetly,
Sleep sweetly,
Let nothing affright ye;
In calm contentments lie.

2
Dream, fair virgins, of delight
And blest Elysian groves,
Whiles the wandering shades of night
Resemble your true loves.
Lulla lullaby!
Your kisses,
Your blisses,
Send them your wishes
Although they be not nigh.

3
Thus, dear damsels, I do give
Goodnight, and so am gone.
With your heart's desires long live
Still joy and never mean.
Lulla lullaby!
Hath pleased you
And eased you,
And sweet slumber seized you
And now to bed I hie.

Mothers, Fathers, and Mastery

> [T]he artist's work is to shew us ourselves as we really are. Our minds are nothing but this knowledge of ourselves; and he who adds a jot to such knowledge creates new minds as surely as any woman creates new men. In the rage of that creation he is as ruthless as the woman, as dangerous to her as she to him, and as horribly fascinating. Of all human struggles there is none so treacherous and remorseless as the struggle between the artist man and the mother woman. Which shall use up the other? that is the issue between them.
>
> George Bernard Shaw, *Man and Superman: A Comedy and a Philosophy*
> (1901–3)

If the mother or nurse was responsible for early exposure to sound and music, formal training generally lay with male masters of the art. As Austin and his contemporaries emphasized, women's skill in music was considered natural and aural, belonging to the same transitory realm as the song of birds or of infancy itself. Parallel to the academic language of Latin, taught by stern masters with their rods and birches, the most vital intellectual skills of music were those of rules and writing. Literate composers and theorists of art-music learned from men to govern the unruly, ephemeral materials of their discipline to bring forth enduring products. The famous introductory passage to Thomas Morley's *Plaine and Easie Introduction to Practicall Musicke*, which presents music as a necessary skill for would-be gentlemen, emphasizes that what is vital is a combination of the abilities to "examine" and "confute" musical arguments through an understanding of learned theory, and the ability to read from a notated partbook.[35] These were not the "natural" skills of crooning nurses or the mother's lullaby. Socially elite amateur performers of both sexes, university men who studied music, professional minstrels from the guild and apprentice-ship systems, and those who learned music as an adjunct to liturgical training, usually studied with qualified masters in the relevant aspect of the art.[36]

Entry into the public world of professional discourse and disciplinary mastery in all fields took place in the years after maternal instruction. Formal education was often a male prerogative, and tended to be more limited for girls than for boys of the same social status. Most girls remained under the tutelage of their mothers, who taught them the survival skills necessary to their gender and class even when they received more formal schooling. Boys were sent to learn more advanced intellectual or pragmatic skills from men with special training, as befitting their class, rank, and professional expectations. During the sixteenth century, as the nuclear family became increasingly institutionalized, educational structures adopted its hierarchical patterns. In the home, children were subject to the wills of their parents, who enforced their utter subjection. In schools and places of apprenticeship, masters filled the patriarchal role as strict guide, disciplinarian, and ultimate authority.[37] Such pedagogues were responsible for the minds, souls, and bodies of their charges *in loco parentis*, and took over the role of enforcing authority through brutal corporeal punishment if need be.[38]

Not only was the father considered the more important parent biologically, but, because only maternity was ever certain, male contract for right over a child was vital. "The son is not only my work, like a poem or an object, nor is he my property," writes Emmanuel Levinas across historical time and metaphorical barriers, "Paternity is a relation with a stranger who while being Other ... *is* me."[39] Such cross-generational narcissism, with its dissolution of the boundary between creation and procreation, was particularly evident in the metaphysical father–son relation of early modern artists and intellectuals. The reciprocal love commanded between parent and child was reflected in the master–student bond, in which the stranger was truly a work of the self like a poem or an object. "There be two whose benefites to us can never be requited: God, and our parents," writes Thomas Morley in a dedication to his mentor William Byrd,

> the one for that he gave us a reasonable soule, the other for that of the[m] we have our beeing. To these the prince & (as *Cicero* tearmeth him) the God of the *Philosophers* added our maisters, as those by whose directions the faculties of the reasonable soule be stirred up to enter into contemplation, & searching of more then earthly things: whereby we obtaine a second being, more to be wished and much more durable the[n] that which any man since the worlds creatio[n] hath received of his parents ... The consideration of this hath moved me to publish these labors of mine under your name both to signifie unto the world, my thankfull mind: & also to notifie unto your selfe in some sort the entire love and unfained affection which I beare unto you.[40]

Morley's younger contemporary, Thomas Ravenscroft, refers to those who trained him at Gresham College, London, as "kinde nursing fathers" in a venerable metaphor of male nurturance.[41] Indeed, the music teacher became strongly equated with a figurative biological "father" in a widespread early modern musical discourse through which professional skill was passed on as an inheritance from master to pupil.[42]

But yet the mother was not entirely absent from this realm of the reasonable soul and its contemplative products. According to the complete metaphor for creativity, this durable second being, gift of the master, required a passive feminine presence. "The trace of the mother cannot be 'successfully' contained," writes Andrea Liss in a modern critique of the maternal body.[43] The place in which early modern men created enduring mind-children was not without the fantasy mother who could at once nurture, be nurtured, and arouse erotic desire like some sort of transitional object between the remembered comforts of their own childhood and the "more durable being" endowed by their masters. Modern developmental psychology acknowledges that boys who are cared for primarily by individuals other than their mothers tend to idealize her, and all children may first identify with the maternal body which nurtures them before boys learn to be boys and desire to possess and return to the mother.[44]

The embodied topos of Music as woman may have been especially appealing to musicians trained from a young age in a homosocial environment, particularly in Protestant countries whose church-related choir-schools had lost their Virgin Mother. Ravenscroft dutifully acknowledges his boyhood choir-master, Edward Pearce as "a man of singular eminency in *his Profession*" in the preface to his theoretical treatise of 1614. However, in the Apologie which precedes the work, he calls himself a "dutiful childe" to his "*Mother Musicke*." Master Pearce is presented as a powerful authority over his pupils and his materials, an expert teacher of voice and instrument, and a productive composer whose diverse and excellent "fruits can bear him witnesse." Mother Music, on the other hand, is a figure of passion and pathos, the body to Pearce's intellect. Where he is a real individual man, she is the imagined embodiment of the art which gave birth to his. Her son enjoys an oddly sadistic and erotic relationship with her, even as he becomes her savior; the boy desires and repudiates the absent mother. Ravenscroft's initial image, which opens the work, is borrowed from the pseudo-Plutarchian treatise *On Music*, which presents a comedian's verbal portrait of the body of Music "pitteously scourged and mangled" by composers who abuse her with unruly modern music. But Ravenscroft goes beyond his source, and lingers on how much she has been "dilacerated, dismembered, and disjoynted," and what his fellow musicians might find "if we did search into her whole *Body*." He finally speaks "as a dutiful childe to condole, and (to my power) to minister a Medicine to *Her* Maladies," using the capacities of his music to revive hers. His own creative abilities have progressed beyond hers, more like his (real) master-father's, by which he becomes able to "make knowne unto the world all her *Spurious* and Illegitimate *Children*, that doe thus unnaturally oppose themselves against *Her*."[45] Like any grown early modern son, he now becomes her caregiver. She is the raw material in whom his infant skills had gestated, but now, come to manhood and mastery, he has become superior. She is a fleshly fantasy of misogynist desire, the lost mother returned as abused daughter-lover in need of succor. One wonders about the visions of gender and sexuality inculcated by such imagery in the homosocial environment of such choir-schools as produced Ravenscroft.[46] Here indeed the artist-man has used up the mother-woman, usurped the qualities which he must give back to her. But this is the most violent of many stock images of Mother Musica. In contrast, for example, stands Lucas Cranach's "Fraw Musica," which opens Martin Agricola's German musical treatise of 1545 in the respectful tradition of Martin Luther (Fig. 14.1). Clad in exquisite garments and surrounded by the instruments of her craft, as described at length in the work, the title figure plays the lute and gazes coyly at the viewer. Above her hang numerous grapes from their leafy arbor, early modern signifiers of the paradox of virgin, wife and mother in one, and often associated with the Virgin.[47]

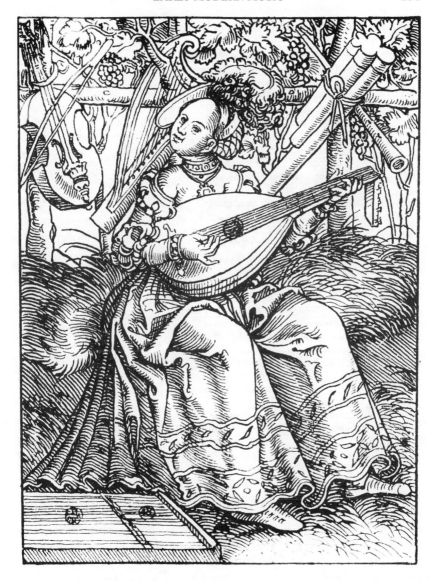

Fig. 14.1   Lucas Cranach, *Fraw Musica*, from *Musica Instrumentalis Deudsch* by
Martin Agricola, 1545

The Lady Musick: Fantasies of Embodiment

> Oh, it breaks my heart to see those stars
> Smashing a perfectly good guitar,
> I don't know who they think they are
> Smashing a perfectly good guitar.
> It started back in 1963,
> His mama wouldn't buy him that new red Harmony.
> He settled for a Sunburst with a crack,
> Now but he's still trying to break his mama's back.
> Oh, it breaks my heart to see those stars
> Smashing a perfectly good guitar,
> I don't know who they think they are
> Smashing a perfectly good guitar.
> He loved that guitar just like a girlfriend,
> But every good thing comes to an end,
> Now he just sits in his room all day,
> Whistling every note he ever played.
>   …
> Oh, it breaks my heart to see those stars
> Smashing a perfectly good guitar,
> I don't know who they think they are
> Smashing a perfectly good guitar.
> Late at night, the end of the road,
> He wishes he still had that old guitar to hold,
> He'd rock it like a baby in his arm,
> Never let it come to any harm.
> Oh, it breaks my heart to see those stars
> Smashing a perfectly good guitar,
> I don't know who they think they are
> Smashing a perfectly good guitar.
>
>   John Haitt, "Perfectly Good Guitar" (1994)

Images of Music as desirable or nurturing woman proliferated and become more portrait-like from the thirteenth century onward, following an increased self-awareness of "musician" as a profession, an increase in limits imposed on real women's participation in music, a fusion of the cult of the Virgin with the secular beloved of *amour courtois*, a proliferation of maternal imagery in medieval texts, and the greater focus on the erotic and the maternal in images of Mary.[48] Music as caregiver was particularly embodied in images that showed her in maternal poses with infantile figures, or emphasized her breasts. In such depictions, the feminine attributes of music as an agent of order and care blended with the maternal body until the two became almost inseparable. Filippino Lippi's famous allegory of the powers of music over eternity and the unseen world from the Strozzi Chapel in Santa Maria Novella, Florence (Fig. 14.2) presents the figure of a young woman in antique garments whose name suggests connections with the Virgin. An embodiment of the heavenly power of music who holds an antique lyre, she gently assists one babyish putto

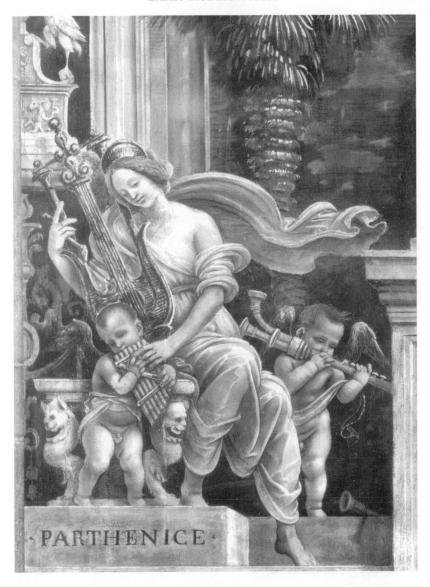

Fig. 14.2   Filippino Lippi, *Allegory of Music (Parthenice)*, Strozzi Chapel, Santa
Maria Novella, Florence (detail)

with a syrinx whose seven pipes allude to the seven planets and the harmony of the universe. His fellow likewise requires her instruction in order to play the fantastical wind instrument that he cannot manage on his own. The abstract world of eternal harmony setting the universe in motion is here embodied by motherly gesture that still remains virginal by its verbal signifer and the unearthly putti.[49]

Early modern family portraiture emphasized the comforting, harmonious effects of music by elevating the mother or the product of her chaste married love into a living image of Musica and her powers. Girolamo Forni's "Musical Family in the North of Italy" of 1600 (Fig. 14.3) presents the mother as an embodied "Lady Music," playing her lute much like Cranach's woodcut "Musica." The family patriarch at the center of the painting gestures toward her with his right hand. Her daughter, a future bride and mother, holds her notes in front of her, waiting for her own chance to maintain a household in harmonious care. Completing a diagonal line across the portrait sits the eldest woman in the lower left, holding a silent harp that could provide support for the lute in consort. A second lute points toward the group of women, its rounded belly visually suggesting the fecundity that clearly blesses the family. Gottfried von Wedig's portrait of "Gertrude Wintzler and her Daughters" of 1616 (Fig. 14.4) likewise presents the musical mother as representation of domestic harmony. She plays for her nine offspring on a harpsichord whose motto further emphasizes the salving role of music within the household: *Musica componit pellitque iram ardores*. Nicolaus Knupfer's mid-seventeenth century Dutch "Portrait of a Family," (Fig. 14.5) perhaps the artist's own, plays with this idea of feminine embodiment of music's nurturing capacities. In this case, where the family performs together "so d'ouden songen, so pipen de jongen" ("as the old ones sing, so pipe the young"). At the center, blowing on a tiny, high-pitched pipe, is revealed the baby daughter, bathed in light "like a little Venus in her dazzling childish nudity," the living product of the domestic concord symbolized and brought about through music.[50] An immature little Musica, she is a reminder of the music in love, and the love in music, the ultimate auditory gift of the art and the metaphor assigned to lovers. "The loved one – called a child or an animal – is also she who holds the highest note. Whose voice carries the farthest, the finest, the strongest," writes Julia Kristeva in an acoustic tribute to the power of productive love.[51]

Just as the maternal instinct has long been bound up in the breast, the early modern image of musical nurturance emphasized the same swelling mound. Like the belly, the breasts serve at once as a primary object of erotic fantasy and of perfect nourishment for the newborn. Like tears, breast-milk has long served as a metaphor for primal, non-linguistic communication, particularly associated with the power of the Virgin Mother.[52] In a culture that repeatedly emphasized the importance of breastfeeding in a myriad ways, human milk

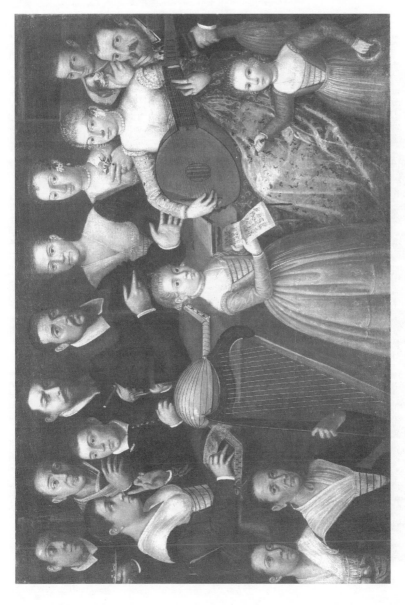

Fig. 14.3 Girolamo Forni, *Musical Family in the North of Italy (Portrait of a Family)*, 1600

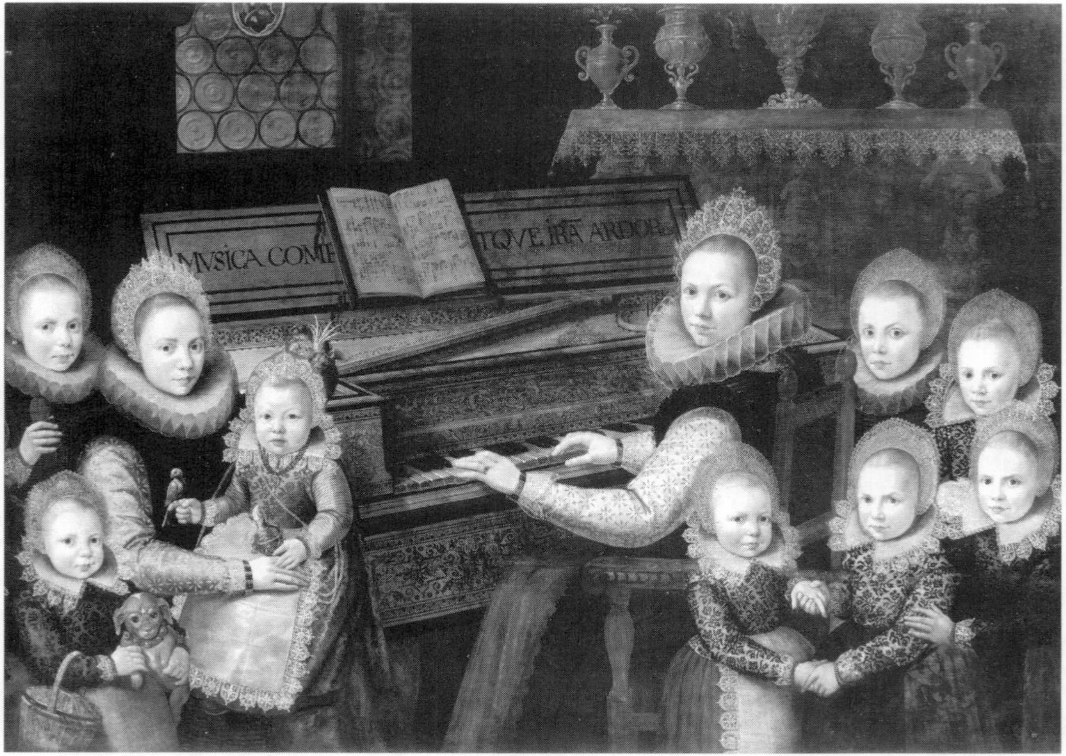

Fig. 14.4   Gottfried von Wedig, *Familie Christoph Wintzler (Gertrude Wintzler and her Daughters)*, 1616

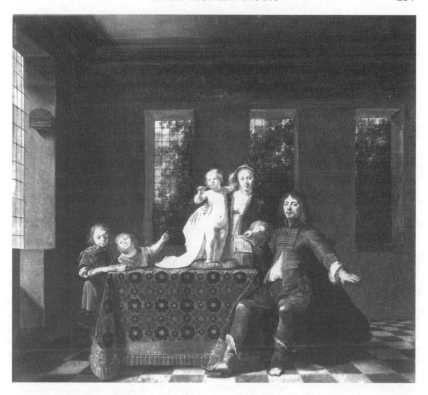

Fig. 14.5   Nicolaus Knüpfer, *Portrait of a Family*, c. 1650

took on its own miraculous powers. "[T]here is no *milke* (whatsoever) so *nourishing*, and cherishing in *effect*, nor *so sweet* and *honied* in *taste* as that of a *Woman*," writes William Austin,

> So that, seeing shee is compared in *Ecclesiasticus*, to a *possession*: and in the *Proverbs*, preferred before a *possession*: she may well be *likened* to that holy habitation and *possession*, (the land of *Promise*) hich *flowed with milke and hony*[.][53]

More importantly, "Moreover, from the *Milke* of the *Breasts*, proceeds not only nourishment to children, but *helpe* and *medicine*, both to the *eyes* and body of man: yea even to dumb and reasonlesse creatures."[54] With its association with non-linguistic communication, of which music is one sort, it is hardly surprising to find breastmilk linked to early modern musical creativity and inspiration; after all, Dante had presented the allegory of the muse inspiring the creative mind with her milk in *Purgatorio* XXII. Giulio Cesare Capaccio presents an image of the siren Parthenope, mythical founder of the city of

Naples when her body washed ashore after her ill-fated encounter with Ulysses, nourishing a "dumb and reasonlesse" lira as part of a metaphor for concord (Fig. 14.6).[55] This unusually benign siren, emblem of her city, squeezes milk from her full left breast, the one over her heart, onto the passive instrument, giving it her magical nourishment.

The most widely influential storehouse of visual imagery of the early modern era, Cesare Ripa's *Iconologia*, presents the most important representation of lactation in the service of music. Its emblem of Poesia reinforces the inseparability of music and poetry during his era by presenting the art as a beautiful young girl dressed in celestial blue, around whom either fly or are placed three young winged boys with musical instruments. Most importantly, "le mammelle piene di latte," the left bared in the woodcut that accompanies the text (Fig. 14.7), signify the fecundity of ideas and inventions which are the soul of poetry.[56] This emblem exerted an inestimable influence on allegories and musical portraiture for over a century and a half. An anonymous sixteenth-century Flemish allegory of inspiration (Fig. 14.8) shows the laurel-crowned woman expressing milk onto the lira which she hands to a downcast male musician. In Bernardo Strozzi's life-like portrait of an anonymous female musician (Fig. 14.9), whom Ellen Rosand has suggested might be the Venetian composer Barbara Strozzi (no relation), the subject clutches a bass viol and its bow in her left hand as a violin points outward toward the viewer, inviting him to grasp it and join her in a duet.[57] Her lush left breast spills over her bodice in obvious homage to Ripa's emblem, and she gazes boldly at the viewer. Laurent de la Hire's "Allegory of Music" of 1649 (Fig. 14.10) presents a neo-Classical musician tuning a theorbo, full left breast exposed above its curvature, and mirroring the rounded belly of the lute before her. Beside her right shoulder sits a tiny nightingale, borrowed from one of Ripa's emblematic descriptions of music and further linked to the same sensuous, instinctual realm as women's music.[58]

Perhaps the most eloquent and maternal of all of these images brings together several aspects of music as nurture. In Francois Boucher's "Allegory of Music" of 1764 (Fig. 14.11), the title figure, clad in soft blue draperies over a loose white shift, reclines in motherly repose with two chubby "young winged boys." The air-borne one proffers a recorder and holds a laurel-wreath. The other climbs on her knee not like a putto from a distant allegory, but like a baby, holding out a lyre as if to invite her to play for his delight. A pair of doves nestle against half-open roses and a music-book, cast in the same brilliant light that illuminates her bare left breast. A third one flutters beside the flying child. Opposite the tender tableau, in the lower left corner of the painting, lie the arms of Mars, discarded beneath a storm-cloud. These manly, destructive things have no place in this nurturing world of music. Here, Venus and the virgin mother merge to embody the beneficial, healing aspects of music, sweet salve for every

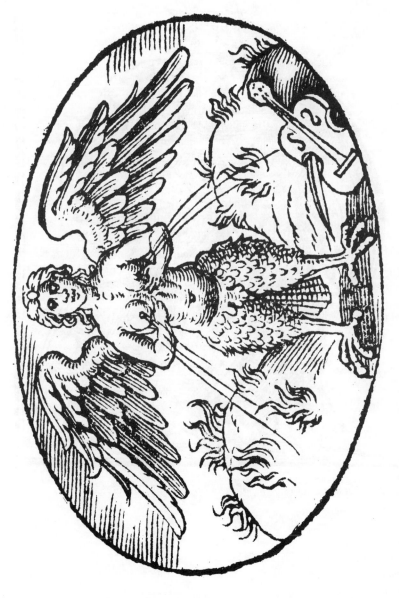

Fig. 14.6 *Parthenope* from *Delle imprese trattato* by Giulio Cesare Capaccio, fol. 23v

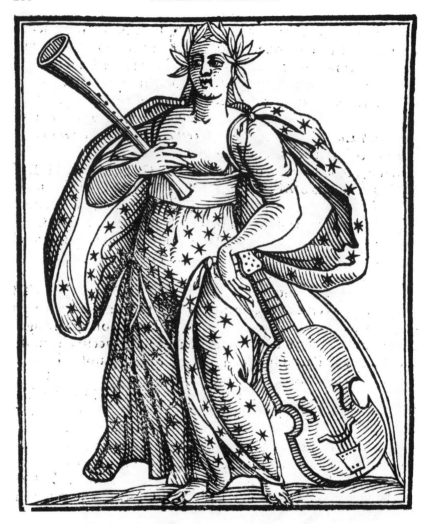

Fig. 14.7　*Poesia* from *Cesare Ripa, Della Novissima Iconologia*, page 519

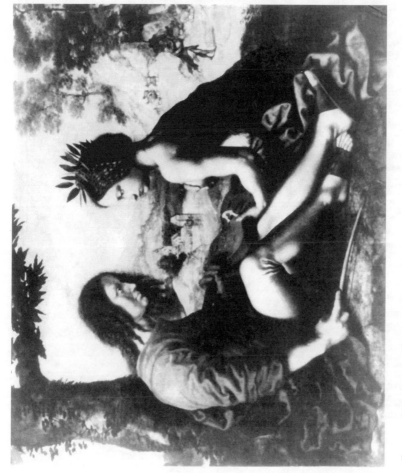

Fig. 14.8   Anon., *Allegory of Inspiration*, Flemish, 16th century

261

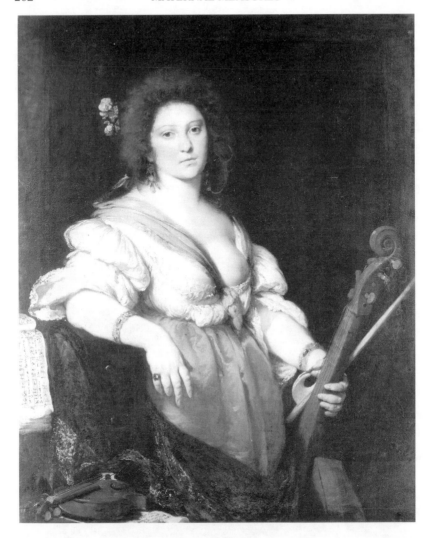

Fig. 14.9   Bernardo Strozzi, *Female Musician with Viola da Gamba*

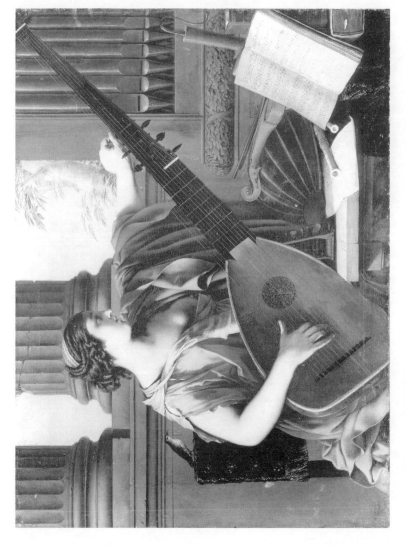

Fig. 14.10 Laurent de la Hire, *Allegory of Music*

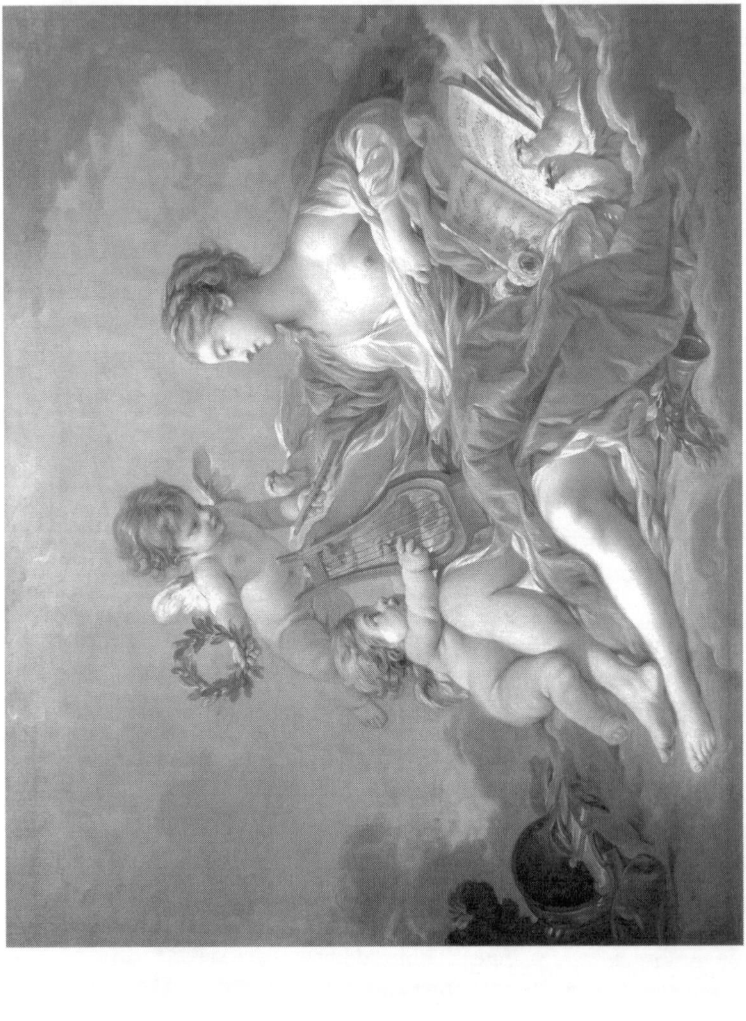

Fig. 14.11 François Boucher, *Allegory of Music*

mind. Like the mother's gentle touch or her nutritious milk, this music drives away all cares and envelops the listener in a warm cocoon of comfort.

Codetta

Might women have also enjoyed a more active role in this scheme of musical nurture than that afforded by still, silent, closed-mouthed imagery? Perhaps the answer lies in the underexplored fields of women's patronage, composition, and performance. A patroness provides a precise sort of protection and materiality to those who labor under her name, and certainly embodies her chosen art in a particular allegorical manner. And a woman performer or composer, breasts and womb a living duplicate of her metaphorical mother's, would have a far different relationship with the "milk of inspiration" than the sons of the art. She had not just the potential to be a harmonious source of order and comfort to her children like Elizabeth Grymeston or Gertrude Wintzler, but the physical capacity to be a mother, any mother. "[A] woman becoming a mother will be *the Mother*, totally identified with maternity," writes Luce Irigaray,

> She will be her mother and yet not her mother, nor her daughter as mother, *with no closure of the circle or the spiral of identity*. Endlessly encircling the speculum of a primal place. Passing from inside to outside without ever, simply, being resolved, resorbed, reflected. And with this extra turn, this extra return, this additional twist, both open and closed, imprinted by each new 'birth' – that is and is not identified with her mother, with maternity – she would no doubt be able to 'play' her role of mother without being totally assimilated by it. In this way provision would be made for the subsistence of her female sexual desire.[59]

In 1655, Barbara Strozzi (1619–after 1664) dedicated her collection of devotional songs for high solo voice to her patroness Anne of Austria (Anna de'Medici), Archduchess of Innsbruck. The collection opens with a work in honor of St. Anne, her patroness's namesake and the mother of the Virgin. Addressed not to "saint" Anne, or "most holy" Anne, but to "mother" Anne (Mater Anna), it serves as a reminder that images of the saint and her Daughter often emphasized the latter's debt to the former for her learning, or the idea that the raw material and means to achieve perfection is something conveyed by mother to daughter.[60] Strozzi's jubilant piece is of a sort often intended for domestic performance (Ex. 14.3). Published when she herself had become a mother four times over, it is full of rising melismas, harmonic and melodic changes of direction, ecstatic "extra turns" and "additional twists" before it returns not quite to its beginning.[61] It is a virtuostic vehicle for solo female voice, an invocation of the sweet, listening mother of the Mother to "hear us." It is also the creative vehicle of one made in the image of sacred and secular mothers all the way back through Mary to Eve, to her patroness, each linked in

Ex. 14.3   Barbara Strozzi, *I Sacri Musicali Affetti*. Da Capo Press, © 1988

A S. ANNA

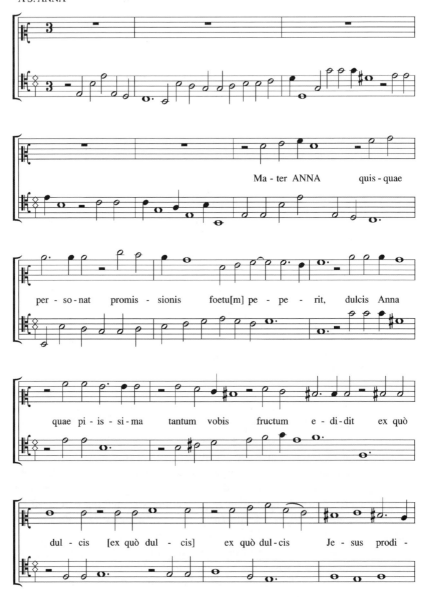

Ex. 14.3 continued

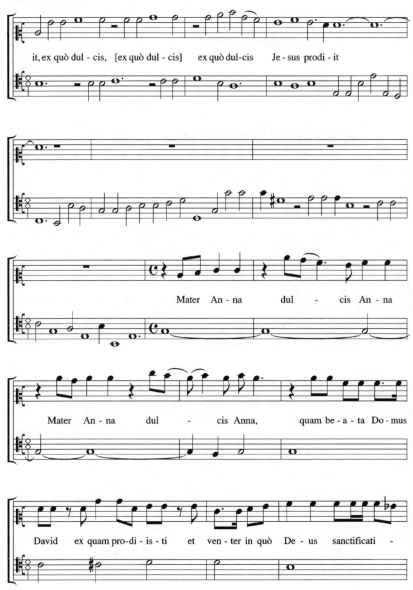

Ex. 14.3 continued

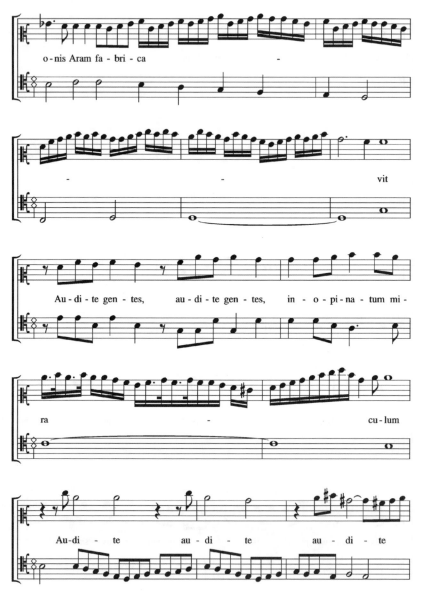

Ex. 14.3 continued

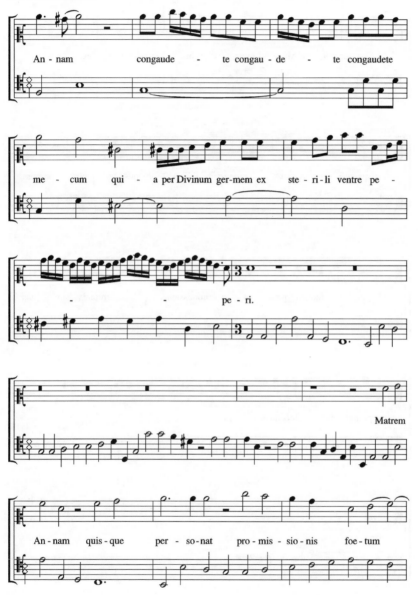

Ex. 14.3 continued

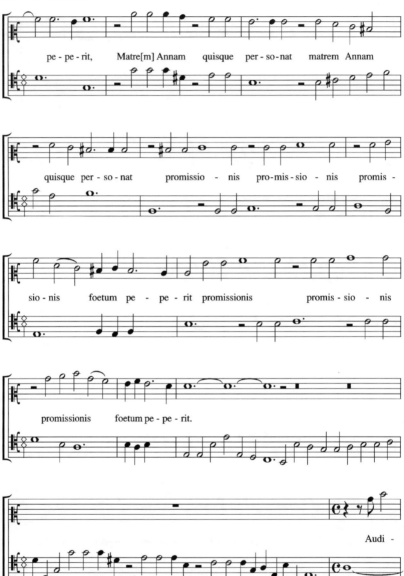

pe - pe - rit, Matre[m] Annam quisque per - so - nat matrem Annam

quisque per - so - nat promissio - nis pro-mis - sio - nis promis -

sio - nis foetum pe - pe - rit promissionis promis - sio - nis

promissionis foetum pe - pe - rit.

Audi -

Ex. 14.3 continued

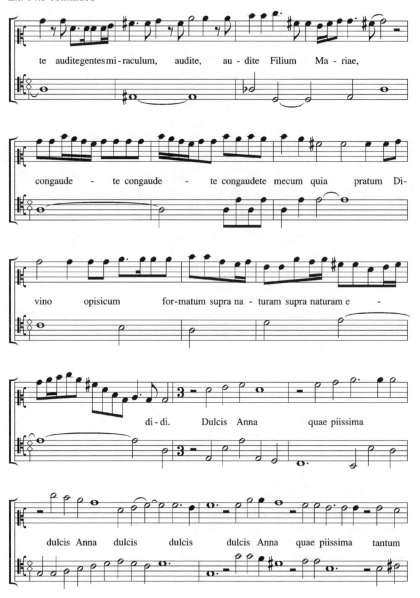

Ex. 14.3 continued

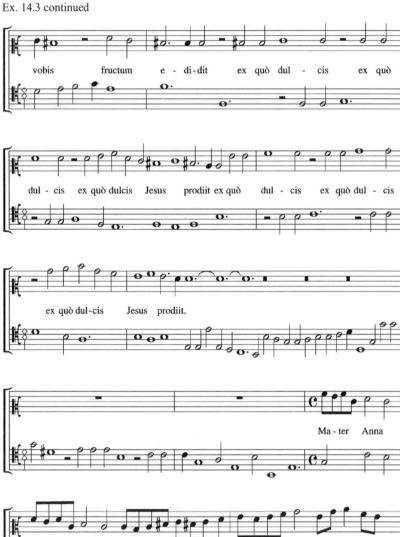

Ex. 14.3 continued

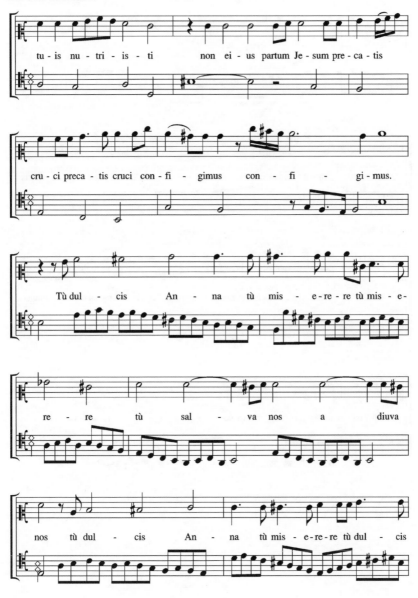

Ex. 14.3 concluded

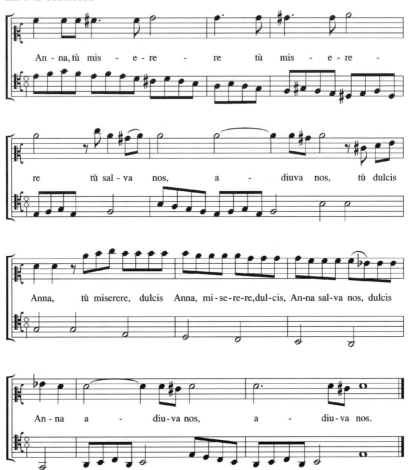

her own way to music. The skills of the artist-man have been subsumed by the mother-woman, the powers of music completely embodied in the form of the ultimate caregiver.

Notes

1. Plato, *The Banquet* [*Symposium*], transl. Percy Bysshe Shelley (Chicago: Way and Williams, 1895), p. 92.
2. Ibid., p. 99.
3. *The Praise of Musicke* (Oxenford: Joseph Barnes, 1586), pp. 3–4
4. John Case, *Apologia Musices* (Oxford: Joseph Barnes, 1588), sig. A4.
5. John Wing, *The Crowne Conjugall, or the Spouse Royal* (London: John Beale for Robert Mylbourne, 1632), pp. 28–9.
6. On this process of allegorization and exegesis in relation to the female body, see Joan M. Ferrante, *Woman as Image in Medieval Literature* (New York and London: Columbia University Press, 1975), p. 38.
7. See Roland Barthes, "The Grain of the Voice," in Barthes, *Image, Music, Text*, transl. Stephen Heath (New York: Farrar, Strauss, and Giroux, 1977), pp. 179–89; Caroline Bynum, "Why All the Fuss About the Body? A Medievalist's Perspective," *Critical Inquiry* 22 (Autumn 1995), pp. 13–14; Thomas Clifton, *Music as Heard: A Study in Applied Phenomenology* (New Haven and London: Yale University Press, 1983), p. 289; Sharon A. Farmer, "Introduction" to Paula M. Cooey, Sharon A. Farmer, and Mary Ellen Ross, eds., *Embodied Love: Sensuality and Relationship as Feminist Values* (San Francisco: Harper and Row, 1987) pp. 1–4; and David Summers, *The Judgment of Sense: Renaissance Naturalism and the Rise of Aesthetics* (Cambridge: Cambridge University Press, 1987), p. 247.
8. See Howard Mayer Brown, "St. Augustine, Lady Music, and the Gittern in Fourteenth-Century Italy," *Musica Disciplina* 38 (1984): 25–65; Thomas Connolly, *Mourning into Joy: Music, Raphael, and Saint Cecilia* (New Haven and London: Yale University Press, 1994), pp. 60–78 and 151–95; Sophie Drinker, *Music and Women* (New York: Coward-McCann, 1948; reprint ed., Washington, DC: Zenger Publishing Co., Inc., 1977), pp. 263–72; Robert Herrick, *Hesperides* (London: John Williams and Francis Eglesfield, 1648), p. 116; John Hilton, *Catch That Catch Can* (London: John Benson and John Playford, 1652), sig. A2; John Hollander, *The Untuning of the Sky* (Princeton: Princeton University Press, 1961), pp. 337; Richard Luckett, "St. Cecilia and Music," *Proceedings of the Royal Musical Association* 99 (1972–73), pp. 24–6; Kimberly Marshall, "Symbols, Performers, and Sponsors: Female Musical Creators in the Late Middle Ages," in Marshall, ed., *Rediscovering the Muses: Women's Musical Traditions* (Boston: Northeastern University Press, 1993), pp. 156–7; and Albert Pomme de Mirimonde, *Sainte-Cecile: métamorphoses d'un thème musical* (Geneve: Editions Minkoff, 1974), pp. 4–8.
9. See Ferrante, *Woman as Image in Medieval Literature*, pp. 18–35 and 42–3; and Gaytari C. Spivak, "Displacement and the Discourse of Woman," in M. Krupnick, ed., *Displacement: Derrida and After* (Bloomington: Indiana University Press, 1987), p. 169.
10. On several contrasting uses of this topos in early modern Europe, see Linda Phyllis Austern, "'Sing Again Siren': the Female Musician and Sexual Enchantment

in Elizabethan Life and Literature," *Renaissance Quarterly* (1989): 431–45; Suzanne Cusick, "Gendering Modern Music: Thoughts on the Monteverdi-Artusi Controversy," *Journal of the American Musicological Society* 46 (1993): 3–9; Richard Leppert, "Music, Representation, and the Social Order in Early Modern England," *Cultural Critique* (1989): 53–4; and Susan McClary, "Constructions of Gender in Monteverdi's Dramatic Music," in McClary, *Feminine Endings* (Minneapolis: University of Minnesota Press, 1991), pp. 39–46.

11. See Clarissa W. Atkinson, *The Oldest Vocation: Christian Motherhood in the Middle Ages* (Ithaca and London: Cornell University Press, 1991), pp. 29–30 and 238; Bynum, "Why All the Fuss About the Body," pp. 16–17; Bynum, *Jesus as Mother: Studies in the Spirituality of the High Middle Ages* (Berkeley and Los Angeles: University of California Press, 1982), pp. 115–16; Joseph Campbell, *The Hero With a Thousand Faces* (Princeton: Princeton University Press, 1942; 2nd edn., 1968), p. 113; Brenda O. Daly and Maureen T. Reddy, "Introduction: Narrating Mothers: Theorizing Maternal Subjectivities," in Brenda O. Daly and Maureeen T. Reddy, eds., *Narrating Mothers: Theorizing Maternal Subjectivities* (Koxville: University of Tennesee Press, 1991), p. 4; Ferrante, *Woman as Image in Medeival Literature*, pp. 19 and 41; Elizabeth Grosz, *Sexual Subversions: Three French Feminists* (New South Wales, Australia: Allen and Unwin, 1989), pp. 79–80; Julai Kristeva, "Stabat Mater," transl. Arthur Goldhammer, in Susan Rubin Suleiman, ed., *The Female Body in Western Culture* (Cambridge: Cambridge University Press, 1986), p. 100; Thomas Laqueur, *Making Sex: Body and Gender from the Greeks to Freud* (Cambridge, MA: Harvard University Press, 1990), pp. 29–30; Emmanuel Levinas, *Totality and Infinity: An Essay on Exteriority*, transl. by Alphonso Lingis (The Hague: Martinus Nijhoff Publishers, 1979), p. 267; Erich Neumann, *The Great Mother: An Analysis of the Archetype*, transl. Ralph Manheim (Princeton: Princeton University Press, 1955; 2nd edn., 1963), pp. 31–2 and 62–3; Mary O'Brien, *The Politics of Reproduction* (Boston and London: Routledge and Kegan Paul, 1981), p. 125; Plato, *Timaeus* in *Timaeus and Critias*, transl. A.E. Taylor (London: Methuen and Co., Ltd., 1929), pp. 49–50; and Shari L. Thurer, *The Myths of Motherhood: How Culture Reinvents the Good Mother* (Boston: Houghton Mifflin Company, 1994), pp. 102–6.

12. See Sue Best, "Sexualizing Space," in Elizabeth Grosz and Elspeth Probyn, eds., *Sexy Bodies: The Strange Carnalities of Feminism* (London and New York: Routledge, 1995), pp. 181–5; and Luce Irigaray, *Speculum of the Other Woman*, transl. Gillian C. Gill (Ithaca: Cornell University Press, 1985) p. 239.

13. Johannes Cochlaeus, *Tetrachordium Musices [1511]*, transl. Clement Miller (N.P.: American Institute of Musicology, 1970), p. 33; Heinrich Glarean, *Dodecachordon*, (N.P.: American Institute of Musicology, 1965), vol. 2, p. 286; and Henrici Glarean, *Isagoge in musice* [Basilae: N.P., 1516], sig. E3.

14. Robert Heath, *Clarastella* (London: Humph[rey] Moseley, 1650), p. 19. See also Humfrey Gifford, *A Posie of Gillowflowers* (London: John Perin, 1580), fol. 76^V; and Robert Herrick, *Hesperides* (London: John Williams and Francis Eglesfield, 1648), p. 115.

15. Johannes Tinctoris, *Concerning the nature and propriety of Tones (De Natura et Proprieatate Tonorum)*, transl. Albert Seay (Colorado Springs: Colorado College Music Press, 1967), pp. 1–2; and *The Praise of Musicke*, sig. *ij^V. See also Thomas Tomkins, *Songs of 3. 4. 5. and 6 Parts* (London: Matthew Lownes, John Browne and Thomas Snodham [1622]), Cantus partbook, sig. A2.

16. Atkinson, *The Oldest Vocation*, pp. 242–3; Patricia Crawford, "The Construction and Experience of of Maternity in Seventeenth-Century England," in Valerie

Fildes, ed., *Women and Mothers in Pre-Industrial England* (London and New York: Routledge, 1990), pp. 11–13; Coppelia Kahn, "The Absent Mother in *King Lear*," in Margaret W. Ferguson, Maureen Quilligan and Nancy J. Vickers, eds., *Rewriting the Renaissance: The Discourses of Sexual Difference in Early Modern Europe* (Chicago: University of Chicago Press, 1986) p. 39; and Lawrence Stone, "The Rise of the Nuclear Family in Early Modern England: The Patriarchal Stage," in Charles E. Rosenberg, ed., *The Family in History* (Philadelphia: University of Pennsylvania Press, 1975), p. 53.

17. Baldessare Castiglione, *The Courtyer*, transl. Thomas Hoby (London: Wyllyam Seres, 1561), sig. Jii^V; and Henry Peacham, *The Compleat Gentleman*, 2nd. edn. (London: Francis Constable, 1634), p. 98.

18. Castiglione, *The Courtyer*, sig. Jiii. See also *The Praise of Musicke*, pp. 42–3; and John Jones, *The Arte and Science of preserving Bodie and Soule in Health* (London: Henrie Bynneman, 1579), which discusses the most effective musical repertory for a nursing woman to sing to her charge.

19. Franchinus Gaffurius, *Practica musicae*, transl. Clement Miller (N.P.: American Institute of Musicology, 1968), pp. 14–15; Ruth Kelso, *Doctrine for the Lady of the Renaissance*, pp. 118–19 and 129; and Peacham, *The Compleat Gentleman*, p. 103.

20. Dorothy Leigh, *The Mother's Blessing*, 10th edn. (London: Robert Allott, 1627), p. 11. See also Hufton, *The Prospect Before Her*, pp. 208–9; Suzanne W. Hull, *Chaste, Silent and Obedient: English Books for Women 1475–1640* (San Marino, CA: Huntington Library, 1982), pp. 101–4; David Leverentz, *The Language of Puritan Feeling: An Exploration in Literature, Psychology and Social History* (New Brunswick, NJ: Rutgers University Press, 1980), p. 84; Maclean, *The Renaissance Notion of Woman*, pp. 59 and 64; Christopher Newstead, *An Apology for Women* (1620), as edited in Kate Aughterson, *Renaissance Woman: A Sourcebook* (London and New York: Routledge, 1995), p. 116; and Betty Travitsky, "The New Mother of the English Renaissance: Her Writings on Motherhood," in Cathy N. Davidson and E.M. Broner, eds., *The Lost Tradition: Mothers and Daughters in Literature* (New York: Frederick Ungar Publishing Co., 1980), pp. 37–40.

21. Nic[h]olas Yonge, *Musica Transalpina. The Second Booke of Madrigalles* (London: Thomas Este, 1597), Bassus partbook, sig. A2.

22. Berny Grymeston, "A Madrigal Upon the Conceipt of His Mother's Play to the Former Ditties," in Elizabeth Grymeston, *Miscelanea. Meditations. Memoratives.* (London: Melch. Bradwood for Felix Norton, 1604; reprint edn., London: George Elde for William Aspley [1608?]), sig. D2.

23. Hull, *Chaste, Silent and Obedient*, p. 36; and Mary Prior, Foreward to Prior, ed., *Women in English Society 1500–1800* (London and New York: Methuen, 1985), pp. 12–13.

24. Herrick, *Hesperides*, pp. 106–7. See also Castiglione, *The Courtyer*, sig. Jii; Gretchen L. Finney, "'Organical Music' and Ecstasy," *Journal of the History of Ideas* 8 (1947): 283; [relevant forthcoming essays in] Penelope Gouk, ed. *Musical Healing in Cultural Contexts* (Aldershot, Hants, England: Ashgate, 2000); Hollander, *The Untuning of the Sky*, pp. 266–72; *The Praise of Musicke*, p. 61; and Thomas Robinson, *The Schoole of Musicke* (London: Thomas Este for Simon Waterson, 1603), sig. B.

25. Giorgio Vasari, *Lives of the Most Eminent Painters, Sculptors, and Architechts*, transl. Gaston de Vere (London: Philip Lee Warner for the Medici Society, 1912–14), p. 240.

26. Thomas Morley, *A Plaine and Easie Introduction to Practicall Musicke* (London:

Peter Short, 1597), p. 195. See also Linda Phyllis Austern, "Musical Treatments for Lovesickness: The Early Modern Heritage," in Peregrine Horden, ed., *Music as Medicine* (Aldershot, Hants, England: Ashgate, 2000); William R. Bowen, "Love, the Master of all the Arts: Marsilio Ficino on Love and Music," in Kenneth R. Bartlett, Konrad Eisenbichler, and Janice Liedl, eds., *Love and Death in the Renaissance* (Ottawa: Dovehouse Editions, 1991), pp. 51–7; Hollander, *The Untuning of the Sky*, pp. 199–200; and Robin Headlam Wells, *Elizabethan Mythologies* (Cambridge: Cambridge University Press, 1994), pp. 83–4 and 170–75.

27. Elizabeth Grymeston, *Miscelanea. Meditations. Memoratives* , sig. A3. Dorothy Leigh further explains that "every man knowes that the love of a Mother to her children, is hardly contained within the bonds of reason," *The Mother's Blessing*, pp. 11–12. See also Crawford, "Construction of Maternity," pp. 27–8; Hufton, *The Prospect Before Her*, pp. 173, 193 and 208–9; Leverentz, *Puritan Feeling*, p. 85; and Newstead, *An Apology for Women*, p. 116.

28. William Austin, *Haec Homo, Wherein the Excellency of the Creation of Woman is Described* (London: Richard Olton for Ralph Mabb, 1637), pp. 125 and 132–3.

29. See Austern, "'Alluring the Auditorie to Effeminacie': Music and the Idea of the Feminine in Early Modern England," *Music and Letters* 74 (1993): 350–51; Henry Alden Bunker, Jr., "The Voice as (Female) Phallus," *The Psychoanalytic Quarterly* 3 (1934), p. 392; Chantal Chawaf, "Linguistic Flesh," transl. Yvonne Rochette-Ozello, in Elaine Marks and Isabelle de Courtivron, eds., *New French Feminisms* (Amherst: University of Massachusetts Press, 1980); pp. 177–8; Sharon A. Farmer, "'Softening the Hearts of Men: Women, Embodiment, and Persuasion in the Thirteenth Century," in Cooey *et al.*, eds., *Embodied Love*, pp. 115–6; Luce Irigaray, "The Fecundity of the Caress," in Richard A. Cohen, ed., *Face to Face with Levinas* (Albany: State University of New York Press, 1986), pp. 249–51; McClary, "Constructions of Gender in Monteverdi's Dramatic Music," pp. 38–9; Thomas Pavel, "In Praise of the Ear (Gloss's Glosses)," in Sulieman, ed., *The Female Body in Western Culture*, pp. 46–51; and John Shepherd, *Music as Social Text* (Cambridge: Polity Press, 1991), pp. 154–8.

30. See A.C. Crombie, "Theories of Perceiver and Perceived in Hearing," in Jean Céard, Marie-Madelaine Fontaine and Jean-Claude Margolin, eds., *Le Corps à la renaissance* (Paris: Aux Amateurs de Livres, 1990), pp. 382–7.

31. See Philippe Ariès, *Centuries of Childhood*, transl. Robert Baldick (London: Jonathan Cape, 1962), pp. 62–3 and 79–80; and Kelso, *Doctrine for the Lady of the Renaissance*, pp. 118–9.

32. Austin, *Haec Homo*, pp. 125, 126, and 133.

33. See Jessica Benjamin, "The Omnipotent Mother: A Psychoanalytic Study of Fantasy and Reality," in Donna Bassin, Margaret Honey and Meryle Mahrer Kaplan, eds., *Representations of Motherhood* (New Haven and London: Yale University Press, 1994), pp. 129–32; Thomas Clifton, *Music as Heard: A Study in Applied Phenomenology* (New Haven and London: Yale University Press, 1983), p. 289; Robin Maconie, *The Concept of Music* (Oxford: Clarendon Press, 1990), pp. 11–13; Guy Rosolato, *Essais sur le symbolique* (Paris: Gallimard, 1969), pp. 291–2; and David Schwartz, *Listening Subjects: Music, Psychoanalysis, Culture* (Durham and London: Duke University Press, 1997), pp. 7–8.

34. See Irigaray, "Fecundity of the Caress," pp. 248–9; Kristeva, "Stabat Mater," p. 108; Judith Roof, "'This is Not for You': The Sexuality of Mothering," in Daly *et al.*, *Narrating Mothers*, p. 159; Guy Rosolato, "La Voix: entre corps et language," *Revue Française de Psychanalyse* 38 (1974), p. 81; Schwartz, *Listening Subjects*,

pp. 7–8, 15–16, and 21; and Kaja Silverman, *The Acostic Mirror* (Bloomington: Indiana University Press, 1988), pp. 84–5.

35. Morley, *A Plaine and Easie Introduction to Practicall Musicke*, p. 1.

36. For further information on the diversity and patterns of the era's formal musical education, see Nan Cooke Carpenter, *Music in the Medieval and Renaissance Universities* (Norman: University of Oklahoma Press, 1958), pp, 128–371; Jane Flynn, "the Education of Choristers in England During the Sixteenth Century," in John Morehen, ed., *English Choral Practice 1400–1650* (Cambridge: Cambridge University Press, 1995), pp. 180–99; Kristine Forney, "'Nymphes gayes en abray du laurier': Musical Instruction for the Bourgeois Woman," *Musica Disciplina* 49 (1995), pp. 158–79; David G.T. Harris, "Musical Education in Tudor Times," *Proceedings of the Royal Musical Association* 65 (1938–39), pp. 109–40; and Jessie Ann Owens, *Composers at Work: The Craft of Musical Composition 1450–1600* (Oxford: Oxford University Press, 1997), pp. 11–33.

37. See Ariès, *Centuries of Childhood*, pp. 331 and 365–75; Crawford, "Construction of Maternity," p. 13; Hufton, *Prospect Before Her*, pp. 213–5; Ann Laurence, *Women in England 1500–1760: A Social History* (New York: St. Martin's Press, 1994), pp. 165–71; Stone, "Rise of the Nuclear Family," pp. 24–36 and 53–4; and Merry E. Wiesner, *Women and Gender in Early Modern Europe* (Cambridge: Cambridge University Press, 1993), pp. 100–106 and 117–32.

38. See Ariès, *Centuries of Childhood*, pp. 252–4 and 258–61; Hufton, *Prospect Before Her*, 207–8; and Stone, "Rise of the Nuclear Family," pp. 37–49. Some former schoolboys were so traumatized by excessive, brutal corporeal punishment by sadistic masters that they felt compelled to write of it later in graphic terms; see William Hornbye, *Hornbyes Hornbook* ([London:] Aug. Math. for Thomas Bayly, 1622), sigs. B7^V–C^V.

39. Levinas, *Totality and Infinity*, p. 277. See Crawford, "Construction of Maternity," pp. 27–8; and Carole Pateman, *The Sexual Contract* (Stanford: Stanford University Press, 1988), p. 217.

40. Morley, *A Plaine and Easie Introduction to Practicall Musicke*, sig. A. For comparison to the construction of reciprocal parental love, see also William Gouge, *Of Domesticall Duties* (London: John Haviland for William Bladen, 1622), pp. 429–30.

41. Thomas Ravenscroft, *A Briefe Discourse of the true (but neglected) use of Charact'ring the Degrees* (London:Edw[ard] Allde for Thomas Adams, 1614), sig. q2^V. See also Bynum, *Jesus as Mother*, pp. 114–20; and Debora Kuller Shuger, *Habits of Thought in the English Renaissance* (Berkeley and Los Angeles: University of California Press, 1990), pp. 220–27

42. See Paula Higgins, "Musical 'Parents' and Their 'Progeny': The Discourse of Creative Patriarchy in Early Modern Europe," in Jessie Ann Owens and Anthony Cummings, eds., *Music in Renaissance Cities and Courts: Studies in Honor of Lewis Lockwood* (Michigan: Harmonie Park Press, 1997), pp. 170–85.

43. Andrea Liss, "The Body in Question: Rethinking Motherhood, Alterity and Desire," in Joanna Frueh, Cassandra L. Langer, and Arlene Raven, eds., *New Feminist Criticism: Art, Identity, Action* (New York: HarperCollins, 1994), p. 94.

44. See Ann Dally, *Inventing Motherhood: The Consequences of an Ideal* (New York: Schocken Books, 1983), p. 93; Irigaray, *Speculum of the Other Woman*, pp. 40–41; and Eve Feder Kittay, "Womb Envy: An Explanatory Concept," in Joyce Trebilcot, ed., *Mothering: Essays in Feminist Theory* (Totowa, NJ: Rowman and Allanheld, 1984), pp. 94–7 and 100–110.

45. Thomas Ravenscroft, *A Briefe Discourse of the true (but neglected) use of*

Charact'ring the Degrees (London:Edw[ard] Allde for Thomas Adams, 1614), sigs. q4–q4^V and A2–A2^V. See also Andrew Barker, ed., *Greek Musical Writings, Volume I. The Musician and His Art* (Cambridge: Cambridge University Press, 1984), pp. 93–7, 205 and 236–7; and Plutarch, *The Philosophie, Commonly Called, The Morals*, transl. Philemon Holland (London: Arnold Hatfield, 1603), pp. 1248 and 1257–8.

46. For information on the sort of training Ravenscroft received, see Linda Phyllis Austern, "Thomas Ravenscroft: Musical Chronicler of an Elizabethan Theater Company," *Journal of the American Musicological Society* 38 (1985), pp. 241–6; Flynn, "The Education of Choristers in England During the Sixteenth Century," pp. 180–99; and Michael F. McDonnel, *A History of St. Paul's School* (London: Chapman and Hall, 1909), pp. 20 and 29–31.

47. Martinum Argicolum, *Musica Instrumentalis Deudsch* (Wittemberg: Georg Rhaw, 1545). See also Luckett, "St. Cecilia and Music," pp. 24–5; and Edy de Jongh, "Grape Symbolism in the Paintings of the Sixteenth and Seventeenth Centuries," *Simiolus* 7 (1974), pp. 174–7 and 185–90.

48. See Bynum, *Jesus as Mother*, pp. 138–9; Marshall, "Symbols, Performers, and Sponsors," pp. 142–3; Tilman Seebass, "Lady Music and her *Protégés* From Musical Allegory to Musician's Portraits," *Musica Disciplina* 42 (1988): 23–61; and Thurer, *Myths of Motherhood*, pp. 109–13.

49. For an analysis of the musical meaning of this image and the iconography of the wall on which it appears, see Emanuel Winternitz, *Musical Instruments and Their Symbolism in Western Art* (London: Faber and Faber Ltd, 1967), pp. 166–81.

50. See Pieter Fischer, "Music in Paintings of the the Low Countries in the Sixteenth and Seventeenth Centuries," *Sonorum Speculum* 50/51 (1972): 112–4.

51. Irigaray, "Fecundity of the Caress," p. 248.

52. Françoise Borin, "Judging by Images," transl. Arthur Goldhammer, in Natalie Zemon Davis and Arlette Farge, eds., *A History of Women in the West, Volume III: Renaissance and Enlightenment Paradoxes* (Cambridge, MA: Harvard University Press, 1993), pp. 204–10; and Kristeva, "Stabat Mater," 109.

53. Austin, *Haec Homo*, p. 122.

54. Ibid., p. 135. For further information on the deep psycho-cultural roots this sort of magical attribution to human milk, see Mary Douglas, *Purity and Danger: An Analysis of the Concepts of Pollution and Taboo* (London: Routledge and Kegan Paul, 1966; reprint edn., 1980), pp. 120–21.

55. Giulio Cesare Capaccio, *Delle impresse trattato* (Napoli: Gio. Carlino & Antonio Pace, 1592), fol. 23^V.

56. Cesare Ripa, *Novissima iconologia* (Padova: Donato Pasquardi, 1630), pp. 518–9. For further information on the wealth of musical imagery included in this work, see Nicoletta Guidobaldi, "Images of Music in Cesare Ripa's *Iconologia*," *Imago Musicae* 7 (1990): 41–68, which mysteriously omits the importance of the breasts in this image. The large-breasted figure was associated with fertility, piety, credulity and other maternal attributes from the Middle Ages on; see Danielle Jacquart and Claude Thomasset, *Sexuality and Medicine in the Middle Ages*, transl. Matthew Adamson (Princeton: Princeton University Press, 1988) pp. 143–4.

57. Ellen Rosand, "The Voice of Barbara Strozzi," in Jane Bowers and Judith Tick, eds., *Women Making Music: The Western Art Tradition* (Urbana and Chicago: University of Illinois Press, 1986), pp. 184–5. See also Beth Glixon, "New Light on the Life and Career of Barbara Strozzi," *The Musical Quarterly* 81 (1997), p. 322.

58. See Linda Phyllis Austern, "Nature, Culture, Myth, and the Musician in Early Modern England," *Journal of the American Musicological Society* 51 (1998): 18–24; and Ripa, *Novissima iconologia*, pp. 501–2.

59. Irigaray, *Speculum of the Other Woman*, p. 76.

60. Hufton, *The Prospect Before Her*, p. 212.

61. For information concerning Strozzi and her children, see Glixon, "New Light on the Life and Career of Barbara Strozzi," pp. 319–20.

CHAPTER FIFTEEN

Marian Devotion and Maternal Authority in Seventeenth-Century England

Frances E. Dolan

Many seventeenth-century English writers, Protestant and Catholic, male and female, defended or attacked Mariolatry as a central practice in English Catholicism, as a paradigmatic example of where Catholics invested power and directed adoration, and as a telling analogy to the distribution of power in the Caroline court and in recusant households. They thereby contested women's authority as mothers as much as they did the Virgin Mary's claims on devotion. The Madonna who stands at the center of these debates, while powerful and controversial, does not stand alone. Her relationships, to God the father, and especially to Jesus, are at issue. As described by attackers and defenders alike, she cradles an infant Jesus in her arms, and she stands between believers and their God.

While Protestant writers tend to assume that women should be humble handmaidens, and that a woman elevated to the Virgin Mary's position in Catholic worship, is, of necessity, proud, ambitious, vengeful, and bossy, Catholic writers are less resistant to the very idea of female power. "Great is the force undoubtedly of the mother of God; who not only was and is able to combate with the devil, but to crush him, & domineere over him, as over a poor worme," writes Robert Chambers.[1] Chambers also interprets Mary's response to the annunciation, "fiat," or "let it be," not as submission, but as an assertion of agency equal to God's creation of the world: "By his *Fiat*, he made the world and man, by her Fiat, God entred into the world, and became man."[2]

These debates over Mary's merits, like the medieval and early Reformation discussions that anticipated them and have received more attention, had mixed results for women. Members of Mary's cult amplify her power and exalt her status, but they do so by distinguishing her from other women. With the author of *The Widdowes Mite*, a devotional treatise, they insist that she did not deliver

Jesus "after the same laborious, vulgar, and uncomly manner to which other women are subject by their descendence from Eve."[3] Indeed, many join Thomas Price in condemning any assertion "that Mary the Mother of Christ is no better than other women."[4] Protestant writers seeking to deflate her status insist that while she may have been "advanced ... above all other women," as Andrew Willet concedes, she remained a woman like other women in most respects.[5] They repeatedly point to the paucity of scriptural reference to Mary, and, particularly, to the lack of any scriptural foundation for Mary's "immaculate conception" (which would have distinguished her as the only human conceived after the fall without original sin) or for her "assumption" (which would have distinguished her as the only human assumed directly into heaven, without undergoing corporeal decay, or a separation of soul from body, perhaps without undergoing bodily death).[6] Both sides in the debate, then, view Mary's resemblance to other women as a disparagement, a "foule comparison," as John Floyd says, which serves Protestant, but not Catholic, purposes.[7] Although Mary seems to offer an unattainable ideal to other women,[8] mothers might find in the Virgin a model of their own importance and influence, if not of their bodily experience of intercourse, pregnancy, and labor; they might also turn to her for succor in childbed.[9]

Whether or not Mary is viewed as a remarkable exception, the sustained and passionate public debate over her status in seventeenth-century England did not take place in a vacuum, remote from other contests over women's authority and agency, or from historical women. Because many writers weighed in both pro and con, and over many decades, this debate offered one popular discursive site for a more general discussion of female authority and influence. The stature of Mary in Catholic belief and practice, proof of the excessive power Catholics were willing to invest in women, served as a starting point for attacks on actual Catholic women, such as Henrietta Maria; it also informed Protestant, mainstream assumptions about and responses to Catholic women, especially mothers.[10]

The fear of, fascination with, and hostility toward maternal power in early modern English culture motivated attempts to understand and control, even repudiate it in medical treatises about reproduction, prescriptive writings on breastfeeding and other maternal conduct, legal constructions of infanticide, and witchcraft discourses and prosecutions. These discursive contests never corresponded neatly with women's actual experience of maternity, or their lived opportunities to exercise maternal authority. Nor were the constructions of maternal power consistent, even at a given site. Instead, across a strikingly wide range of locations and genres, early modern English culture fiercely debated the extent and value of maternal authority. The varied perspectives available demonstrate that, as Mary Beth Rose has argued, in sixteenth- and seventeenth-century England, "motherhood was very slowly beginning to be construed as a problematic status, and that the perceived conflicts center on parental power and authority."[11] Discussions of the Virgin Mary's apparently exceptional status participate in this more widespread construction of maternal power as a problem.

Addressing three crucial, and controversial, stages in a mother's relationship to her child – pregnancy, lactation, and adulthood (the most troublesome) – attacks on and defenses of Mary suggest that the problems begin in her blessedly fruitful womb. Certainly, Mary's situation is extraordinary; during her miraculous pregnancy, conceived without sexual intercourse, she contained and nurtured within her body "him whome Heaven cannot containe." According to *The Widdowes Mite*, Mary is not only the woman cloathed by the sun "but [she] didst also cloath the Sunne of Justice, whilest [her] immaculate flesh and bloud was imparted to the Sonne of [her] womb."[12] Three-dimensional images of Mary that opened to reveal an infant, or a crucifix, or the Trinity in their bellies reflect the frank Catholic acceptance of Mary's role as corporeal enclosure, and Jesus's status as son "covert."[13] Yet Mary's pregnancy, however unusual, reveals that motherhood always embodies "coverture" at its most literal; the mother of a son, let alone the son of God, inverts the expected operations of coverture in particularly threatening ways. Whereas, on the one hand, *The Lawes Resolutions of Womens Rights* describes a wife or feme covert as "veiled, as it were, clouded and overshadowed," *The Widdowes Mite*, on the other hand, explains that, during Mary's conception and gestation of her son, "the vertue or power of the most High was to environe, and overshaddow her, whereby she might be enabled to enclose, and as it were again to overshaddow the Sonne of God."[14] Thus, during pregnancy, Mary, like other mothers, "overshadows," covers, or subsumes her fetal son. The Holy Spirit must first "overshadow" her to empower her to do so, as a wife must submit to her husband before she gains her status as wife and mother. Yet under the cover of these enabling, to a large extent conceptual subsumptions, the mother then engages in a concrete subsumption of the unborn son which reverses and undermines the gender hierarchy on which marriage (and Christian theology) depend.

When Mary's attackers describe the errors of Marian devotion, they use quite similar imagery, although they interpret it differently. From their perspective, Mary also "overshaddows" Jesus, but the result is an apocalyptic eclipse. As *The Widdowes Mite* presents this Protestant view, Mary "sinned by exceeding her boundes, and by intruding her selfe so far, as that she might chance to have obscured the glory of Christ thereby."[15] William Crashaw suggests that *The Widdowes Mite* did not overstate the case when he warns that "wee must take heede we so inlarge not the excellencie of the Mother, that wee diminish the glorie of the sonne."[16] Here, as in so many prescriptions for household order and marital harmony, mother and son, like husband and wife or master and servant, compete for a finite amount of power; as a consequence, to enlarge the mother is, of necessity, to diminish the son. Descriptions of Mary as a vessel attempt to redress this maternal empowerment and inverse coverture. If Mary encloses and overshadows Jesus, she does so only temporarily, serving rather than subordinating him. When he exits her body, he leaves no residue of the divine. As *The Widdowes Mite* complains, such arguments treat the Virgin as "a saffron bagge" which is of no value once its precious contents are gone.[17] This counters a more disturbing possibility: that Mary is not a vessel, but a parthenogenetic mother who does not need a human father. As Anthony Stafford marvels in *The Femall Glory*, "it is a miracle that in the forming of such, and so great an issue [Jesus] the aide of man should be utterly excluded, and that as he was man, he was onely made of the pure bloud of the Virgin."[18]

Such opposing interpretations of Mary's contribution to Jesus' incarnation – as "saffron bagge" or sole human creator – participate in discussions of whether Mary is a vessel or an efficient cause. The subtle distinctions between Catholic and Protestant positions on this issue reveal that both sides operate within the same theological logic – which subordinates human initiative to divine providence – and the same ideological logic – which particularly constrains women's capacity for effectively and positively intervening in history. Yet there is a crucial difference. In however qualified a way, Catholic writers attribute efficacy to Mary, while Protestant writers vehemently deny it. Protestant attacks on Mariolatry insist that Mary simply cannot contribute as well as submit to the processes of incarnation and redemption, because, as Willet declares, "Christ onelie was the efficient cause and meritorious worker of our redemption, the Virgin *Marie* was a chosen vessell and instrument only of his holy incarnation."[19] George Hickes concurs that Mary is "a chosen vessel, but nevertheless a woman, who hath not changed her nature."[20] Since she is like other women, a fallen creature, she does not deserve to be worshipped as a creator, an "efficient cause," a goddess.

Obviously, those Catholic writers who exalt Mary's power always emphasize that God confers it on her, that it is a reward to her for her service, and that she acts as God's agent. But they emphasize the operation of Mary's will, and the extent of her powers, rather than her humility. Answering the Protestant charge that Mary may be praised only "as an instrument ... not ... as an agent," Catholic defenders of Mary concede her instrumentality while yet attempting to infuse it with agency.[21] *The Widdowes Mite* explains that God "is the fountaine, she is the streame; he is the great Artificer and primary cause, and she a most elevated Instrument; he is the Sunne, and she the Beame, whereby he hath communicated his light, and heat to this darke & frozen world of ours."[22] The imagery here resembles explanations of the relationship between husband and wife, in which the husband is the "*primus motor*," and the wife the tributary who submerges herself in the larger river, thus losing her separate identity.[23]

This passage also offers a variation on the sun and moon analogy so prevalent in prescriptions for marriage. Here Mary is not the moon, borrowing her light from the sun, but a part of the sun itself, its beam. By describing Mary as a beam and an "elevated Instrument," this text can confer some efficacy on her without positioning her as God's equal or rival.

Furthermore, Mary's defenders insist that she deserves credit for her role in Christ's incarnation because she freely consented to serve. According to *The Widdowes Mite*, "our B. Lady did whatsoever she did with perfect liberty of will, though prevented [i.e., anticipated] and assisted by the rich grace of God, to the very last point whereof, she did most eminently cooperate as a most elevated, active, and lively instrument; and was not of no more use unto her selfe then a very stocke, or stone could be."[24] According to this Catholic view, although Mary may be represented by "a very stocke, or stone," she was an "active and lively instrument," that is, both agent and instrument, cause and vessel, in the processes of incarnation and redemption. As a consequence, according to Catholic belief, the images of Mary might borrow some of this efficacy, channeling Mary's own power in order to work miracles in the contemporary world.

Descriptions of miracles enacted by images of Mary seem to have inspired many of the most vituperative denunciations of Mariolatry. In accounts of these miracles, Mary's status as symbolic representation and effective agent conjoin disturbingly, for, in the miracle-working images, symbolic preeminence becomes agency. Images of Mary made of "stock or stone" reinforce her connection to materiality, the flesh, the mortal, the transient; for most Protestant writers, these associations conjoin with feminine gender to disparage Mary, proving that she is a human creature of the earth, not a goddess or creator in heaven, that she is associated with the lowly flesh, not the transcendent spirit. But images that are simultaneously passive matter and miraculously agential confuse that neat hierarchy. Associated with the material world, these images may yet intervene in and change it. "Marionettes" seem to have derived their name from the "little Mary" or automated figure of Mary in creche scenes, suggesting how closely connected Mary was to animate images which disturbed the distinction between passivity and action, body and spirit.[25]

Protestant attacks on Mary's miraculous images draw on a tradition, fully developed and widely deployed in early modern England, which denigrates women's agency by associating or conflating it with violence. One particularly virulent attack on Marian devotion, William Crashaw's *The Jesuites Gospell* (published in 1610 and 1621, then in 1641 as *The Bespotted Jesuite*), insists that Catholics believe that "all the miracles must be wrought by her, and at her picture, as though either he [Jesus] could not, or in his mothers presence would not" work miracles himself. In response, John Floyd jests that Crashaw "might add with as great truth, that we say that he [Jesus] dare not, for shee

being a *shrew*, would rappe him on the fingers, did he stretch out his hand
to do any Myracle before her."[26] Floyd's joke – that Crashaw depicts the
"commaunding mother" Mary as a "shrew" – is an astute one. As in the vast
range of depictions of shrews in medieval and early modern discourses,
Crashaw's ridicule of Marian devotion assumes that women's exercise of
power is invariably presumptuous, arbitrary, and laughable. There is something
funny about a bossy woman, even when she is God's mother. As Floyd intuits,
this comic tradition for exaggerating, censuring, and mocking women's
exercise of authority also links their self-assertions to violence. The Virgin
tenderly nursing her baby might "rappe him on the fingers" at any moment.

One of Crashaw's defenders, Sir Edward Hoby, shares this assumption that
female authority erupts into violence. In Hoby's dialogue, *A Curry-Combe
for a Coxe-Combe*, one interlocutor, a minister, refers to Our Lady of Halle, a
purportedly vengeful image, as "a hard-hearted Saint." Remarking on the claim
that the Virgin Mary repaid iconoclasts with the same mutilations they inflicted
on her, he scoffs: "I never heard before that a milde Ladie did cut off so manie
Gentlemen's noses." If images are so vengeful (and powerful), he wonders,
how did it come to pass "when Popish Idols were suppressed in *England*, that
no man lost his nose, nor received any harme, though many such wooden
Ladies then lost their heades?"[27] In Hoby's analysis, as in depictions of shrews'
violence in ballads, jokes, and other popular discourses, the woman's violence
reveals that she does not deserve power, and that she will abuse whatever power
she usurps; her violence does little lasting damage to anything other than her
own credibility and authority.

While women's violence was usually depicted in these terms, it might also
be understood positively. Mothers, for instance, could legitimately administer
punishment.[28] In addition, children might appeal to their mothers, and the
faithful, by analogy, might appeal to the Virgin Mary, for protection against
paternal violence. As Alexis de Salo writes, "Having then a Mother in heaven
so powerful as she, let us have recourse to her, as children to … their Mothers
when they fly their Fathers wrath."[29] Like the anxious jokes about the shrew
who is also a mother, de Salo's appeal offers a reminder of mothers' perceived
power both to inflict harm and to defend against it.

Representations of Mary as a nursing mother, cradling or suckling an infant
Jesus, became another focus both for Catholic reverence for and defenses of
Mary's power, and for Protestant attacks on it. Although Marina Warner, for
instance, argues that "the image of the Virgin suckling Christ represented
women's humility in accepting the full human condition," seventeenth-century
English debates over Mariolatry construct the suckling mother as a very
powerful figure, whether in negative or in positive terms.[30] Infants' dependence
on and symbiosis with their lactating mothers provoked controversy in
other discursive registers in seventeenth-century England. On the one hand, a

range of medical and moral texts sought to persuade elite women that they should nurse their own infants, rather than farming them out to wet nurses; identifying maternity with lactation, such texts also, it has been argued, worked to identify women with mothers and with bodily needs, and to limit women's mobility and independence. Some also emphasized the erotic pleasure and intimate attachment mother and child might both derive from breastfeeding as an incentive. On the other hand, pamphlets, demonological treatises, and published trial narratives that describe witches suckling their familiars at displaced teats promote these same identifications – women=mothers=nursing – but only to demonize and criminalize women.[31] However great their differences, both discourses participated in a larger movement to subordinate women and restrict them to a more narrowly defined domestic sphere by promoting a maternity of service, and criminalizing a maternity of power.[32] Controversy over Mariolatry reveals that if mothers had been identified as a problem, that the problem had not yet been resolved. For both Catholic and Protestant writers, the nursing Virgin, so confusingly combining service and power, nurture and eros, was not a humble figure but a threatening one.

Protestant writers censure the image of Mary as suckling mother for exaggerating her power and diminishing Jesus's. Most concretely, these images depict Mary as physically larger than Jesus. Crashaw, always the most colorfully virulent attacker of Mary, complains that Catholics infantilize Christ, dwelling on him as a "suckling child in his mothers armes," "an Infant governed, and an obedient child," "in *wardship* and under age"; "Nay that is nothing, they make him an underling to a woman."[33] Even after 1,600 years, Crashaw complains, Catholics refuse to allow Jesus to grow up. Mary

> must still bee a commanding Mother, and must shew *her authority over him*, and he *must receive our prayers by her meanes*, and still she must beare him in her armes; or lead him in her hand, and her Picture must worke all the miracles, but his none; and she must be saluted as a Lady, a Queene, a Goddesse, and he as a Child.[34]

In Crashaw's view, to depict or imagine Christ as an infant is to degrade him; to confer command and authority onto Mary is to wrench them away from both God the Father and his Son: "The *Christ* of God and of his Church, is God equall to the father, and can do all things himselfe: the Christ of the Romish Church is a child inferiour to his mother and may deny her nothing."[35] Floyd countered that to depict Jesus as an infant is not to diminish his majesty but to emphasize his humanity. The Christ who is a babe in arms, sucking on the Virgin's breasts, is "though not in bignes of body, yet in Majesty, power, wisdome, sanctity, both as God and man ... equall to himself bleeding on the Crosse."[36] Those who think of Jesus as a child do not imagine that he presently is one, but remember that he once was one. Floyd presents this memory as a comfort, a reminder that even the savior shares human mortality and fragility.

Such a memory was not inevitably comforting, however. For many Protestant writers, this remembrance of infant dependency, Jesus' or their own, announces the return of the repressed. One way to cope with this memory, made so concrete in Catholic iconography, was to grow up and away from the mother, to grow bigger and more powerful than she. Another strategy was to free Jesus and unmother Mary through iconoclasm, wrenching the infant from her arms. John Stowe, for instance, describes how a virgin at the cross in west Cheap was "robbed of her son, and her armes broken, by which she staid him on her knees."[37]

Catholic depictions of the relationship between Mary and Jesus were disturbing not only because they seemed to freeze Jesus in infancy, or to compel him back into it, but also because they suggested that he remembered his early dependency and revered his mother as a consequence, that her early nurturance of him translated into later authority over him. Robert Chambers, for instance, locates Mary's power not just in God's grace, but in her intimacy with her son. With Jesus, Mary "had not onely domestical familiaritie for many yeares, but had motherly authoritie over him, for he was obedient unto her, yea subject unto her, yea subject to Joseph for her sake, which truly was a power above all power, a miracle above all miracles, to have in pious and reverend subjection the high Majestie of heaven, the author and supreme worker of all miracles." This passage asserts not only Mary's maternal authority, but her precedence over her husband, Joseph. Jesus is subject to Joseph only "for her sake"; obviously, her contribution is much more important than Joseph's and therefore her power and prestige are far greater. "In his life tyme," Jesus "alwaies yelded unto her authoritie."[38] As a consequence, according to *The Widdowes Mite*, "she cannot without blasphemy be denyed to have beene for many yeares Superiour to the true, only, & begotten Sonne of God, who is the Lord both of Saints and Angells." Mary's power, then, stems from her maternal authority over Jesus: "it is infinitly a greater dignity to have God for her Son, and her subject, then to be the Superiour and Empresse of all things created."[39] This geneology of Mary's power assumes that mothers inevitably exercise authority over their offspring, not only in childhood, but into adulthood.

Although Chambers claims that the reverence for mothers "is a law meerely natural, & consequently indispensable," such reverence for mothers was not at all a given in either medieval or early modern English culture, as many scholars have recently demonstrated.[40] Thus, while Catholic apologists base their defenses of the Virgin Mary's power on her authority as a mother, those who question devotion to Mary begin by questioning that founding premise. As Willet states, "it is great presumption to thinke, that the Virgine *Mary* may commaund her Sonne in heaven, seeing she had no authoritie to commaund him upon earth, in any thing pertaining to his office."[41] Many early modern political theorists refer to women's lack of maternal authority, whether natural or cultural, to explain why they cannot and do not rule. John Knox, for instance, proposes that, just as men's power as fathers is an analogy to or source of their power over other men as rulers, so women's lack of authority as mothers, especially over their sons, explains why they cannot rule: "those that will not permit a woman to have power over her owne sonnes, will not permit her (I am assured) to have rule over a realme."[42] Almost a century later, Thomas Hobbes offers a more complicated version of the same argument. He claims that maternal and paternal power cannot be equal, as mothers' and fathers' mutual participation in the act of generation and equal ability to kill might suggest, because "no man can obey two Masters." Hobbes here uses the phrase frequently employed to describe the untenable position of Catholic subjects in a Protestant state to describe the dilemma of the child whose parents are equals; in his formulation, the mother who vies for power with the father is analogous to the Pope who competes with the sovereign and divides the subject's allegiances. Hobbes resolves the child's dilemma by subordinating or excluding the mother. He concedes that, by "Nature," "Dominion is in the Mother," but goes on to insist that in a commonwealth which has risen out of and above this state of Nature, maternal power is subordinated to paternal power; through a generational contract with their sons, men govern both the household and the commonwealth.[43] Knox and Hobbes, then, represent the two alternatives that Rose has identified in discourses which are more explicitly about sexual and familial life: "male-authored sexual discourse either denies maternal authority altogether or acknowledges and then erases it."[44] Yet Catholic defenders of Marian devotion suggest a third possibility – a male-authored discourse that assumes and even extends maternal authority.

Notes

1. Robert Chambers, "Epistle Dedicatorie" to Philippe Numan, *Miracles Lately Wrought by the Intercession of the Glorious Virgin Marie, at Mont-aigu*, trans. Chambers (Antwerp, 1606), sig. C4.
2. Chambers/Numan, *Miracles Lately Wrought*, sig. C4v.
3. A. G., *The Widdowes Mite. Cast into the Treasure-house of the Prerogatives, and Prayses of our B. Lady*, (St. Omer, 1619), sig. Fv.
4. Thomas Price in his translator's preface to Orazio Torsellino, *The History of Our B. Lady of Loreto* (St. Omer, 1608), sig. **4.
5. Andrew Willet, *Synopsis Papismi, that is, a Generall View of Papistrie* (London, 1614), sig. Zz3v.
6. Elizabeth's "Immaculate Conception" of Mary, which should be distinguished from Mary's "Virgin birth" of Jesus, did not become dogma until 1854; the assumption did not become dogma until 1950.
7. Floyd, *Overthrow of the Protestants Pulpit-Babels* (St. Omers, 1612), sig. D2v.
8. Marina Warner, *Alone of All Her Sex: The Myth and the Cult of the Virgin Mary* (New York: Knopf, 1976), p. 153. On the persistence of contests over Mariolatry,

see Jaroslav Pelikan, *Mary Through the Centuries: Her Place in the History of Culture* (New Haven: Yale University Press, 1996).

9. On the positive values assigned to motherhood and to Mary in the medieval period, see Caroline Walker Bynum, *Jesus as Mother: Studies in the Spirituality of the High Middle Ages* (Berkeley: University of California Press, 1982), chap. 4; and Merry Wiesner, "Luther and Women: The Death of Two Marys," in *Disciplines of Faith: Studies in Religion, Politics, and Patriarchy*, ed. Jim Obelkevich, Lyndal Roper, and Raphael Samuel (London and New York: Routledge and Kegan Paul, 1987), pp. 295–308, esp. p. 303. Patricia Crawford observes "the high esteem of maternity in Catholic popular culture" (*Women and Religion in England, 1500–1720* [London and New York: Routledge, 1993], pp. 47, 61).

10. In chapter 3 of *Whores of Babylon: Catholicism, Gender, and Seventeenth-Century Print Culture* (Ithaca: Cornell University Press, 1999), from which this essay is drawn, I link debates over Marian devotion to the controversy surrounding Henrietta Maria's influence over her husband and sons, to penal laws directed at Catholic mothers, and to Elizabeth Cary's motherhood.

11. Mary Beth Rose, "Where Are the Mothers in Shakespeare? Options for Gender Representation in the English Renaissance," *Shakespeare Quarterly* 42.3 (Fall 1991): 290–314, esp. p. 296. Motherhood continued to be viewed as problem into the eighteenth century (Toni Bowers, *The Politics of Motherhood: British Writing and Culture, 1680–1760* [Cambridge: Cambridge University Press, 1996]).

12. A. G., *Widdowes Mite*, sigs. B8v, L3.

13. Michael Camille, *The Gothic Idol: Ideology and Image-making in Medieval Art* (Cambridge: Cambridge University Press, 1989), 232.

14. T. E., *The Lawes Resolutions of Womens Rights* (London, 1632), sig. I7; A. G., *Widdowes Mite*, sig. B5.

15. A. G., *Widdowes Mite*, sig. Fv.

16. William Crashaw, *The Sermon Preached at the Crosse, Feb. xiiii, 1607* (London, 1608), *Sermon*, sig. H4v, quoting Bonaventure.

17. A. G., *Widdowes Mite*, sig. F; cf. Samuel Harsnett, *A Declaration of Egregious Popish Impostures* (London, 1603), sig. V2.

18. Anthony Stafford's *The Femall Glory* (London, 1635), p. 87. Because this was an Anglican text, it was highly controversial. See Anthony Milton, *Catholic and Reformed: The Roman and Protestant Churches in English Protestant Thought, 1600–1640* (Cambridge: Cambridge University Press, 1995), pp. 67–8.

19. Willet, *Synopsis Papismi*, sig. Zz5.

20. George Hickes, *Speculum Beatae Virginis. A Discourse of the Due Praise and Honour of the Virgin Mary* (London, 1686), sig. F.

21. Willet, *Synopsis Papismi*, sig. Zz5.

22. A. G., *Widdowes Mite*, sig. G6r–v.

23. T. E., *Lawes Resolutions of Womens Rights*, sigs. O6v, I6v–I7.

24. A. G., *Widdowes Mite*, sig. C7.

25. Scott Cutler Shershow, *Puppets and "Popular" Culture* (Ithaca: Cornell University Press, 1995), pp. 40–2.

26. Crashaw, *The Jesuites Gospell* (London, 1621), sig. E4; Floyd, *Purgatories Triumph Over Hell* (St. Omer, 1613), sig. X3.

27. Sir Edward Hoby, *A Curry-Combe for a Coxe-Combe. or Purgatories Knell* (London, 1615), sigs. Ee2v, Gg3v. For the claim that those who neglect or dishonor the Virgin fall into "poverty, misery, and disreputation, and confusion" see A. G., *Widdowes Mite*, sig. K5v.

28. Dolan, "Household Chastisements: Gender, Authority, and 'Domestic Violence,'"

in Patricia Fumerton and Simon Hunt, ed., *Renaissance Culture and the Everyday* (Philadelphia: University of Pennsylvania Press, 1999).

29. Alexis de Salo, *An Admirable Method to Love, Serve, and Honour the B. Virgin Mary*, trans. R. F. (Rouen, 1639), p. 314.

30. Warner, *Alone of All Her Sex*, p. 204.

31. Gail Paster, *The Body Embarrassed: Drama and the Disciplines of Shame in Early Modern England* (Ithaca: Cornell University Press, 1993), chaps. 4 and 5; and Deborah Willis, *Malevolent Nurture: Witch-Hunting and Maternal Power in Early Modern England* (Ithaca: Cornell University Press, 1995).

32. See Jodi Mikalachki's brilliant *Legacy of Boadicea: Gender and Nation in Early Modern England* (London: Routledge, 1998), chap. 4.

33. William Crashaw, *Jesuites Gospell*, sigs. A3, I3, I2, A3.

34. Ibid., sig. F2v.

35. Ibid., sig. K.

36. Floyd, *Overthrow of the Protestants*, sig. F.

37. John Stow, *A Survey of London* (1603), ed. Charles Lethbridge Kingsford, 2 vols. (Oxford: Clarendon Press, 1971), 1:266, 267.

38. Chambers/Numan, *Miracles Lately Wrought*, sig. C5; see also, A. G., *Widdowes Mite*, sig. C3.

39. A. G., *Widdowes Mite*, sigs. C5 (mismarked A5), E4v.

40. Chambers/Numan, *Miracles Lately Wrought*, sig. C5v. On ambivalence toward mothers in medieval and early modern culture, see Janet Adelman, *Suffocating Mothers: Fantasies of Maternal Origin in Shakespeare's Plays, "Hamlet" to "The Tempest"* (New York and London: Routledge, 1992); Clarissa W. Atkinson, *The Oldest Vocation: Christian Motherhood in the Middle Ages* (Ithaca: Cornell University Press, 1991); Valerie Fildes, ed., *Women as Mothers in Pre-Industrial England* (London and New York: Routledge, 1990); and Mikalachki, *Legacy of Boadicea*, chap. 4.

41. Willet, *Synopsis Papismi*, sig. Zz3.

42. John Knox, *First Blast of the Trumpet against the Monstruous Regiment of Women* (Geneva, 1558), sigs. B4v–B5.

43. Thomas Hobbes, *Leviathan*, ed. C. B. Macpherson (Harmondsworth: Penguin, 1983), II.21.253–4. See Carole Pateman, *The Sexual Contract (Stanford: Stanford University Press, 1988); and Mikalachki, Legacy of Boadicea*, pp. 47–9.

44. Rose, "Where Are the Mothers in Shakespeare?," p. 312.

CHAPTER SIXTEEN

Mother Love: Clichés and Amazons in Early Modern England

Kathryn Schwarz

> To you your father should be as a god,
> One that composed your beauties; yea, and one
> To whom you are but as a form in wax,
> By him imprinted, and within his power
> To leave the figure, or disfigure it.
>
> (*A Midsummer Night's Dream*, 1.1.46–52)

> WHO'S THE FATHER?
> CALL 1–800–DNA–TYPE
>
> (Billboard overlooking Interstate 40, Knoxville, TN)

I will begin by quoting two highly conventional claims. The first, from *The Womans Doctour*, describes a natural relationship between female bodies and domestic space. "Women were made to stay at home, and to look after Houshold employments, and because such business is accompanied with much ease, without any vehement stirrings of the body, therefore hath provident Nature assigned them their monthly Courses."[1] The second, from Samuel Purchas's *Purchas his Pilgrimage*, comments on accounts of Amazons. "The Amazons are still one nation further then the relaters or their authors have traveled. In two places of Asia, two of Africa, two of America; the Amazons have bin, till that men came there and found none."[2] Taken together, these quotations suggest the doubled logic that structures early modern theories of domesticity: femininity confines women to the home, and women who act outside the home are excluded from domestic structures, an exclusion strikingly figured in the Amazons' absence from any known or knowable space. "The sixteenth-century aristocratic family was patrilinear, primogenitural, and patriarchal," writes Lawrence Stone;[3] such a system, if it cannot dispense with women entirely, can at least define them in terms that make virtue and agency mutually exclusive. Real women and Amazons may be juxtaposed, but they never meet.

And yet, in a culture that often seems perfectly willing to accept Amazons themselves as real, descriptions of unnatural women and the rhetoric of domesticity intersect, even as the conventionally male prerogative of definition relies on a gap between them. This essay considers the implications of that intersection for conventions of maternity. As a number of scholars have demonstrated, the processes of conception, pregnancy, birth, and child-rearing are highly contested in early modern England, bringing together the conviction that women lack power and the fear that mothers might have too much control. Stories about Amazons provide a vocabulary for this tension, and give narrative shape to anxieties concerning maternity more generally. Imagined in a simultaneously intimate and disruptive relationship to domestic structures, Amazons as mothers both are and are not other. At its most unnatural, amazonian maternity is oddly predictable, a logical outcome of the fear that, even within the safe space of the home, women may be dangerous to men. But even as Amazon myth intersects and comments on domestic conventions, it poses a radical alternative to the assumptions about sexual and social power on which male control of those conventions depends.

In *Fashioning Femininity*, Karen Newman writes, "In the early modern period, the female body is the site of discourses that manage women: by continually working out sexual difference on and through the body, the social is presented as natural and therefore unchangeable, substantiated, filled with presence."[4] Women's bodies, and in particular women's reproductive bodies, become metonyms for the ways in which patriarchy works. As a process carried out by women and governed by men, maternity is an embodied sign; the operations that produce children give physical form to social theory, incorporating the abstractions that shape sexual hierarchy. But if this is the story of a wish-fulfillment, it is not the whole story, and early modern discourses of maternity reflect a suspicion that it may be difficult to give women significance without at least lending them agency. Fear that women might not only enable sexual reproduction, but control it, produces narratives in which that reproduction displaces rather than demonstrates the potency of men. Maternity threatens to become a version of the supplement, that doubled figure of which Jacques Derrida writes, "It adds only to replace. It intervenes or insinuates itself *in-the-place-of*; if it fills, it is as if one fills a void. If it represents and makes an image, it is by the anterior default of a presence."[5] Rather than metonymically illustrating patriarchal hierarchies, women might signify an altogether different structure in which female bodies refer to female power. Such a possibility informs early modern versions of Amazon myth, which fantasize a self-sufficient reproductive economy populated entirely by women. But the conditions of that fantasy are already present in conventional accounts of maternity; stories about Amazons represent an extreme, but it is a *logical* extreme.

If, as some texts from the period insist, women are merely vessels for the processes through which men reproduce themselves in their own image, maternity shouldn't be a problem at all. Described by Thomas Laqueur as "the idea that conception is the male having an idea in the female body," this theory relegates mothers to a strictly material role;[6] women provide both a physical shelter for and the physical substance of the child, but at the moment of sexual intercourse the important conceptual work has already been done. Female children are either mistakes or unfortunate biological necessities; the collection of popular ideas titled *The Problems of Aristotle* explains, "[B]ecause Nature doth always tend to that which is best, therefore she doth always intend to beget the male and not the female, because the female is only for the males sake, and a monster in nature."[7] Women, like hermaphrodites and other natural accidents, may be facts of life, but that does not change the idea that maleness is an end in itself.

And yet maternity notoriously *is* a problem, generating fears of excessive female power that become clichés as soon as they find articulation. Mary Beth Rose has suggested that a growing tendency to define women in public, rather than strictly private, terms creates anxiety about their maternal function: "Once construed in the 'public' rhetoric of authority, as well as in the 'private' vocabulary of nurture and desire, motherhood presents a test case for female power, making visible the destabilizing contradictions that that power comprises in English Renaissance society."[8] Maternity is both a site and a symptom of conflict, becoming as much a struggle between women and men as a way in which men ensure their own exclusive continuity. And in early modern gynecological texts, conception, the process through which the child's form is determined, might not be about exclusively male agency at all. Instead, accounts such as Thomas Vicary's emphasize the need for mutual contribution: "[A]s the Renet and Milke make the Cheese, so both the Sparme of man and woman make the generation of Embreon."[9] Conception results here from a constructive union of substances, but not all versions of female participation are so benign. Nicholas Culpeper describes not mutuality but competition: "The reason why sometimes a *Male* is conceived, sometimes a *Female*, is, The strength of the Seed; for if the Mans Seed be strongest, A Male is conceived; if the Womans, a Female: The greater light obscures the lesser by the same rule; and that is the reason weakling men get most Girls, if they get any."[10] Male and female seed fight a pitched battle in the womb, and losing that battle, for men, compromises not only the sex of their children but their own effective performance of gender.

Heterosexual conflict thus invades not only the protected space of the domestic but the female body itself. Battles between men and women, comfortably exiled to the margins of geography, society, and epistemological likelihood as elements of Amazon myth, here implicate the generative principles of patriarchy itself. Sexual reproduction might be less a tool in the perpetuation of ideology than a space of resistance, a level playing field on which women complicate and even contest the autogeny of men. It is in this context that *The Nobilitie of Women* articulates a homology between being a mother and being an Amazon: "As for strengthe we rede of the Amasones and manye other that wer wont to go to batteyll and have braught home manye tryumphs and victoris and yf this use were in o[u]r daies we shoulde see what ye strengthe of wymen coulde doe. and nature hathe allso preferred them in the order of generac[i]on ffor Gallen and Auicen sayethe, that the woman hathe the pryncypall office to conserve and conceyve the seede whearby the more parte of chyldren be lyke theyre mothers."[11]

If Barker does not argue that all mothers are Amazons, he does suggest that both versions of female power prove the same point. Other texts go farther, defining Amazons in terms of their conjugal and maternal potential; the apparently counterintuitive idea of amazonian domesticity has a powerful hold on the early modern imagination. The Amazon stories that circulate most freely in this period are not those that end in Amazonomachy – the utter destruction of all Amazons popular in classical myth – but those that end in marriage. Theseus marries Hippolyta, Artegall marries Britomart, Philoclea marries Cleophila (who is "really" Prince Pyrocles, but that is another story), Achilles wants to marry Penthesilea, and wishes that he had not killed her first. If such stories were contained within the genres of epic and chivalric romance, they might be in some sense extra-social, examples of the extraordinary rather than patterns for the quotidian. But in fact they appear repeatedly in texts designed to model social order itself. Conduct manuals and exemplary catalogues invoke Amazons to make arguments about how women should act. In *The Renaissance Notion of Women*, Ian Maclean suggests that female agency is always mediated and attenuated by moralizing texts. "The heroic exploits of exceptional women are noted, but moralists do not advise emulation of them, but rather their translation into domestic and private terms."[12] The Amazons of exemplary texts are indeed translated, or at least boiled down: Penthesilea often exemplifies chastity, and Anthony Gibson, in *A Womans Woorth*, describes Hippolyta in hyperbolically submissive terms, adjuring Theseus to be grateful "to have faire *Hippolyta*, / So worthy noting every way, / In thy house to waite on thee."[13] But the process of translation is at best incomplete. Hippolyta, Gibson informs his readers, defeated Theseus in battle before making him her husband "on meere grace"; Penthesilea kills men, as in Spenser's reference to "bold *Penthesilee*, which made a lake / Of *Greekish* bloud."[14] In *An Apologie for Women*, William Heale relies on his readers' awareness of such violence, arguing that, since a man might imaginably find himself married to an Amazon, it is inadvisable to beat one's wife.[15]

Amazons in the early modern period are thus implicated in both the history of heterosexual violence and the rhetoric of heterosexual domesticity. One sixteenth-century author claims that killing men is a prerequisite of amazonian marriage, writing, "To none of the Amazons was graunted liberty to marry, escepte that she had in warre valiauntly vanquished an enemy."[16] As they stretch the boundaries of what "marriage" can be imagined to mean, amazonian narratives entangle martial women in social conventions without mitigating or obscuring their essentially antisocial effect. The idea of Amazons as mothers takes shape through a convergence of domesticity and violence, based in a version of home life in which masculinity is controlled by women and has no natural connection to husbands or sons. Like the medical texts that imagine conception as a battle in the womb, accounts of amazonian generation stage a conflict between male and female agency in a space that is by definition women's home ground. And also like those medical texts, narratives about Amazons who have children imagine a potentially monstrous result.

Let me begin by focusing, as both Amazon narratives and responses to them have tended to focus, on the boys. Early modern claims concerning amazonian treatment of boy children follow two versions of classical myth, the first of which is summarized in Strabo's *Geography*: Amazons, Strabo writes, join their neighbors the Gargarians for two months each spring, having sexual intercourse with them at random at night, "and the females that are born are retained by the Amazons themselves, but the males are taken to the Gargarians to be brought up; and each Gargarian to whom a child is brought adopts the child as his own, regarding the child as his because of his uncertainty."[17] Strabo's account not only draws on anxiety surrounding the uncertain connection of father to child, but institutionalizes it, obscuring the mother's identity "in secrecy and darkness" and leaving each father to find himself in his son. The second version of the myth withholds even this dubious consolation; as recounted in the *Bibliotheca Historica* of Diodorus Siculus, amazonian maternity produces a body permanently excluded from the social world of men. "The men-children that among theym were borne, there thyes and armes were forthwith so embrosed that ever aftre they were croked and nevermore apt unto the warre, but as unwildye and lame people."[18] William Painter repeats this in *The Palace of Pleasure*, adding the alternative of a body that is literally as well as effectively a corpse: "If by chaunce they kept any [male children] backe, they murdred them, or else brake their armes and legs in sutch wise as they had no power to bear weapons."[19] Abandoned, maimed, or killed, the son who is valueless to his mother is made useless to his father; one early exploration narrative even conflates these various possibilities, making explicit the might-as-well-be-dead sentiment that attends any version of the amazonian son. "Afterwards, when the time came for [the Amazons] to have children, if they gave birth to male children, they killed them and sent them to their fathers."[20] In writing out the link of the recognizable and reliably possessed maternal body, Amazon myth exposes the contingency of the connection between father and son.

Despite its elaborate claims to shock value, then, the doubled narrative of Amazon boy-children tells us nothing new. In his analysis of *A Midsummer Night's Dream*, Louis Montrose writes, "Amazonian mythology seems symbolically to embody and to control a collective anxiety about the power of the female not only to dominate or reject the male but to create and destroy him."[21] The fantasy of control may characterize narratives that end in Amazonomachy, narratives, that is, in which all the Amazons end up dead. But in their fascination with the space *between* – between conquest and murder, between courtship and corpse – early modern texts bring amazonian domesticity close to home. For these texts, talking about Amazons works less as therapy than as symptom. In its tropes of abandonment and violence, amazonian maternity mirrors the conventional understanding of *all* maternity as a constant struggle between too little and too much. From the moment of conception, through an excess of involvement or through its lack, women's bodies might always do damage to the bodies of their sons. In *Suffocating Mothers*, Janet Adelman describes the sense in which maternity both forms and threatens to deform the male child: "Culturally constructed as literally dangerous to everyone, the maternal body must have seemed especially dangerous to little boys: fed *in utero* on her menstrual blood and then on the milk that was its derivative, he had too much of her blood in him … Until the little boy came of age as a man, he was dangerously close to the maternal body."[22] That closeness is materialized in the child's attachment to the maternal breast, an attachment implicating issues that range from the social practice of wet-nursing to the psychological processes of successful self-differentiation. The bodies of mothers and those of amazonian mothers converge most clearly in this question of the significance of the breast: as material links between mothers and sons, as symbols of nurture and signs of sexual difference, breasts promise and threaten at the same time, and the single-breasted Amazon makes visible that doubleness of need and loss. Amazonian monomasty, a "fact" obsessively recounted and analysed in early modern texts, materializes not only a fear of maternal inadequacy but the female bodily agency that gives that fear its force. As Gail Kern Paster writes of the amazonian body, "[I]t only too clearly instantiates the good breast/bad breast dichotomy so crucial to the developing infant's focal object relation, with this proviso: that even the Amazon's one 'good' breast is, by virtue of its anomalous, threatening, *grudging* singularity, perhaps none too good."[23]

I have argued elsewhere that early modern representations of the breast metonymically figure conventions of socialized femininity, and that fantasies surrounding the amazonian practice of breast mutilation make explicit the points at which those conventions and their failure intersect.[24] Here I want to suggest that invoking Amazons as figures of maternity illuminates the shiftiness of the breast as a signifier, and in so doing exposes a concern that the agency of interpreting female bodies might change hands. "While the boy's sense of *self* begins in union with the feminine, his sense of *masculinity* arises against it," writes Coppélia Kahn.[25] In such a reading masculinity, constituted through the move from *with* to *against*, takes shape in the gap between tropes: between metonymy as the sign of contiguity and metaphor as the sign that immediacy has been lost. But if, in this developmental narrative, the missing breast is a figure for the usefulness of that loss, in amazonian narratives it is a physical fact; stories about amazonian maternity are not about how the child interprets but about what the mother does. Loss here is useful only to Amazons, who sacrifice a breast in order, as Heywood writes, "that with the more facilitie they may draw a Bowe, thrill a Dart, or charge a Launce."[26] Representations of amazonian monomasty literalize lack without referring it to disempowerment, shifting emphasis from the child's perception to the mother's choice, asking what happens if the things the boy child imagines about his mother are *true*, the products not of his ideas but of her acts. The result is a story about the mother's bodily agency rather than the child's imaginative power, a story that separates sons from their mothers without enabling masculine independence. Left to the agency of Amazons, the process of disjoining at once goes too far and stops short.

Claims that Amazons kill or maim their sons demonstrate a fear that maternal instincts might not be exclusively benign, a fear that in the early modern period catalyzes increased legislation against infanticide. But the breaking and killing of amazonian boy children also reflects the conviction that maternity itself is potentially a form of violence against men. Rose writes of early modern mothers, "Their potential threat resides neither in their limited educative powers nor even in their possible neglect of nurture but rather in their overindulgence of love."[27] For medical texts from the period, the primary threat is perhaps rather an overindulgence of *thinking*: mothers may make their children effeminate by loving them too much after they are born, but they can make them monsters by thinking about them too much before. If mistakes of nature can be produced by women who have too much to do with conception – Ambroise Paré explains hermaphrodites in this way, writing, "Now for the cause, it is that the woman furnished as much seed as the man proportionately" – then still greater alterations might occur when the woman is left alone with the developing child.[28] In his analysis of women's imaginative power, Culpeper writes,

> So also you may read of some, that brought forth a Blackmore, the woman beholding the Picture of a Blackmore hanging in her Chamber: and of a woman at Pisa, that brought forth a child ful of Hair like a Chamel, because she was so superstitiously wise to kneel every day to the Picture of *John the Baptist* cloathed in Chamels-Hair. Also I my self know a woman this day living, that in the time of her Conception fixed her Eyes and Mind much upon a Boy with two Thumbs on each Hand, sitting at Dinner by her, brought forth a Boy with as many her self: this I say, may be the cause of some deformity.[29]

If a woman looks at or thinks about the wrong thing, her child will become that thing. Such causalities appear throughout early modern medical texts, their popularity suggesting a kind of intuitive connection between what women intend and what their children are; even those who claim to pursue a strictly physical reading of what *Aristotle's Works Compleated* calls "the Agent or Womb" cannot resist the story of the Moor's picture.[30] In this context, in which women can by an accident of thought or sight give birth to children who are black or hairy or have birthmarks or scars or the wrong number or kind of genitals or limbs, the violence of Amazons against their infant sons seems only a selective example, the result of a more constant preoccupation.

This returns us again to epistemological violence, to the erasure of patrilinearity implicit in the relationship of amazonian sons to their fathers. Descriptions of that relationship suggest that a father's claim on an Amazon's son requires a blend of optimism and recognition, that the mother's anonymity threatens to impose the same condition on her child. This, as I suggested earlier, is a logical extreme of paternal uncertainty; female separatism makes explicit the opacity of men's generative function. The argument that women are vessels, that fathers form children in all the ways that matter, is after all a compensatory fantasy, an antidote for the "secrecy and darkness" in which children – and not only amazonian children – are conceived. And in early modern theories of women's imaginative power, even a child's resemblance to its socially appropriate father may prove nothing about paternity. In response to the question "Why are children oftener like the father than the mother?" – a question most optimistically answered in terms of the relative strength of the seed – *The Problems of Aristotle* gives the following reply. "That proceedeth of the imagination of the mother, which thinketh of the disposition of the father in the act of carnal copulation, & therefore by reason of the strong imagination in the time of conception, the children get the disposition of the father."[31]

This explanation, made still more extraordinary by its matter-of-fact tone, gives the father's body no agency but that of the mother's imagination. If a woman thinks of a man at the moment of conception, her child will resemble him, in a way no more potent or privileged than the way in which that same child might come to resemble a Moor or a four-thumbed boy or a camel's-hair coat. *Aristotle's Works Compleated* pursues this argument to its disconcerting conclusion: "So that the children of an Adulteress, by the Mother's Imaginative Power, may have the nearest Resemblance to her own Husband, though begotten by another Man."[32] Faithful wives, who look at their husbands when they conceive, may generate a less obvious patrilineal connection than adulterous wives who fear that their husbands may be looking at them. In such explanations as among Amazons, women control the conditions of conception and birth, and even the children men have may not have the value that paternal desire seeks to assign to them.[33] Like Strabo's Gargarians, men in the early modern period perpetually scrutinize their sons, looking for a resemblance which, even when found, may not signify.

In all its variations, then, Amazon myth models the fear that mothers and their sons may be basically at odds, and that in this area women's power, or at least male conceptions of it, may exceed the naturalized agency of men.[34] But I want to turn here from the contested position of male subjects to a differently symptomatic reading, considering not the anxieties of male lack reflected in Amazon myth but the structural alternative that that myth proposes. Despite its apparent preoccupation with sons, the narrative of amazonian mothering does not universalize an experience of rejection and loss. Boys are deprived literally of their mothers and epistemologically of their fathers; girls become like their mothers in the effective absence of their fathers. Amazon mothers, in other words, divide the doubled concerns of early modern maternity along lines of sex: paternity anxiety is played out in the experience of Amazon boy-children, while fear that the mother may identify with the child too closely is materialized in Amazon girls. The effects of maternal violence illustrate the relationship between gender and agency: the maiming of boy-children makes them unlike men, while the mutilation of girl-children makes them just like Amazons. As Painter writes, "And for as mutch as these Amazons defended themselves so valiantly in the warres with bowe, and arowes, and perceyved that their breastes did very mutch impech the use of that weapon, and other exercises of armes, they seared up the right breasts of their yonge daughters."[35]

It is easy to read past the Amazon daughters; their fate is at once less extravagant and less obviously interesting than that of their male counterparts. They are a laconic coda to a catalogue of horrors, as in Thevet's account: "They kil their male children inco[n]tinently after they are delivered, or else they deliver him to the ma[n], to whom they think it doth pertain. If it be a female, they retaine it to them selves."[36] But I want to pause for a moment on this afterthought, and to consider its result: the reproduction of a sexually separatist society in its own image. Even as the amazonian disposition of sons exposes connections among men as fragile, Amazon daughters are material signs of successful social parthenogenesis. Promising an endlessly self-generating supply of Amazons, they appropriate a fantasy of self-sufficient reproduction more familiarly associated with men; as Laqueur writes, "[T]o be a father is to produce the substance, semen, through which blood is passed on to one's successors. Generation seems to happen without women at all."[37]

Ultimately, this is a social rather than a sexual fantasy. David Halperin describes the way in which female reproductive bodies provide a logic for the perpetuation of male homosociality, writing of Plato's Diotima that "her presence endows the paedegogic processes by which men reproduce themselves culturally – by which they communicate the secrets of their wisdom and social identity, the 'mysteries' of male authority, to one another across the generations – with the prestige of female procreativity."[38] Montrose reaches a similar conclusion, describing *A Midsummer Night's Dream* as "formulat[ing] in poetic discourse, a proposition about the genesis of gender and power: men make women, and make themselves through the medium of women."[39] Male homosocial power not only excludes women from generation but appropriates their reproductive role. So Richard Brathwait, in *The English Gentlewoman*, advises his female readers to submit themselves to men: "Contest not with your *head* for preeminence: you came from him, not he from you, honour him then as he cherisheth the love he conceives in you."[40] The tautology here is perfect, as women come from men who in turn reconceive themselves in women. Female bodies are tools, female procreativity a male possession, female agency an impossible fiction.

And yet male parthenogenetic fantasies are themselves vulnerable to the charge of fictionality, for if power is generated among and through men, children are not. Biblical myths of origin notwithstanding, women are more self-evidently the producers than the products of men. For the parthenogenetic story to work, social reproduction must obscure the sexual reproduction on which it is based, and the constellation of anxieties and desires surrounding maternity suggests the difficulty of that project. The centrality of women to the male scheme of self-replication becomes homosociality's open secret, and it is this gap in patriarchal logic, this necessary intervention of female bodies, which amazonian maternity illuminates and rewrites. As it posits female homosocial power as the consequence of female sexual production, this parthenogenetic fantasy achieves a seamlessness inaccessible to men. Male bodies appear as *only* bodies, playing a strictly technical role in the processes of conception. Claims about women as vessels attempt this distinction between bodies that matter and bodies that don't, only to complicate it by representing reproduction as a mutual effort or a contest of wills; the mother, however thoroughly repressed, always returns. But in Amazon myth heterosexuality is reduced to a merely material fact to an extent that male homosociality, with its variously idealizing and demonizing cults of maternity, cannot approximate. It is worth noting that, in the early modern period, telling stories about Amazons is an almost exclusively male preoccupation: if men cannot quite imagine themselves disposing of women, they can easily imagine women dispensing with men. In one instance of this ruthless utilitarianism, Diodorus records that Amazons dedicate their youth to war in order to preserve their chastity; then, he explains, "when the nyse and tikkilly yeres of wanton coraige be wele overpassed and renne, they mary theym-self and gete theym husbondes not for then-norishyng of the fleshly lust and carnall appetite, but oonly for generation and bicause to have children."[41] The separation of desire from sexuality and of sexuality from considerations of person, the excision of men from any meaningful responsibility for children, produces a kind of efficiency unimaginable in the sentimental and contested heterosexuality defined by men. As Diodorus's description suggests, there is no cult of paternity among Amazons.

Again Amazon myth plays out what patriarchal ideology can only imagine. And if the effects of amazonian maternity on male children directly reflect conventional fears, the story of Amazon daughters is a mirror image of inversion. Narratives of amazonian maternity are structured by the familiar idea that the homosocial bonds that matter are reproduced through heterosexual connections that do not in themselves signify, but here homosocial bonds are formed between women rather than between men. The bodies of women validate the connections among women, requiring neither fictions of exclusion nor discreet silence. Adopting an attitude toward heterosexuality that is at once utilitarian and violent, amazonian narratives construct a self-sufficient female generative economy that efficiently enacts the fantasy of self-creation. The reproductive processes ascribed to Amazons exploit rather than masking or attempting to rewrite the causal relationship between sexual and social reproduction, using heterosexuality to produce a female separatist state within which women and the bonds between them can be parthenogenetically reconceived. In Amazon myth as in early modern theory, the mother's imagination has the power to form the child, and by extension to re-form the conditions of social convention; but in Amazon myth the image the mother conceives and perpetuates is her own. As Helen Diner writes in *Mothers and Amazons*, "All varieties of Amazon society share the characteristic that they reared only the girls into full-fledged specimens of mankind."[42]

Notes

1. Nicholas Fontanus, *The Womans Doctour, or, An exact and distinct Explanation of all such Diseases as are peculiar to that Sex* (London, 1652), p. 2. I have modernized "u," "v," and the long "s" in all quotations from sixteenth- and seventeenth-century texts. For a detailed discussion of the ways in which early modern medicine presents women as limited by their bodies, see Hilda Smith, "Gynecology and Ideology in Seventeenth-Century England," in *Liberating Women's History: Theoretical and Critical Essays*, ed. Berenice A. Carroll (Urbana: University of Illinois Press, 1976), pp. 97–114.
2. Samuel Purchas, *Purchas his Pilgrimage. Or Relations of the World and the Religions Observed in all Ages and Places discovered, from the Creation to the Present* (London, 1613), p. 334n.
3. Lawrence Stone, *The Family, Sex, and Marriage in England, 1500–1800* (New York: Harper and Row, 1978), p. 7. For readings of women's roles in the early modern period that interrogate and complicate Stone's analysis of patriarchy, see for example Margaret J. M. Ezell, *The Patriarch's Wife: Literary Evidence and the History of the Family* (Chapel Hill: University of North Carolina Press, 1987); Judith Newton, "Making – and Remaking – History: Another Look at

'Patriarchy,'" in *Feminist Issues in Literary Scholarship*, ed. Shari Benstock (Bloomington: Indiana University Press, 1990), pp. 124–40; Susan Dwyer Amussen, *An Ordered Society: Gender and Class in Early Modern England* (Oxford: Basil Blackwell, 1988).

4. Karen Newman, *Fashioning Femininity and English Renaissance Drama* (Chicago and London: The University of Chicago Press, 1991), pp. 4–5.

5. Jacques Derrida, "… That Dangerous Supplement …," in *Of Grammatology*, trans. Gayatri Chakravorty Spivak (Baltimore: The Johns Hopkins University Press, 1974), pp. 144–5.

6. Thomas Laqueur, *Making Sex: Body and Gender from the Greeks to Freud* (Cambridge: Harvard University Press, 1990), p. 35.

7. *The Problems of Aristotle, with other Philosophers and Physitians, wherein are contained, Divers Questions with their Answers, Touching the Estate of Mans Body* (London, 1670).

8. Mary Beth Rose, "Where Are the Mothers in Shakespeare? Options for Gender Representation in the English Renaissance," *Shakespeare Quarterly* 42: 3 (Fall 1991), 291–314; p. 308.

9. Thomas Vicary, *The English-mans Treasure: with the true Anatomie of Mans bodie* (London, 1587), p. 50.

10. Nicholas Culpeper, *A Directory for Midwives: Or, A Guide for Women, In their Conception, Bearing, and Suckling their Children* (London, 1651), p. 57. For a detailed account of the debate over whether men, women, or both contribute the sperm that forms the child, see Laqueur's reading of the early medieval models presented by Isidore of Seville (*Making Sex*, pp. 55–7).

11. William Barker, *The Nobility of Women* (1559), ed. R. Warwick Bond (London, 1904: privately printed), p. 136.

12. Ian Maclean, *The Renaissance Notion of Woman: A Study in the Fortunes of Scholasticism and Medical Science in European Intellectual Life* (Cambridge: Cambridge University Press, 1980), p. 58.

13. Anthony Gibson, *A Womans Woorth, defended against all the men in the world* (London: 1599), p. 37r; p. 37.

14. Gibson, p. 5; Edmund Spenser, *The Faerie Queene*, ed. Thomas P. Roche, Jr. (New York: Penguin Books, 1978, 1987) 3.4.2.5–6.

15. William Heale, *An Apologie for Women* (Oxford, 1609), p. 15.

16. Hieronimus Osorius, *The Five Bookes of the Famous, learned, and eloquent man, Hieronimus Osorius, contayning a discourse of civill, and Christian Nobilitie*, trans. William Blandie (London, 1576).

17. Strabo, *The Geography of Strabo*, trans. Horace Leonard Jones (Cambridge: Harvard University Press, 1956), 5: 237.

18. Diodorus Siculus, *The Bibliotheca Historica*, trans. John Skelton (London: Oxford University Press, 1956), p. 200.

19. William Painter, "The First Nouell: The hardinesse and conquests of diuers stout, and aduenturous women, called Amazones," *The Second Tome of the Palace of Pleasure* (1566, 1575) (London: Reprinted for Robert Triphook by Harding and Wright, 1813), p. 3.

20. Qutd. in José Toribio Medina, *The Discovery of the Amazon*, trans. Bertram T. Lee, ed. H. C. Heaton (New York: Amercian Geographical Society, 1934), p. 221.

21. Louis Montrose, "'Shaping Fantasies': Figurations of Gender and Power in Elizabethan Culture," in *Representing the English Renaissance*, ed. Stephen Greenblatt (Berkeley: University of California Press, 1988), p. 36.

22. Janet Adelman, *Suffocating Mothers: Fantasies of Maternal Origin in*

Shakespeare's Plays, "Hamlet" to "The Tempest" (New York: Routledge, 1990), p. 7.

23. Gail Kern Paster, *The Body Embarrassed: Drama and the Discipline of Shame in Early Modern England* (Ithaca: Cornell University Press, 1994), p. 238.

24. Kathryn Schwarz, "Missing the Breast: Disease, Desire, and the Singular Effect of Amazons," in *The Body in Parts: Fantasies of Corporeality in Early Modern Europe*, ed. David Hillman and Carla Mazzio (New York: Routledge, 1997), pp. 147–70.

25. Coppélia Kahn, *Man's Estate: Masculine Identity in Shakespeare* (Berkeley: University of California Press, 1981), pp. 9–10.

26. Thomas Heywood, *Nine Bookes of Variovs Historie, Onelie concerning Women: Inscribed by the names of the nine Muses* (1624), p. 223

27. Rose, p. 301.

28. Ambroise Paré, *On Monsters and Marvels* (1573), trans. Janis L. Palliser (Chicago: University of Chicago Press, 1982), p. 26.

29. Culpeper, p. 140.

30. *Aristotle's Works Compleated in Four Parts, Containing I. The Compleat Master-Piece; II. His Compleat and Experienced Mid-wife; III. His Book of Problems; IV. His Last Legacy.* I quote here from the London edition of 1733.

31. *The Problems of Aristotle*, D8v.

32. *Aristotle's Master-Piece*, in *Aristotle's Works Compleated*, pp. 95–6.

33. For a discussion of the conflict between male domination of medical science and female autonomy in birth, see Richard Wilson, "Observations on English Bodies: Licensing Maternity in Shakespeare's Late Plays," in *Enclosure Acts: Sexuality, Property, and Culture in Early Modern England* (Ithaca: Cornell University Press, 1994). For an argument concerning the association of female generative power with witchcraft, see Deborah Willis, *Malevolent Nurture: Witch-Hunting and Maternal Power in Early Modern England* (Ithaca: Cornell University Press, 1995).

34. For readings of the representation of maternal power as a male fantasy, see Madelon Gohlke, "'I wooed thee with my sword': Shakespeare's Tragic Paradigms," in *Representing Shakespeare: New Psychoanalytic Essays*, ed. Murray M. Schwartz and Coppélia Kahn (Baltimore: The Johns Hopkins University Press, 1980), pp. 170–87; and Valerie Traub, "Prince Hal's Falstaff: Positioning Psychoanalysis and the Female Reproductive Body," *Shakespeare Quarterly* 40: 4 (Winter 1989), pp. 456–74.

35. Painter, p. 5.

36. André Thevet, *The New Founde Worlde, or Antarctik, wherein is contained wonderful and strange things* (London, 1568), p. 102v.

37. Laqueur, p. 56.

38. David M. Halperin, "Why is Diotima a Woman?," in *One Hundred Years of Homosexuality and Other Essays on Greek Love* (New York: Routledge, 1990), p. 144.

39. Montrose, "'Shaping Fantasies,'" p. 42.

40. Richard Brathwait, *The English Gentlewoman, drawne out to the full Body* (London, 1631), p. 40.

41. Diodorus Siculus, p. 287.

42. Helen Diner, *Mothers and Amazons: The First Feminine History of Culture*, trans. John Lundin (New York: The Julian Press, 1965), p. 127.

CHAPTER SEVENTEEN

Native Mothers, Native Others: La Malinche, Pocahontas, and Sacajawea

Kari Boyd McBride

> My reputación precedes me. I come from a long line of women much maligned.
> Pat Mora, "Malinche's Tips"[1]

Pioneer. Explorer. Adventurer. Discoverer. Linguist. Envoy. Hero. Ambassador. Naturalist. Leader. Trader. Tracker. Hunter. Any of these epithets, and many others, might be appropriate to characterize the work and lives of the three women whose stories form the basis for this study. But the tradition surrounding them has not tended to use these words. Instead, the stories told about them focus on their sexualized bodies and, significantly, on their motherhood.[2]

La Malinche. La chingada. The screwed one. La vendida. La Llorona. Puta. Whore. Traitor. Squaw. Mistress. Siren. Seductress. Nubile princess. Little Wanton. Savage. Earth Mother. These are the names they are known by in the popular historical tradition. Whether demonized like La Malinche or figured as merciful, gentle, pious, meek, refined, and pure[3] like Pocahontas, they are known primarily in their relationship to European and Euro-American men, whom these women, the stories tell us, recognized as members of a superior race (as in the case of Pocahontas) or perhaps even as divine (as the Aztecs in general and La Malinche in particular are said to have viewed the conquistadores).

Doña Marina. Malintzín. Malinal. Malinalli. Tenepal. La Malinche. Pocahontas. Matoaka. Matoa. Amonte. Lady Rebecca. Frenchman's squaw. Janey. Sakakawea. Sah-kah-gar-we-a. Sacajawea. We cannot even get their names right. But they have endured, nonetheless, as cardinal figures in popular American historical narrative. Given the forgetful tendencies of most Western cultures when it comes to women and other Others, it is remarkable that these three indigenous women have been canonized as central to Euro-American founding narratives. Perhaps even more remarkable is the way that their maternity inflects these histories in significant ways. All three were pregnant during the periods that the dominant historical record memorializes their lives, and all three were mythologized, for good or ill, as mothers of a new people, a new dispensation, a new world.

Like women of many eras, they functioned as commodities for the traffic in women, exchangeable chattel, the ultimate gift. All three had been traded, kidnapped, bought, or sold by their own families and people before their lives brought them in contact with the Europeans and Euro-Americans whose stories of them continue to be told. In every way, their lives inhabit what Mary Louise Pratt calls "the contact zone": the "social [space] where cultures meet, clash, and grapple with each other, often in contexts of highly asymmetrical relations of power" – no relation more asymmetrical than that between Euro male and indigenous female.[4] They are, in Clara Sue Kidwell's words, "the first important mediators of meaning between the cultures of two worlds."[5] They existed on the threshold, their maternal bodies bearing children neither white nor "red," belonging neither to the tribe nor to the conqueror – their bodies most liminal of all, inhabiting that space in between. As Diane Purkiss has noted, "the bodies of women are more 'leaky,' permeable and problematic than the bodies of men. This is partly because of maternity, in which the boundaries of a woman's body are broached and the body itself distended and ambiguous during pregnancy, representing an uncertain number of bodies ... The maternal body, though venerated, is also a problematic source of pollution."[6] So the maternal bodies of La Malinche, Pocahontas, and Sacajawea bridge the worlds of colonizer and colonized at the same time that they are fixed within the dominant narrative where they serve – in practice and in the mythology that developed out of that practice – as native (m)others for self-justifying fantasies of both dominance and oppression and, as Pratt has said of La Malinche, as "site[s] for the ongoing negotiation of meaning and self understanding."[7]

The story of La Malinche has been much retold recently, as she has become a symbol for Chicana writers of "androcentric ethno-nationalism," of gender divisive accounts of the conquest of the Aztec empire that lay the blame for the loss of indigenous autonomy and sovereignty at the feet of one woman and make "malinchista" a synonym for traitor: "betrayal," Pratt notes, "is coded in the language as *female*."[8] The work of these Chicana writers has provided a fuller picture of La Malinche, one that offers commentary both on the contemporary accounts from Cortés's party and on the mysogynistic scapegoating that has followed, and has turned her into a symbol of chicana feminist resistance to oppressive signifying systems, "a vital resonant site through which to respond to androcentric ethno-nationalism and to claim a gendered oppositional identity and history."[9] As Pratt, citing Sandra Messinger Cypess, notes, La Malinche is "one of the most complex cultural icons of post-conquest America" by virtue of "her race, her gender, and her historical role":

> Her very presence contradicts, for example, canonical ideologies of conquest and resistance as masculine heroic enterprises, and reductive visions of the conquest as a straightforward relation between victimizers and victims.[10]

As Cypess suggests, she is a palimpsest upon whose body a series of narratives have been written,[11] both by the Aztec chroniclers and the conquistadores, but not, significantly, by La Malinche herself, whose linguistic abilities placed her at the crossroads of history, but whose voice is absent from these records. Miguel León-Portilla assembled the earliest indigenous accounts of the conquest, some of them as early as 1528 (within a decade of the fall of Tenochtitlan), and the reports of Cortés to Charles V survive, as well as that of his secretary and biographer, López de Gómara, and one of Cortés's soldiers, Bernal Díaz del Castillo, who published his *History of the Conquest of New Spain* to correct what he saw as the misinformation of López and others.[12] Reading the narrative about La Malinche that emerges in the space created between these accounts, scholars propose that she was named Malintzín (*tzin* being a Nahuatl suffix indicating respect[13]), born in the first decade of the sixteenth century (just where is unclear), the eldest daughter of a privileged family. She was well educated in her early life, before her fortunes fell with her father's death and her mother's remarriage. The birth of a male child prompted her mother to sell Malintzín into slavery to preserve the family inheritance to the son. Cortés notes, and others confirm, that she had been given to him along with twenty other women, but he called only her his interpreter, "la lengua que yo tengo."[14] So she stood out from her twenty compatriots, a fact that is confirmed by Díaz, who devoted an entire chapter to her and is lavish in his praise of the woman known to the Spanish as Doña Marina:

> Before speaking of the great Montezuma, and of the famous city of Mexico and the Mexicans, I should like to give an account of Doña Marina. Who had been a great lady and a *Cacique* over towns and vassals since her childhood.[15]

Díaz recounts the story of her early years and her having been given to another tribe by her parents, but his focus is on her (Christian) forgiveness of them in later life.[16] Cypess notes that this narrative "corresponded to events during the childhood and adolescence of Amadís de Gaula, the exemplary Christian knight of a fictional work of the same name" as well as to the biblical story of Joseph and the brothers who had sold him into slavery. The "implicit presence of the Spanish subtext of Amadís" and Joseph makes Doña Marina a symbol of indigenous conversion to Christianity and of Christian – and noble – virtues. So Díaz's account repeatedly sets her apart from her people. She is "an excellent person," "a good interpreter," "a person of great importance, and was obeyed without question by all the Indians of New Spain"; indeed, "without

Doña Marina we could not have understood the language of New Spain and Mexico."[17] She was married to "a [Spanish] gentleman," Juan Jaramillo," and reportedly refused local honor, saying that

> God had been very gracious to her in freeing her from the worship of idols and making her a Christian, and giving her a son by her lord and master Cortés, also in marrying her to such a gentleman as her husband Juan Jaramillo. Even if they were to make her mistress of all the provinces of New Spain, she said, she would refuse the honour, for she would rather serve her husband and Cortés than anything else in the world.[18]

She is presented as an idealized Christian woman, faithful wife and mother, in this account, one that represents "the assimilation by Marina of Spanish culture," in Cypess's words – and her assimilation *into* Spanish culture.[19] But the narrative finesses her ties to two men, which would ordinarily be anything but ideal. Gómara comments that "Cortés was criticized for allowing [her to marry Jaramillo], because he [Cortés] had children by her."[20] Indeed, she was given to Jaramillo by Cortés, another episode in her continuing role as gift, the evidence and exchange of masculine and nationalist authority, which passed through La Malinche "between men" in the trafficking of her body and in the Euro-American child that she bore. Yet, as Cypess notes, Gómara neglects to include her name when he lists Cortés's children, suggesting that "Gómara never sees La Malinche as anything more than an objectified extension of the will of Cortés."[21] What is important for Gómara is that Cortés had "three daughters, each by a different mother, all Indians."[22] And, indeed, La Malinche passes out of the contemporary historical record with the birth of that daughter, and nothing is known of her after her marriage to Jaramillo.

La Malinche's role as heroine of the conquest – albeit limited and ambiguous – in the accounts of the Spanish chroniclers made her a likely target for Mexican revisionist history following independence. Gloria Anzaldúa and others have argued that "the Aztec nation fell not because *Malinali (la Chingada)* interpreted for and slept with Cortés, but because the ruling elite had subverted the solidarity between men and women and between noble and commoner."[23] But in the chauvenist narratives that grew out of the independence movement, La Malinche's sexualized and maternal body continues to be the focus, but now for another masculinized nationalist story of dominance. As Cherríe Moraga says,

> Upon her shoulders rests the full blame for the "bastardization" of the indigenous people of México. To put it in its most base terms: Malintzín, also called Malinche, fucked the white man who conquered the Indian peoples of México and destroyed their culture. Ever since brown men have been accusing her of betraying her race, and over the centuries continue to blame her entire sex for this "transgression."[24]

Though La Malinche was, in Verena Stolcke's words, "recognized and represented as the victim of a rape, she is characterized as a consenting and useful tool for Cortés in the service of the conquest."[25] She, like Eve, is the mother of a people, of the mestizo people, but responsible for their troubles: "Viva México, hijos de la chingada" (long live Mexico, children of a fucked woman). Only misogyny can make this expression of "debilitating self-hatred"[26] an expression of even ironic nationalism. La Malinche's liminal maternal body has served, then, as the site for a series of inscriptions; her body has been repeatedly inseminated, in a sense, made to bear a variety of meanings for a series of patriarchal narratives.

Pocahontas, too, has been called the mother of a nation, seen in some romanticized accounts as the counterpart of George Washington.[27] Like La Malinche, Pocahontas has been the useful site for colonizing narratives, but has not left her own record. Like La Malinche, she is known by many names, a situation that Karen Robertson suggests

> exposes an English struggle over the right to name her that her own illiteracy cannot contest but also suggests the perhaps disturbing malleability of her rank and breeding. Unlike her counselor Uttamatomakkin, whose name remains the same despite his travels, Pocahontas's name is translated, from Matoaka, to Pocahontas, to the Lady Rebecca, as her legal affiliation shifts from daughter to wife.[28]

Information about Pocahontas comes from three English accounts, all of which construct Euro-American identity by subsuming her story into existing Euro-American colonialist narratives.[29] She was the daughter of chief Powhatan of the Powhatan tribe, born in the last decade of the sixteenth century and named Matoaca; Pocahontas was a nickname, meaning naughty or spoiled child. The story of her saving John Smith was, in all likelihood, a much later invention by Smith. She would have been only ten or eleven years old at the time (during Smith's winter stay with the Powhatans in 1607), and the story does not appear in Smith's earliest account of his adventures.[30] Further, it is one of three such rescues by women that he relates in later accounts, and the details of Pocahontas's saving Smith accord with a number of rescue stories popular in the late sixteenth and early seventeenth centuries. Green notes that in an old Scottish ballad, entitled "Young Beichan" or "Lord Bateman and the Turkish King's Daughter," an Englishman is similarly rescued:

> [A] young English adventurer travels to a strange, foreign land. The natives are of a darker color than he, and they practice a pagan religion. The man is captured by the King (Pasha, Moor, Sultan) and thrown in a dungeon to await death. Before he is executed, however, the pasha's beautiful daughter – smitten with the elegant and wealthy visitor – rescues him and sends him homeward. But she pines away for love of the now remote stranger who has gone home, apparently forgotten her, and contracted a marriage with a "noble Lady" of his own kind. In all the versions, she follows him to his own land, and in most, she arrives on his wedding day whereupon he throws over his bride-to-be for the darker but more beautiful

Princess. In most versions, she becomes a Christian, and she and Lord Beichan live happily ever after.[31]

Not surprisingly, given the magnetic pull of this narrative (which has parallels in other stories, both before and after Smith's), many fictionalized accounts of Pocahontas have her marrying Smith. But, in fact, she married John Rolfe, after having been kidnapped by the English in 1612 and held at Jamestown for over a year, a political pawn in negotiations between the English and Powhatan peoples. Rolfe took "a special interest"[32] in her. While in captivity, she was given religious instruction and converted to Christianity (the first Native American in Virginia to do so). In 1614, she married John Rolfe, becoming Rebecca Rolfe, and bore a son, Thomas Rolfe. In 1616, she traveled to England, making an appearance at court, on behalf of the colony. The Powhatan-Renape Nation suggests that

> the Virginia Company of London used her in their propaganda campaign to support the colony. She was wined and dined and taken to theaters. It was recorded that on one occasion when she encountered John Smith (who was also in London at the time), she was so furious with him that she turned her back to him, hid her face, and went off by herself for several hours. Later, in a second encounter, she called him a liar and showed him the door.[33]

She died soon after the beginning of her return voyage. (She is buried at Gravesend.) Her son remained in England to be educated, became a militia officer, and returned to command a fort on the James River.

Robertson says of Pocahontas that she "is an overdetermined figure, serving multiple purposes, both then and now."[34] And Rayna Green has documented how Pocahontas is but one manifestation of a series of Indian women who "stand for the New World," an "earthly, frightening, and beautiful paradise."[35] She begins, according to Green, as a "familiar Mother-Goddess figure – full-bodied, powerful, nurturing but dangerous – embodying the opulence and peril of the New World." She re-emerges as "the Princess ... when the colonies begin to move toward independence, and she becomes more 'American' and less Latin than her mother." In contemporary iconography, "[s]he often stands with The Sons of Liberty, or later, with George Washington."[36] Opposed to "the Princess" is "the Squaw," the savage. Whereas the Princess "must save or give aid to white men,"[37] as does Pocahontas in Smith's narrative (or, earlier, La Malinche in the otherwise contrasting narratives of the Spanish and the post-independence Mexicans), the Squaw is a symbol of animal nature, of the debasement of white virtue in succumbing to the delights of exoticized native flesh. The "good Indian," like Pocahontas, is always a princess, always a convert to Christianity who "cannot bear to see [her] fellow Christians slain by 'savages.'" As Green says, "[t]o be 'good,' she must defy her own people, exile herself from them, become white, and perhaps suffer death."[38] A host of such stories of star-crossed and consummated encounters between

European or Euro-American men and Native American women survive from
the seventeenth and eighteenth centuries. Sometimes the white man "goes
native," a plot development that Green notes "add[s] to the exotic and sexual,
yet maternal and contradictorily virginal image of the Indian Princess ...
reminiscent of the contemporary white soldier's attachments to 'submissive,'
'sacrificial,' 'exotic' Asian women."[39] In this vein, we have been blitzed
since 1995 with Disney's *Pocahontas* (and, more recently, in 1998 with
Pocahontas II), a figure one of my students aptly called "Barbie with a suntan."
As the Powhatan-Renape Nation comment (on their web site critical of the
Disney portrayal), "Euro-Americans must ask themselves why it has been so
important to elevate Smith's fibbing to status as a national myth worthy of
being recycled again by Disney," a myth they suggest Euro-Americans "should
find embarrassing."[40] Indeed, as Green notes, Pocahontas "offers an intolerable
metaphor for the Indian-White experience[,] ... unendurable metaphors for the
lives of Indian women."[41]

Like La Malinche, Pocahontas served as palimpsest for colonial narratives,
"a *tabula rasa* awaiting inscription by the bearers of the true word: a savage yet
nubile nymph who longed for the English embrace."[42] Like La Malinche, she is
able to straddle the Madonna-whore dichotomy, both sexualized and idealized
in her maternal body that carries the incarnation of asymmetrical relations in
"the contact zone." Thus, she is portrayed as both innocent and sexualized in
her earliest visits to the Jamestown colony:

> Pochahuntas, a well featured but wanton yong girle Powhatan's daughter,
> sometymes resorting to our fort, of the age then of eleven or twelve yeares, get the
> boyes forth with her into the markett place, and make them wheele, falling on
> their handes, turning their heeles upwardes, whome she would followe, and
> wheele so her self, naked as she was, all the fort over; but being once twelve
> yeares, they put on a kind of semicinctum lethern apron (as doe our artificers
> or handycrafts men) before their bellies, and are very shamefac't to be seene
> bare.[43]

Here the Powhatan dress is subsumed into the European-style apron as a
sign of her movement from savage to "civilized" woman, just as, in the only
contemporary portrait of Pocahontas, painted by the Dutchman Simon van de
Passe in 1616 during her visit to England, she appears in doublet, ruff, and
stylish hat. As a contemporary commented, "Here is a fine picture of no
fayre Lady and yet with her tricking up and high stile and titles you might
thincke her and her worshipfull husband to be sombody."[44] "Englishness," like
Christianity, has been superimposed on her body like a costume, like the person
of her husband, impregnating her with a liminal respectability that does not
ultimately inhere in her. In a wonderful and terrible irony, her voyage to
England signifies this liminal status. Though she left behind her son, she could
not stay there, could not finally be English, but her death just off the coast of

England is a symbol of her inability to return to the Powhatan nation from which she was kidnapped.

Sacajawea, too, inhabits this liminal, miscegenated, maternal space in the contemporary and later accounts of her place in the narrative of colonialist domination and manifest destiny. Born a Shoshone, she was kidnapped by the Minatarees as a young girl and later bought by a French-Canadian trader and guide, Toussaint Charbonneau, becoming one of his two or three Indian wives. Like La Malinche and Pocahontas, she had exceptional linguistic abilities, as well as skill as a guide (evidently greater than that of her "husband"). Sacajawea first appears in the narrative as a young pregnant girl who gives birth just before the Lewis and Clark expedition begins in 1804; she was probably fifteen or sixteen. The child, named Jean Baptiste, but called "Pomp," Shoshone for first-born, made the journey along with his mother, whose worth quickly proved greater to the expedition than that of her husband. Analogous to Charbonneau's relationship with Sacajawea and other Indian women, the expedition was conceived in terms of sexualized conquest. Lewis said of their embarkation, "We were about to penetrate a country at least two thousand miles in width on which the foot of civilized man has never trodden." Sacajawea's presence on the expedition was crucial, not simply because, by both Lewis and Clark's accounts, she was more competent, brave, and quick-thinking than her husband, but because she "mothered" the other members of the expedition by searching out and preparing a wide variety of native food plants, by her "root digging and berry picking, her cooking, sewing, and nursing."[45] She also acted as mediator between the Euro-Americans and many of the tribes they encountered through her interpreting and simply through her presence. As Clara Sue Kidwell notes,

> [s]ince Indian tribes did not take women on war parties, she was a sign that Lewis and Clark came in peace. Indeed, Clark wrote that her presence assured the Indians that the expedition's intentions were peaceful. Her importance in history is to show us how she was valued by two cultures: Lewis and Clark needed her as a translator, but the Indian people whom the expedition encountered saw her as a sign of peace.[46]

Perhaps it is more accurate to say that she was "valuable to" both cultures while belonging, at this point in her life, to neither. After the expedition ended, Clark wrote to Charbonneau inviting him to St. Louis along with "your son [and] your femme Janey" (Clark's nickname for Sacajawea). Clark offered to educate "your little son (my boy Pomp) and to "raise him as my own child."[47] When Charbonneau and Sacajawea later left St. Louis, they left Jean Baptiste behind with Clark.

Like La Malinche and Pocahontas, Sacajawea is known for only a brief period of her life, the one-and-a-half years during which she came into the view of Lewis and Clark, two celebrated Euro-Americans. She exists in the cultural memory on the margins, a mythic mother of a new world who serves the expansionist interest of the colonizers. When she moves out of that dominant spotlight, her story breaks down. The journals of John C. Luttig, secretary to Manuel Lisa, a fur baron, on a trading expedition to the Dakotas in 1812, records the death of "the wife of Charbonneau, a Snake squaw" from "a putrid fever." He comments that "she was a good and the best woman in the fort, aged about twenty-five years." Luttig did not record the "squaw's" name in that entry, but, when the fort was later attacked by Sioux, Luttig noted that he took with him a young girl child, "Sacajawea's Lizette," whose guardian he later became, to be superseded at his death by William Clark.[48] (Even in this final narrative, it is her motherhood – and the surrogate parenthood of two Euro-Americans – that matters.) The Shoshone tradition, however, holds that Sacajawea made her way, on her own, back to the Wind River Shoshone reservation, where she died in 1884.

La Malinche, Pocahontas, and Sacajawea were women from significantly different times and places, inhabiting different stations within their own families and nations as well as within the societies of the colonizers they became attached to and whose children they bore. Yet their roles within the colonial narratives, where they all serve to articulate the relationship between colonizer and colonized, are suspiciously similar and should encourage us to make careful use of the accounts of their lives. Like many women before and after, they were passed between men as the ultimate gift to signify masculine relationships, cement alliances, confirm treaties, and mark and preserve asymmetrical relationships with the contact zones of the Americas – all relationships that were inscribed most saliently on their pregnant bodies. We can read their bodies as texts that bear the marks of these narratives of conquest and assimilation, but we will with difficulty read the narratives to learn about the women, whose stories remain mostly invisible within the womb of myth and history.

Notes

1. Pat Mora, "Cuarteto Mexicano: Talk Show Interviews with Coatlicue the Aztec Goddess, Malinche the Maligned, The Virgin of Guadalupe, and La Llorona: The Wailer," *Agua Santa: Holy Water* (Boston: Beacon Press, 1995), 64.
2. This study is a synthesis, one that would not have been even imaginable apart from the groundbreaking work of Chicana and Native American scholars such as Gloria Anzaldúa, Sandra Messinger Cypess, Rayna Green, Clara Sue Kidwell, Pat Mora, Cherríe Moraga, and Mary Louise Pratt. I am grateful for all they have taught me.
3. Åsebrit Sundquist, in her categorizing of fictional Indian character types, shows the ways in which Pocahontas was figured as an "angel" in the developing tradition. *Pocahontas & Co. The Fictional American Indian Woman in Nineteenth*

Century Literature: A Study of Method (Atlantic Highlands, NJ: Humanities Press; Oslo: Solum Forlag, 1987), 98.

4. Mary Louise Pratt, "Arts of the Contact Zone," *Profession* 91: 34.
5. Clara Sue Kidwell, "Indian Women as Cultural Mediators," *Ethnohistory* 39 (1992): 97.
6. Diane Purkiss, *The Witch in History: Early Modern and Twentieth-Century Representations* (London: Routledge, 1996), 99.
7. Mary Louise Pratt, "'Yo Soy La Malinche': Chicana Writers and the Poetics of Ethnonationalism," *Callaloo* 16 (1993): 859.
8. Pratt, "'Yo Soy La Malinche,'" 860.
9. Pratt, "'Yo Soy La Malinche,'" 861.
10. Pratt, "'Yo Soy La Malinche,'" 859–60.
11. Sandra Messinger Cypess. *La Malinche in Mexican Literature: From History to Myth* (Austin: Univ. Of Texas Press, 1991), 5.
12. Miguel León-Portilla, ed. *The Broken Spears: The Aztec Account of the Conquest of the Mexican Empire* (Boston: Beacon Press, 1962); Hernán Cortés, *Letters from Mexico*, trans. A. R. Pagden (New York: Grossman, 1971); Francisco Lópezde Gómara, *The Life of the Conqueror by His Secretary*, trans. Lesley Byrd Simpson (Berkeley: Univ. of California Press, 1964); Bernal Díaz del Castillo, *The Conquest of New Spain*, trans. J. M. Cohen (Harmondsworth: Penguin, 1963).
13. Cypess, *La Malinche*, 33. La Malinche is "the syncretic, mestizo form," according to Cypess (2). Díaz records La Malinche as the name by which Cortés was known, ironically, through his association with her: "[I]n every town we passed through and in others that had only heard of us, they called Cortes Malinche. ... The reason why he received this name was that Doña Marina was always with him, especially when he was visited by ambassadors or *Caciques*, and she always spoke to them in the Mexican language. So they gave Cortes the name of 'Marina's Captain,' which was shortened to Malinche." *The Conquest of New Spain*, 172.
14. Quoted in Cypess, *La Malinche*, 179, n. 1.
15. Díaz, *The Conquest of New Spain*, 85.
16. Cypess, *La Malinche in Mexican Literature*, 30.
17. Díaz, *The Conquest of New Spain*, 86, 87.
18. Díaz, *The Conquest of New Spain*, 86.
19. Cypess, *La Malinche*, 31.
20. Quoted in Cypess, *La Malinche*, 32.
21. Cypess, *La Malinche*, 32–3.
22. Quoted in Cypess, *La Malinche*, 32.
23. Gloria Anzaldúa, "Entering Into the Serpent," in *Weaving the Visions: New Patterns in Feminist Spirituality*, ed. Judith Plaskow and Carol P. Christ (San Francisco: Harper, 1989), 82.
24. "From a Long Line of Vendidas: Chicanas and Feminism," in *Loving in the War Years* (Boston: South End Press, 1986), 99–100. Rpt. in *Theorizing Feminism: Parallel Trends in the Humanities and Social Sciences*, ed. Anne C. Herrmann and Abigail J. Stewart (Boulder: Westview Press, 1994), 35.
25. Verena Stolcke, "Invaded Women: Gender, Race, and Class in the Formation of Colonial Society," trans. Walden Browne, in *Women, "Race," and Writing in the Early Modern Period* (London: Routledge, 1994), 277. Stolcke notes that "Octavio Paz could thus describe her in *The Labyrinth of Solitude* as the quintessence of indigenous collaborationism."
26. Pratt (following Octavio Paz), "'Yo Soy La Malinche,'" 860.

27. See Philip Young, "The Mother of Us All: Pochahontas Reconsidered," *The Kenyon Review* 24 (1962): 391–441.
28. "Pocahontas at the Masque," *Signs* 21 (1996): 551–83.
29. John Smith's *A True Relation* (1608) and his later *A Map of Virginia* (1612), *Proceedings of the English Colonie in Virginia* (1612), and *The Generall Historie of Virginia* (1624) are reprinted in *The Complete Works of Captain John Smith*, ed. Philip Barbour, 3 vols. (Chapel Hill, Univ. of North Carolina Press, 1986). Ralph Hamor's *A True Discourse of the Present Estate of Virginia* (1615) includes a copy of a letter by John Rolfe about his marriage to Pocahontas. It is reprinted in The English Experience series, no. 320 (Amsterdam: Theatrum Orbis Terrarum, 1971).
30. See the Powhatan-Renape Nation's web site *Pocahontas Myth* for an account of her early life and a rebuttal of the Disney portrayal. http://www.powhatan.org/pocc.html
31. Rayna Green, "The Pocahontas Perplex: The Image of Indian Women in American Culture," *The Massachusetts Review* 17 (1975): 698–9.
32. Powhatan-Renape Nation, *Pocahontas Myth*.
33. Powhatan-Renape Nation, *Pocahontas Myth*. John Smith's account has Pocahontas declaring graciously that "she would consider herself Smith's daughter now that she was in his land, as he had declared himself the son of Powhatan when he had entered her father's land." Quoted in Clara Sue Kidwell, "Indian Women as Cultural Mediators," 101..
34. Robertson, "Pocahontas at the Masque," 556.
35. Green, "The Pocahontas Perplex: The Image of Indian Women in American Culture," *The Massachusetts Review* 17 (1975): 702.
36. Green, "Pocahontas Perplex," 702–3.
37. Green, "Pocahontas Perplex," 703.
38. Green, "Pocahontas Perplex," 704.
39. Green, "Pocahontas Perplex," 709–10.
40. Powhatan-Renape Nation, *Pocahontas Myth*.
41. Green, "The Pocahontas Perplex," 714.
42. John Gillies, "Shakespeare's Virginian Masque," *English Literary History* 53 (1986): 677. Quoted in Robertson, "Pocahontas at the Masque," 556.
43. William Strachey, *The Historie of Travaile into Virginia Britania*, ed. R. H. Major (London: Hakluyt Society, 1849). Quoted in Robertson, "Pocahontas at the Masque," 561.
44. John Chamberlain, *The Letters of John Chamberlain*, ed. Norman Egbert McClure, 2 vols. (Philadelphia: American Philosophical Society, 1939), 2:56–7. Quoted in Robertson, "Pocahontas at the Masque," 554.
45. Harold P. Howard, *Sacajawea* (Norman, OK: University of Oklahoma Press, 1971), 150.
46. Kidwell, "Indian Women as Cultural Mediators," 102.
47. Quoted in Howard, *Sacajawea*, 141, 142.
48. Howard, *Sacajawea*, 158–61.

PART V

MORTALITY

CHAPTER EIGHTEEN

London's Mourning Garment: Maternity, Mourning and Royal Succession

Patricia Phillippy

Unlike the numerous elegies and memorials issued by London publishers in the wake of Queen Elizabeth's death in March, 1603, William Muggins' *Londons Mourning Garment*, published in the same year, mourns the loss to the plague of nearly 38,000 citizens between July and November.[1] Muggins' 87-stanza elegy for London's dead, however, shares with elegies for the queen a preoccupation with the figure of the mother as the central image through which death, its pathos, and its implications – spiritual, social, and political – are negotiated and represented. The frequent casting of Elizabeth as the maternal object *of* lament, "the aged mother of these orphane lands,"[2] finds its complement in the lamenting mothers of Muggins' poem. The narrator, seeking mourners to accompany London in her complaints, dismisses male citizens (as "stronger, sorrowes to begyle") and calls upon the "Dames of London Cittie," (B3) particularly mothers, to mourn the dead:

> Oh, mothers sigh, sit and shed teares a while,
> Expell your idle pleasures, thinke on woes:
> Make not so much as countenance of a smile,
> But with downe lookes, which inward sorrow showes,
> And now a fresh, remember all your throwes,
> > Your gripes your panges, your bodies pincht with paine,
> > As if this instant, you did them sustaine. (B3v)

As this physiology of mourning suggests, Muggins' poem constructs the maternal body as a synecdoche for the city's suffering from the perceived continuity between the "paine yet willing" of "breeding, bearing, and delivery" (B3v) and the unwilling sorrow occasioned by the death of a child. Maternal mourning, predicated on women's physical abilities to bear and breastfeed children, is figured in the poem, and more generally in early modern discourses of death and consolation, as especially violent and immoderate due to the strong affective bond between mother and child – as Muggins puts it, "Mothers love, to Child … fixte so fast" (B4v). Muggins is not alone in seeing maternal grief as a powerful image in which to focus the general suffering of plague-time. Dekker, too, characterizes the horrors of 1603 with the figure of London's "wofully distracted mothers that with disheveld haire falne into swounds … lye kissing the insensible cold lips of [their] breathlesse infants,"[3] while Thomas Brewer's *Weeping Lady* casts plague-ridden London as a mourning Rachel who, seeing death "gorg'd with [her] Sonnes and Daughters" appears "with nothing but grones, Sighs, teares, shreaks, folding of armes; beating of brests, wringing of hands, pale looks, dejected eies, bleeding heart, & most heavy and bitter condolements."[4]

This essay examines the complex role of the maternal mourner in early modern England as an ideologically-charged icon of feminized, immoderate mourning whose troubling presence compromises the political and spiritual teleologies of Muggins' text, of early modern characterizations of the plague as God's punishment of sins, and of post-Reformation mourning more generally. Taking Muggins' poem as a starting point, I examine representations of maternal mourning not only in texts by men – *artes moriendi*, plague literature, and elegies on the death of Elizabeth – but also in early modern women's works. I argue that maternity is constructed in the period as a unique site of affective and emotional license whose suspension of orthodox responses to loss is particularly useful to male authors in scripting difficult or ambivalent social phenomena – the (long-anticipated) death of a female monarch and accession of her male heir, or the descent of the city into the unfathomable darkness of the plague. In such works, the juncture of maternity and mourning enables a conceptual shift from passive to active responses to death, from unproductive excess to profitable moderation – that is, from female to male – that is also the trajectory of royal succession with the death of Elizabeth and accession of James. If male writers make use of the transgressive potential of maternal mourning, suitably contained by masculine orthodoxy, to underwrite this conceptual shift, women writers employ the mother's lament to empower and authorize their textual performances by rooting them within the resistant body of the maternal mourner herself.

* * *

As part of his portrait of inconsolable maternal grief, Muggins encourages London's mothers to recall their experiences of childbirth as liminal moments at which, poised with their children in the threshold between life and death, they glimpse a prolepsis of child loss:

> Againe bethinke you, at that instant hower,
> The little difference, was twixt life and death:

> When as the infant, with his naked power,
> Laboured for life, to have his rightfull birth,
> And with the sickly, Mother gaspt for breath,
>   The one nere death, as nigh to death the other,
>   Sore to the babe, worse Travell for the Mother. (B3v)

Muggins' conflation of women's experiences of the births and deaths of their children reflects the social histories of early modern birth and death, and women's unique roles within them. While the practice of midwifery ensured that, "up to the mid-seventeenth century, the presence of any man at a childbirth was unusual,"[5] the gendering of death and its rituals ascribed to women, prior to the development of the undertaking profession in the late-seventeenth century, not only the task of attending the dying but also the "menial and gendered" work of preparing the body for disposal.[6] Early modern women were the most frequent and immediate attendants on bodies in death, nursing the dying, washing and winding the corpse, "watching" the body during its period of laying-out, lamenting within the home, serving as mourners for funerals, and donning mourning garments according to rules of gender, relation, and class.

A surprisingly large number of texts written by and for early modern women concern themselves explicitly with the matter of death, and bespeak not only the widely-perceived intimacy of women with death's physical ravishments but also the unusual license to write and publish afforded to women in proximity to death, particularly to mothers mourning the loss of their children.[7] Certainly birth and death were conflated in fact, as well as figuratively, for early modern women who survived the deaths of their children, and the effects of these losses are recorded in women's texts.[8] With the chance of death in the first year of life at about 20%, and with another one in five children likely to die before their fifth birthday, child loss was a pervasive and painful fact of life for most women.[9] Thomas R. Forbes' study of mortality in early modern London concludes that "in Shakespeare's day, of every 100 babies born in St. Botolph's parish about 70 survived to their first birthday, 48 to their fifth, and 27–30 to their fifteenth."[10] Assertions by Lawrence Stone and Philippe Ariès of parental indifference to child loss in the period (in Stone's now-infamous words, "parents were obliged to limit the degree of their psychological involvement with their infant children"[11]) have been effectively challenged by social historians and literary and cultural critics engaged in reassessing the evidence provided by female-authored sources.[12] Women's complaints of the death of children in elegies, diaries, and other forms attest to the common affective bond between mothers and children, and record their deep sorrow at and resistance to the severing of that bond. Unlike male-authored elegies, whose compensatory poetics are characterized by "eulogy and transcendence … aris[ing] directly from masculine patterns of competition, separation, and individuation,"[13] maternal mourners tend to concentrate on the physical fact of death and on the corruption, rather than the resurrection, of the beloved body. They often express desires to join departed children in death or to give their lives in place of their children's, suggesting that "maternal severance can only be healed by death – and not by elegy."[14] Sculptures adorning the tomb of Elizabeth Cooke Russell at Bisham, for example, present her as a mother kneeling in the midst of the children she buried in her lifetime – one infant son and five daughters of her two marriages (to Thomas Hoby and John Russell). Lady Russell's epitaphs on the Bisham tombs and on those of the Russell family in Westminster Abbey deeply mourn the loss of these children: in "Verses of the devastated mother Lady Elizabeth Russell on the death of her son," she characteristically complains, "O that I, the mother, lay dead, the light denied me, / and he had first fulfilled my rites!"[15]

Rooted in the physical bond between mother and child forged, according to early modern views, not only during gestation but also through nursing, mothers' stubborn concern with the body of the departed rather than the soul – with irreparable loss rather than spiritual comfort – characterizes maternal mourning in texts authored by both men and women. In 1584, John Soowthern included in his collection of poems, *Pandora*, a series of sonnets written by Lady Russell's niece, Anne de Vere, Countess of Oxford, on the death of her infant son the year before. Throughout four complete poems and two fragments, de Vere presents a mother's inconsolable grief and reluctance to part with the beloved body. "And Destins, and Gods, you might rather have tanne here, / My twentie yeeres; then the two daies of my sonne," she complains, and later collapses the imagery of the tomb and womb to articulate the unique physical link between the living-dead body of the maternal mourner, petrified by sorrow, and the corpse of her offspring:

> Amphion's wife was turned to a rocke. O
> How well I had beene, had I had such adventure.
> For then I might again have been the Sepulchre,
> Of him that I bare in mee, so long ago.[16]

Inscribing within his work the first-person lament of mothers such as de Vere, Muggins also presents his plague mothers, "with lamentations and with Tears good store" (C2), graphically recalling the physical bonds between themselves and their children, now severed by death:

> Ah my sweet Babes, what woulde noe I have done?
> To yeelde you comfort, & maintaine you heere:
> Early and late, no labour would I shun,
> To feede your mouthes, though hunger pincht me neere;
> All three at once, I woulde your bodies cheere.
>   Twaine in my lappe, should sucke their tender Mother,
>   And with my foot, I would have rockt the other.

> Me thinkes I see them still, and heare their cryes
> Chiefly a nights when I on bed am layde,
> Which make fresh teares goe from my watry eyes,
> When I awake and finde I am deceived;
> Sweet pretie Babes, Christ hath your souls received;
> > Faire Babe to me, you nere shall come againe,
> > But where you are, I trust ay to remaine. (C2–C2v)

Despite her acknowledgment that her children are now in heaven, Muggins' maternal mourner refuses consolation, "byd[ing] more sorrowes in this wretched earth" (C2v). The physicality of the maternal bond leads Muggins to a labored description of the nursing of a newborn, in which the mother's pain and tears in breastfeeding explain and prefigure her mourning in child loss:

> And when the Babe doth gather strength amaine,
> Most strongly labouring at his mothers dugge.
> She patiently endureth all the paine,
> Suffering his lippes her nipple still to lugge.
> And with her armes most closely doth it hugge,
> > As she should say, draw childe and spare not mee,
> > My brests are thine, I feele no paine with thee.
>
> Though that poore heart her brest doth ake full sore,
> And inwardly fell prickings she indures,
> Till eyes gush teares, and lippes reach kisses store;
> Which in true mothers gladsome ioyes procures,
> And to more ardent love them still allures. (C1)

As William Gouge explains in his appeal to mothers to nurse their own children, "Together with the milke passeth some smacke of the affection and disposition of the mother: which maketh mothers to love such children best as they have given sucke unto."[17] This affective bond, unfortunately, makes child loss difficult for mothers to bear.

It is intriguing to wonder whether mothers who did not nurse their children (as was frequently the case in upper class and noble families) were considered to suffer as deeply at children's deaths, or conversely, whether wet nurses might be supposed to mourn as profoundly as breastfeeding mothers at the death of a child whom she had nursed, though not her own offspring.[18] Questions such as these illuminate the *naturalization of motherhood* – that is, its essentialist casting as adhering in the physical bodies of women – undertaken by Muggins and others as a performative strategy in which early modern men, as the domestic and social governors of women, had a stake.[19] The view of maternal mourning elaborated by early modern men is similarly essentialized, devoting itself to *constructing* gender on the basis of behaviors and affects which are presented as *describing* it: thus the immoderate mourner *is* female, and the most inconsolable among them are mothers, regardless of the biological facts attending the birth, nursing, or death of an individual child. In the hands of early modern women, this naturalization of motherhood could be turned toward a valorization of women's emotions and their expression: whether or not Anne de Vere nursed her infant, her extreme sorrow at his loss is underwritten by the essentialist reading of maternal mourning as a matter of the body.

Because representations of violent maternal mourning occur in both male- and female-authored works, the gendering of the image requires scrutiny. While the excesses of maternal mourning are commonly depicted as obstinately resistant to the will of God in male-authored works, they are often used by women writers to establish the basis of their authority. Andreas Hyperius' *Practice of Preaching* (1577) typifies the gendering of grief often put forth by early modern *artes moriendi* and consolatory texts in condemning "a wommanish kinde of wayling and shricking" and insisting that, "All that be of sound judgement, do thincke it very uncomly and womannishe to lament without measure, & to take so impaciently the chaunce that happeneth."[20] The frequent assertion of early modern stoicism that men who grieve immoderately are effeminate lends itself to the chastisement of men's mourning through shameful comparisons with women. Erasmus' *De Morto Declamatio*, for instance, admits that death is a "ryght good cause to be hevy," but encourages men to moderate their sorrow with the example of maternal mourning: "For what selye mother doth so extremely bewayle the deth of her childe but that in shorte space of tyme her sorrowe some what asslaketh, and at length is clene forgotten? To have always a stedfast mynde is a token of a perfecte wyse man."[21] Erasmus' comparison, although presented to censure male immoderation, implicitly recognizes the "short space of tyme" in which a mother's excessive lamentation can be expected to occur. The acknowledgment of this site in which orthodox (that is, manly) mourning is suspended – despite men's efforts to limit that "space of tyme" and restrain women's behavior within it – inadvertently authorizes female speech, itself often associated in the period with excess, incontinence, and lack of restraint.[22] The ideological demarcation of mothers' grief as a uniquely volatile emotional site licenses women's textual works of mourning.

This delineation of the site of maternal mourning as one of unusual affective and expressive license offers to male writers, such as Muggins, a unique stage on which to theorize and perform political, poetic, and cultural transformations. As an image of debilitating pathos, the maternal mourner frozen in grief and dedicated to the dead rather than the living (as Henry Peacham describes it, the mother bereft of her daughter "would faine / Even with her fingers dig her up againe"[23]) is a potent figure for cultural, political, and artistic forms at a dead end and in need of resuscitation, correction, or abandonment. Although *Londons Mourning Garment* lingers over the figure of the maternal mourner, milking it (as it were) of its pathetic power, the poem cannot permanently fix its telos of plague and salvation in that static image. Rather, Muggins begins and ends his poem with gestures of welcome to the new monarch, poising the text chronologically between James' entry into London in May, when crowds were "so greedy ... to behold the countenance of the King that, with much unruliness, they injured one another," and his much-delayed triumphal progress through the city, intended to accompany his coronation on July 25 but postponed due to the virulence of the plague until March of the following year.[24] With the nostalgic recollection of James' May entry and the optimistic vision of his long-anticipated progress, Muggins closes his poem:

> My crowned Cesar and his Peerlesse Queene,
> Comes not tryumphing with their princely sonne,
> Deck't with rich robes the like was never seene,
> Nor never none more welcome to London,
> Me thinkes I see the people how they runne,
>> To get them roome this happy sight to see,
>> That this may come say all Amen, with mee. (D2v)

The condition of this triumph – figured not only as a political arrival but also as a resurrection, a triumph over death – is the cessation of the plague. This, in turn, would signal a triumph over sin, since *Londons Mourning Garment* shares with other examples of plague literature from the period an understanding of the epidemic as a scourge of God, visited upon Londoners as a punishment for sins. Minister James Balmford, for example, urges his parishioners, "when it shall please God to remove this heavy judgment, let us never forget this visitation."[25] Lady Margaret Hoby records in her diary for October 23, 1603, "it was reported that, [at] London, the number was taken of the Livinge and not of the deed: Lord graunt that these Judgmentes may cause England with speed to tourne to the Lord."[26] Wednesdays were designated as days of fasting "appointed by the Kinge to be heald thorowe the wholl Realme in regard of the generall mortalitie," and were occasions for repentance, charity, and prayer.[27] The portrait of London as a mourning mother in Brewer's *Weeping Lady* is explicitly offered as a recollection of God's punishment and a call to virtue to avoid its recurrence:

> My intent in erecting this poore Monument of Misery, was, to make this Ladies Teares out-live her Teares: that, when by the infinite Mercies of God they shall bee wip'd off, and all her Sores made whole; we may ... re-view them; in them those infinite Mercies; and in both, be made mindfull of them, and eternally thankfull of them: which God grant.[28]

For Muggins, the agent of this reform is neither King James himself, whose political marriage to London-as Bride (B1v) is the result rather than the means of her recovery, nor the maternal mourner, whose tears are called "the onely Physicke, women can bestow" (B4v). It is London's male magistrates, rather, who are responsible for relieving the strokes of God's "heavie rod" (C4) by enforcing the moral behavior of citizens:

Reforme these things, you heads of London Citie,
Punish lewd vice, let vertue spring and grow:
Then Gods just wrath, now hot will turne to pittie,
And for his children, you again doe know:
Your former health, on you he will bestow,
　　The Plague and Pestilence, wherewith he visites still,
　　To end or send, are in his holy will. (D2)

Recalling them to their duties (often necessary during plague-time due to high numbers of city officials fleeing their posts for fear of infection),[29] Muggins encourages the magistrates to "Remember likewise, God hath plac't you heere, / To be as nursing fathers to the poore" (D1v).

The movement in *Londons Mourning Garment* from nursing-mothers-turned-mourners, petrified in sorrow, to this masculinist appropriation of nursing (by way of Isaiah 49:23, "And kings shall be thy nursing fathers; and their queens thy nursing mothers") converts breastfeeding from an emblem of maternal sacrifice to a figure for male government. It replaces maternal tears, "the onely Physicke, women can bestow," with active paternal "rulers, of each publycke charge" (D1v) in whose hands the city finds not sterile complaint but productive remedy for its losses.[30] This conceptual shift from passive mourning to active government presents a gendered politics of the plague that parallels the gendering of early modern mourning, in which the unproductive excesses of maternal grief – a living death distracting the mourner from God's providential design – is corrected by "wyse" masculine mourning in moderation. The essentialist location of the stubborn stasis of maternal mourning in the physiology of birth and breastfeeding enables the *construction* of the nursing father, or moderate male mourner, as a sublimation and improvement of "natural" maternal instincts.

While the maternal mourner enables the movement from passive to active responses to death in Muggins' text, from domestic sorrow to public policy, and from maternal to paternal nourishment, she nonetheless is a resistant, transgressive presence in the poem and in early modern literatures of death and consolation more generally. Mothers' stubborn emphases on the body's physical demise at the expense of spiritual transcendence challenge not only the decorum of post-Reformation mourning but also the teleology of death and resurrection fundamental to Christian consolation.[31] Muggins' maternal mourners – striking in their powerful, passionate suffering – are the figures that remain in the reader's mind when the text is over: like Brewer's "Monument of Misery," their "Ladies Teares out-live [their] Teares," but with a transgressive pathos that cannot easily be accommodated by Brewer's, or Muggins', teleology of the plague. The refusal of consolation embodied by the maternal mourner is symptomatic not only of the suspended, deferred closure of Muggins' text – able only to hope for rather than guarantee the city's political and spiritual triumph over death – but also of the uncertainties attending death itself, where faith may hope for, but not yet know, salvation.

* * *

The replacement of static female mourning by potent male government in *Londons Mourning Garment* takes place in the shadow of the death of Elizabeth I and imitates the political replacement of a female monarch by her male successor. Muggins never mentions the queen in his poem, eliding her death in the pithy phrase, "With springing March, the tidings of a king" (B1). Mourning for Elizabeth is quickly overtaken by more pressing events, and is both pre-empted by the triumphant image of James and displaced into the poems' maternal mourners. This elision suggests the ambivalence and uncertainty that attended both the queen's death and the king's accession. Lady Anne Clifford's report that, "King James was proclaimed in Cheapside by all the Council with great joy and triumph" since "this peaceable coming of a king was unexpected of all parts of the people,"[32] attests to the anxiety over succession in the latter part of Elizabeth's reign and the general relief at a peaceful transfer of power. But, as Steven Mullaney suggests, noting the merger of mourning and misogyny in responses to Elizabeth's death, "The advent of an orderly and Protestant succession does not in itself account for such a celebratory spirit; in fact, it was a significant transformation in the body politic, a reincorporation and regendering of monarchy, that was being heralded."[33]

The "nation almost begotten and borne under her"[34] mourned Elizabeth as its mother: "And forasmuch as the Scripture calleth kings *nursing fathers, and Queenes nursing mothers* of the church and common wealth," Radford Mavericke's *Mourning Weede* asks, how can her subjects not mourn, "being not lately weaned for any longer sucking the sweete and tender paps of our late most dearest beloved Queene, who living, loved us as dearely (doubtles) if not more dearly, then ever any nurse or mother loved her beloved babe."[35] Mavericke's literalization of the biblical image emphasizes Elizabeth's maternal essence, but disturbingly casts her death as the occasion of the nation's weaning, revising the natural process of maturation with the unnatural severance of the mother–child bond. He exploits, chiasmically, the affective bond utilized in Muggins' teleology of the plague in his description of the providential succession of a male monarch. Weaned by death from the "Pelicanlike" body of Elizabeth,[36] the infantile body politic turns to its "nursing father," James. As Richard Mulcaster's *Comforting Complaynt* concludes, "though [God] tooke our Queene, a King he gave / To play the fathers part in mothers losse."[37] The over-arching argument of Mavericke's work, like that of all of the 1603 elegies for the queen, is that this shift – from mother to father, from literal to metaphoric nursing, from sex to gender – is both necessary and beneficial. The nation must mourn moderately, avoiding excess, for political rather than spiritual reasons: expanding on Psalms 30:5, "Weeping may abide at Evening, but Joy cometh in the morning," Mavericke exchanges the dark night of Elizabeth's demise for the joyful ascension of James. Elizabeth's elegists invariably translate sorrow to joy, often celebrating the James' kingship at far greater length than they devote to eulogizing the queen[38] and employing a version of seasonal, moderate mourning which effectively short-circuits lamentation and renders their texts "attempt[s] to establish in the popular mind the new king's legitimacy."[39]

As a response to royal succession, excessive mourning – understood here as both mourning *of* and *for* the mother – threatens to disable the smooth transfer of power, valorizing past over future, Tudor over Stuart, and female monarch over male. As in *Londons Mourning Garment*, feminine stasis must give way to masculine productivity; the feminine preoccupation with the material body must surrender to the masculine metaphorics of the body politic. While elegies for Elizabeth work to season mourning with joy, the career of the genre itself suggests that the tenacity of mourning predicated upon maternity would reinsert the body of Elizabeth into the nation's heart and imagination. Although the number of elegies written for the queen in 1603 is impressive, it falls well short of the number of works published either on the occasion of Sir Philip Sidney's heroic death in 1586, or at the death of Prince Henry in 1612.[40] Noticeably absent from the ranks of her elegists are the major poets of the era – an absence suggesting an ambivalence about Elizabeth's successor that is at least as great as that surrounding the death of the queen herself. Drayton's complaint that in the wake of Elizabeth's death, "cowardyse had tyed up every tongue, / And all stood silent"[41] articulates a curious reluctance to advance the Stuart claim to power, but, significantly, does so by casting it in terms which align the speechless poet with the mourning woman – both silent, static, unable to leave behind the corpse of Elizabethan monarchy. So indefatigable is that resilient, resistant corpse that nearly 30 years later, amid growing dissatisfaction with James' heir, Diana Primrose would publish an idealized elegy to "Queene Elizabeth, of Glorious Memory" which rewrites the nursing mother as a figure not of passive maternal mourning, but of threatening female power over life and death: in the stream emitted by her "Nectar-flowing Veine," Elizabeth "able was to drowne a World of men, / And drown'd, with sweetnes to revive agen."[42] Although delayed, the elegy finds a woman writer exploiting the provocative, productive merger of maternity and mourning to embalm the powerful female body as the enabling icon of women's political, and textual, authority.

Notes

1. William Muggins, *Londons Mourning Garment, or Funerall Teares: worne and shed for the death of her wealthy Citizens, and other her inhabitants* (London: Ralph Blower, 1603). Further citations will appear parenthetically. A bill of mortality appended to Muggins' poem numbers the deaths in London and its suburbs "of all diseases, since the first beginning of this visitation" at 37,717 (E2). See also F.P. Wilson, *The Plague in Shakespeare's London* (Oxford: Oxford University Press, 1927), 88–115.

2. Thomas Byng, "Offering," in *Sorrowes Joy, or A Lamentation for our late deceased Soveraigne Elizabeth, with a triumph for the prosperous succession of our gratious King James, &c.* (Cambridge: John Legat, 1603), 10.

3. Thomas Dekker, *The Wonderfull yeare 1603: Wherein is shewed the picture of London, lying sicke of the Plague* (London: Thomas Creede, 1603), C3–C3v.

4. Thomas Brewer, *The Weeping Lady: Or, London Like Ninivie in Sack-Cloth* (London: B.A. and T.F. for Mathew Rhodes, 1629), B1v and A2v.

5. Patricia Crawford, "The Construction and Experience of Maternity in Seventeenth-Century England," in *Women as Mothers in Pre-Industrial England: Essays in Memory of Dorothy McLaren*, ed. Valerie Fildes (London: Routledge, 1990), 21.

6. David Cressy, *Birth, Marriage and Death: Ritual, Religion, and the Life-Cycle in Tudor and Stuart England* (Oxford: Oxford University Press, 1997), 429. On the development of professional undertaking, see Clare Gittings, *Death, Burial and the Individual in Early Modern England* (London: Croom Helm, 1984), 96, and Paul S. Fritz, "The Undertaking Trade in England: Its Origins and Early Development, 1660–1830," *Eighteenth-Century Studies* 28:2 (1994–5): 241–53.

7. See Diane Bornstein, "The Style of the Countess of Pembroke's Translation of Philippe de Mornay's *Discours de la vie et de la mort*" in *Silent But For the Word: Tudor Women as Patrons, Translators, and Writers of Religious Works*, ed. Margaret Patterson Hannay (Kent: Kent State University Press, 1985), 127, and Mary Ellen Lamb, *Gender and Authorship in the Sidney Circle* (Madison: University of Wisconsin Press, 1990), 115–41. Mother's legacies offer good examples of how a woman's nearness to death could be used, by her or her publisher, to authorize her work: see Elaine V. Beilin, *Redeeming Eve: Women Writers of the English Renaissance* (Princeton: Princeton University Press, 1987), 266–85. Rachel Speght's *Mortalities Memorandum* takes the occasion of her mother's death to authorize the daughter's publication: see *The Polemics and Poems of Rachel Speght*, ed. Barbara Lewalski (New York: Oxford University Press, 1996). Mothers who published elegies for children or lamented child loss in other written forms include: Anne de Vere, Elizabeth Cooke Russell, Katherine Philips, Gertrude Thimelby, Mary Carey, Alice Thornton, and Lady Elizabeth Egerton. On de Vere and Russell, see below. On Philips, see Celeste Schenck, "Feminism and Deconstruction: Re-Constructing the Elegy," *Tulsa Studies in Women's Literature* 5 (1986): 14, and Kate Lilley, "True State Within: Women's Elegy, 1640–1740," in *Women, Writing, History, 1640–1740*, ed. Isobel Grundy and Susan Wiseman (Athens: University of Georgia Press, 1992), 84–6. On Thimelby, see Donna J. Long, "'She Endeavoured to Relieve Her Owne Emotions': Gertrude Thimelby's Elegies," unpublished paper presented at Shakespeare Association of America, Cleveland, March, 1998. On Carey, Thornton, and Egerton, see Kathryn McPherson, "'I thought my all was given

before': Women's Lamentations in Seventeenth Century England," in *Great-Bellied Women: Religion and Maternity in Seventeenth-Century England*. Diss. Emory University, 1998.

8. Space does not permit a thorough review of *paternal* complaints of child loss in the period, but they should not be overlooked. In general, these are fewer in number than mothers' elegies and complaints (itself a startling fact given the greater access to print enjoyed by men in the period), and support a gendering of grief which casts the stoic acceptance of death as manly and excessive mourning as effeminate. Dekker balances his portrait of maternal mourning, quoted above, with the figure of the mourning father, but portrays him as "basely descend[ing] into brutish & unmanly passions" (C4v). See also Philippe de Mornay, *Philip Mornay, Lord of Plessis his Teares for the Death of his Sonne. Unto his Wife Charlotte Baliste*, trans. John Healey (London: G. Eld, 1609), and Edward Vaughn, *A Divine Discoverie of Death* (London: William Jones for Richard Boyle, 1612), 184.

9. See Roger Schofield and E.A. Wrigley, "Infant and Child Mortality in England in the Late Tudor and Early Stuart Period," in *Health, Medicine and Mortality in the Sixteenth Century*, ed. Charles Webster (Cambridge: Cambridge University Press, 1979), 61–96; Lawrence Stone, *The Family, Sex and Marriage 1500–1800* (New York: Harper & Row, 1977), 68–9; Peter Laslett, *The World We Have Lost: England Before the Industrial Age* (New York: Charles Scribner, 1965), 125; and Patricia Crawford, "From the Woman's Point of View: Pre-industrial England," in *Exploring Women's Past: Essays in Social History*, ed. Patricia Crawford (Sydney: George Allen & Unwin, 1983), 71.

10. Thomas R. Forbes, "By What Disease or Casualty: The Changing Face of Death in London," in *Health, Medicine and Mortality in the Sixteenth Century*, ed. Charles Webster (Cambridge: Cambridge University Press, 1979), 139.

11. Stone, 70. See also Philippe Ariès, *Centuries of Childhood: A Social History of Family Life*, trans. Robert Baldick (New York: Vintage Books, 1962), 39.

12. See, for example, Crawford, "From the Woman's Point of View," 62; Cressy, 393; and Anne Laurence, "Goodly Grief: Individual Responses to Death in Seventeenth Century Britain," in *Death, Ritual, and Bereavement*, ed. Ralph Houlbrooke (New York: Routledge, 1989), 62–76.

13. Schenck, 20.

14. Lilley, 90. See also Schenck, 16–18.

15. Quoted in Louise Schleiner, *Tudor and Stuart Women Writers* (Bloomington: Indiana University Press, 1994), 49. See also 205–12 for the texts of the poems at Bisham.

16. "Foure Epytaphes, made by the Countes of Oxenford after the death of her young Sonne, the Lord Bulbeck," in John Soowthern, *Pandora* (1584) (facs. New York: Columbia University Press, 1938), C4v. Critical opinion has been divided on how the poems found their way to print and on the possible identification of Soowthern as their author. For discussion, see Ellen Moody, "Six Elegiac Poems, Possibly by Anne Cecil de Vere, Countess of Oxford," *ELR* 19 (1989): 152–70, Steven May, "The Countess of Oxford's Sonnets: A Caveat," *ELN* 29 (1992): 9–19, and Schleiner, 85–93. Elizabeth Russell employs the same image in mourning two of her daughters: "Together in one tomb, thus I your mother wanted you, / Whom I, with joy and crying, carried in one womb." Quoted in Schleiner, 209.

17. William Gouge, *Of Domesticall Duties* (London: John Haviland for William Bladen, 1622), 512.

18. On breastfeeding in the period, see Crawford, "The Construction and Experience of Maternity," 22–7.

19. See Judith Butler, *Gender Trouble: Feminist Theory and Psychoanalytic Discourse* (New York: Routledge, 1990), 136.

20. Andreas Hyperius, *Of Framing of Divine Sermons, or Popular Interpretation of the Scriptures* (*The Practice of Preaching*), trans. John Ludham (London: Thomas East, 1577), Z4 and Z3–Z3v.

21. Erasmus, *A treatyse perswading a man paciently to suffer the death of his freende* (London: Thomas Berthelet, 1531), A2v–A3.

22. See Wendy Wall, *The Imprint of Gender: Authorship and Publication in the English Renaissance* (Ithaca: Cornell University Press, 1993), Karen Newman, *Fashioning Femininity and English Renaissance Drama* (Chicago: University of Chicago Press, 1991), and Gail Kern Paster, *The Body Embarrassed: Drama and the Disciplines of Shame in Early Modern England* (Ithaca: Cornell University Press, 1993).

23. Henry Peacham, *Thestylis astrata: or, A Funerall Elegie upon the Death of the Right Honourable, most Religious and Noble Lady, Frances, Countess of Warwicke* (London: J.H. for Francis Constable, 1634), B1v.

24. T.M., *The True Narration of the Entertainment of His Royal Majesty*, quoted in Wilson, 88.

25. James Balmford, *A Short Dialogue Concerning the Plagues Infection* (London: Richard Boyle, 1603), A3v–A4.

26. Margaret Hoby, *Diary of Lady Margaret Hoby, 1599–1605*, ed. Dorothy M. Meads (London: Routledge, 1930), 207.

27. Ibid, 206. See Wilson, 3–6 and 99–103.

28. Brewer, A3.

29. See Balmford, 71. Muggins explicitly addresses the problem: "Though feare of sicknesse drive you hence as men,/ Yet leave your purse, and feeling heart with them" (D1).

30. Balmford also adapts this image to describe male government in plague-time, urging his parishioners to suspend charitable visits to the sick by reminding them that since "Kings and Queenes ought to be nursing fathers and nursing mothers to the Church," James "should (out of fatherly care) preserve [his] subjects from destruction" (6). When the 1603 Plague Orders sought to isolate the sick by prohibiting visits to houses known to be infected, the morality of this prohibition was widely debated.

31. A similar argument appears in Sarah Stanbury's "The Virgin's Gaze: Spectacle and Transgression in Middle English Lyrics of the Passion," *PMLA* 101 (1991): 1083–93.

32. Lady Anne Clifford, *The Diaries of Lady Anne Clifford*, ed. D.J.H. Clifford (Wolfeboro Falls, NH: Alan Sutton, 1990), 21.

33. Steven Mullaney, "Mourning and Misogyny: *Hamlet, The Revenger's Tragedy*, and the Final Progress of Elizabeth I, 1600–1607," *Shakespeare Quarterly* 45 (1994): 139. See also Christopher Haigh, *Elizabeth I* (New York: Longman, 1988), 160–8.

34. Dekker, B2.

35. Radford Mavericke, *Three Treatises Religiously Handled, and named according to the severall subject of each Treatise: The Mourning Weede. The Mornings Joy. The Kings Rejoicing* (London: John Windet, 1603), C2v and B3v.

36. Ibid, C4v.

37. Richard Mulcaster, *The Translation of Certaine Latine Verses Written Uppon her Majesties Death, Called A Comforting Complaynt* (London: Edward Aggas, 1603), A2.

38. The oxymoronic titles of many of these works suggest their double purpose to eulogize Elizabeth and praise James: see, for example, *Sorrowes Joy*; H.S., *Queen Elizabeths Losse and King James his Welcome* (London: T.C. for John Sythicke, 1603); and Joseph Hall, *The King's Prophecie, or Weeping Joy* (London, 1603).

39. Dennis Kay, *Melodious Tears: The English Funeral Elegy from Spenser to Milton* (Oxford: Clarendon, 1990), 82.

40. Ibid, 78 and 90.

41. Quoted Ibid, 78.

42. Diana Primrose, *A Chaine of Pearle, or A Memoriall of the peerles Graces, and Heroick Vertues of Queene Elizabeth, of Glorious Memory* (London: Thomas Paine by Philip Waterhouse), C1v.

CHAPTER NINETEEN

Early Modern Medea: Representations of Child Murder in the Street Literature of Seventeenth-Century England

Susan C. Staub

> I have given suck, and know
> How tender 'tis to love the babe that milks me;
> I would, while it was smiling in my face,
> Have pluck'd my nipple from his boneless gums,
> And dash'd the brains out, had I so sworn as you
> Have done to this.

(Macbeth, I, vii, 54-9)

As familiar as these lines are, Lady Macbeth's vivid perversion of motherly nurturance maintains its power to shock listeners because it runs counter to everything traditionally associated with the good mother. Lady Macbeth provides a terrifying example of the mother who abuses maternal power by exchanging her mother's milk for gall and violently destroying her imaginary baby. This horrible picture of motherhood is not unique to Shakespeare or to the period. Lady Macbeth's lines participate in a pervasive cultural anxiety about motherhood. Historically, mothers have occupied an ambivalent position as both sexual object/nurturer and mistress/servant within the family structure. But during the early modern period, the construction of the mother seems especially problematic and becomes enmeshed with other anxieties as well, anxieties about family relations, religion and economics.

The figure of the murdering mother appears repeatedly in early modern dramas, broadsheets and news pamphlets and became popular at the same time that domestic literature was busily redefining the mother's role. Conduct books, domestic manuals and sermons increasingly emphasized the intellectual and spiritual duties of the mother in addition to her physical obligations. In the words of one writer, mothers were to "nourish [their children's] bodies as the pelican" and "suckle [their] minds with the milk of good manners, training [them] up … in religion and learning."[1] These responsibilities conferred an authority on the early modern mother heretofore unmatched within the household.[2] Recent research suggests further that some mothers possessed very real economic power, playing significant roles in arranging their sons' marriages and making decisions about wills and property.[3] It is not surprising, then, that early modern writings on motherhood attempted to contain maternal power by insisting on the mother's intellectual and moral weakness at the same time that they affirmed her special place within the household.

The mother's role was ambiguous at best. Her authoritative position as mother conflicted with her subordinated position as wife. Although she seemed to have a unique power within the domestic sphere, she was pictured as subject to her husband. She might be the steward of the household in the husband's absence, but in his presence she remained his subordinate. As we might expect, the increasing importance given to the mother in the late sixteenth and early seventeenth centuries opens up a potential site of conflict between motherly authority and wifely submission. Clearly, as Mary Beth Rose points out, "motherhood presents a test case for female power, making visible the destabilizing contradictions that that power comprises in English Renaissance society."[4] In fact, any woman involved in the nurturing and upbringing of the child, from pregnancy through breaching, could be suspect.[5]

Like the domestic tracts, the street literature participates in the ambivalent construction of motherhood during the period. And like domestic literature, the popular pamphlets are concerned with maternal duty. For the most part, however, these writings concentrate on instances when motherhood goes awry, on those cases when maternal nurture transmutes into maternal violence. The emphasis on violence in these texts is part of the criminalization of female agency posited by several scholars to take place during this period.[6] Since women's power in early modern England is almost wholly within the household, the violence depicted is largely domestic, and at least in the case of married mothers, most often occurs at the point where motherly authority and wifely submission collides.

Newsbooks and cheap pamphlets issued after a crime or an execution sought both to capitalize on the public's appetite for the sensational and, ostensibly, to spread official ideas about behavior, crime and punishment. Although these pamphlets purport to deal with actual crimes, much of what they present is clearly fictional. They were not written to be great literature, but to report on, respond to, even exploit the concerns and anxieties of a general readership. Precisely because of their ephemeral status, they more clearly reflect the period's often contradictory attitudes about women than more aesthetically and carefully written literature might. At the same time that domestic texts and conduct books valorized motherhood, dubbing it "the salvation of [the female] sex," the popular press criminalized mothers. Although the method might be different, the end result was the same: to limit maternal authority.

Despite the prevalence of "spinsters" in the court cases involving infant and child murder, the popular press rarely treated unmarried infanticides, choosing instead to represent married women (and sometimes widows) who murdered their children, apparently because their crimes suggested a potential disruption of the marital structure and were thus more threatening. Child murder by married women was rare, and presumably even more notorious given its infrequency. As Malcolmson notes, "Documented instances of infanticide within marriage are exceptional ... women from genteel or middle-class families were seldom accused of infanticide, almost all of the women involved appear to have been from labouring, mechanic, or farming backgrounds."[7] Infanticide committed by unmarried mothers, while not condoned, was at least understandable; the murder of infants and children by married mothers was not. The very fact that it occurred evoked the horrible power of the mother that conduct books, prescriptive literature and even medical manuals tried to suppress. Because middle class married women were generally not committing infanticide to maintain their socio-economic status, their actions more clearly indicted the patriarchal definition of domesticity and necessitated an examination of the motivation behind their crimes. In their recounting of these crimes, these texts explore the definition of the good mother and expose contradictions and anxieties about maternal authority.

Where it does treat unmarried infanticides, the street literature represents these women as decidedly unnatural, monstrous, and sexually promiscuous.[8] In contrast, the majority of the pamphlets dealing with married mothers do not sexualize the mothers and are at least partially sympathetic in their critiques of them. Because they are socially and religiously sanctified wives, these women are granted a measure of respect not typically given to the unmarried women. Their crimes are not an attempt to avoid the shame of motherhood; in fact, most of these women commit their crimes out of their sense of duty as mothers. For the most part, they do not define themselves against the social order, but completely within it. This literature focuses precisely on those sites where the mother is deemed to have the most power – over the physical, spiritual and mental well being of her children. In a perversion of the responsible mother of the conduct manuals, these mothers kill their children in order to save them from religious falsehood, from starvation, and occasionally, from the mother's own desperate psychological state. As such, while mothers' manuals and conduct books limit maternal power by emphasizing paternal governance, these pamphlets seek to undermine that authority by constructing it as dangerous and violent.

As noted earlier, one of the mother's chief responsibilities was to instill proper faith in her children, a responsibility that grants the mother an enormous amount of power not just over the child's earthly life but over its eternal soul. Although in many ways the Reformation replaced the parish priest with the godly father who had ultimate responsibility for the spiritual instruction of the family, the mother's influence was also widely recognized. William Gouge in *Of Domesticall Duties*, for instance, lists religious instruction as one of the special duties of mothers, a duty that most women seem to have taken quite seriously. In *The Mother's Legacie to her Unborn Child*, one of the few places where we actually hear a mother's voice, Elizabeth Jocelin fears that her death in childbirth will prevent her "from executing that care I so exceedingly desired, I mean [the] religious training of our Childe."[9]

Always looking for a sensational angle, several popular pamphlets treat the disastrous repercussions of misdirected and excessive religious piety, thus playing on cultural anxieties about Catholicism and other religious sects. *A Pittilesse Mother*, for one, tells the story of Margaret Vincent, a mother who murders her children out of an obsessive concern for the salvation of their souls when her husband refuses to allow them to be baptized in the Catholic Church (Fig. 19.1). Her crime is not one of anger or hatred, but rather, stems from her concept of what it means to be a good mother. By defining good mothering as raising and educating her children in her true faith, Vincent sees no recourse but to kill them in order to deliver them from eternal damnation. This pamphlet is more openly propagandistic than other texts of this kind (though one could argue that virtually all of this literature has a propagandizing intent), and the story is told in large measure to warn of the dangers of Roman Catholicism. Addressed specifically to the "good Gentlewomen" whom the pamphlet depicts as particularly vulnerable to the machinations of the Catholic church, the text is "both anti-Papist and misogynistic," according to Betty Travitsky.[10] Just as women fall easily victim to Satan's wiles, so too are they easily swayed by false religion; they are, in the pamphlet writer's words, "the weak sex they [Roman Catholics] continually make prize of."[11] Margaret Vincent is transgressive and dangerous not just as mother but in her recusancy as well, "both of which provided her with some grounds for resisting domestic patriarchy."[12] Although the pamphlet basically constructs Vincent as religiously misguided, it also defines her actions as a resistance to husbandly authority by defining her in opposition to her less gullible husband, a "good Gentleman" who accounted her persuasions "vaine and frivolous and she undutifull to make so fond an attempt" (A3).

As the pamphlet begins, the author takes great pains to establish Vincent as a model of wifely and motherly gentleness, describing her as "discreet, civil, and of modest conversation" and "much esteemed of all that knew her for her modest and seemly carriage." Married for 12 or 14 years in comfort and concord, this "good soul," this "unfortunate gentlewoman," falls into the clutches of "Roman Wolves" who entangle the "sweet Lamb" with their subtle

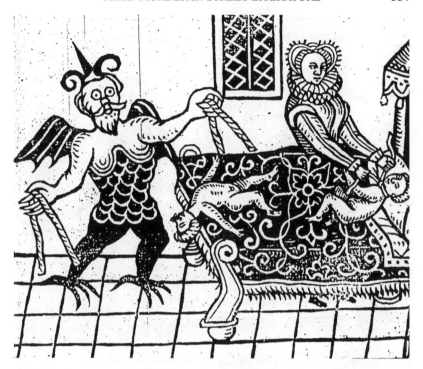

Fig. 19.1 *A Pittilesse Mother.* Title page from a pamphlet, STC 24757

persuasions. For the most part, Vincent is portrayed as an innocent victim without agency, bewitched by the deceptive allure of the Catholic Church. The Catholic Church is presented as a seductive lover, offering such charming inducements that "hardly the female kinde can escape their inticements" (A2v). The depiction of the woman as easily swayed by false doctrine builds on a long held tradition of women as intellectually and morally weaker than men and lends support to the argument that men should retain dominance over the household. The text illustrates the woman's limited power over her husband as she tries futilely to persuade him to convert, feeling that "she was appointed by the holy Church to shew him the light of true understanding" (A3). Interestingly, though, the husband seems at least partially culpable and is described as snubbing Vincent with unkind speeches. Further, one place in the text suggests that the issue is not only religion but also the struggle for power within the household. "Oh Margret, Margret, how often have I perswaded thee from this damned Opinion, this damned Opinion that hath undone us all," the husband moans. Flouting her role as submissive wife, Vincent, sounding oddly like Chaucer's Wife of Bath, admonishes her husband for not giving her

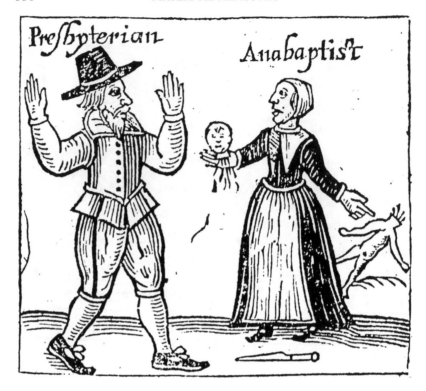

Fig. 19.2   *Bloody Newes from Dover*. Title page from a pamphlet

sovereignty in the marriage: "Oh, Jarvis, this had never beene done if thou hast been ruld and by me converted" (A4v). Although it is only suggested in this text, the conflict can be read as centering in parental power and authority; the father contends with the mother for control of the children. The woodcut on the title page, however, glosses over this bit of wifely intransigence, showing the mother less in control of her actions, being goaded by the devil to strangle her babies. Despite the mother's formidable power over her children, then, she is still the weaker sex, subject to all of the errors of the flesh and spirit, and in need of the close supervision of her husband.

A similar pamphlet from the mid-seventeenth century, *Bloody Newes from Dover* (1647), also exploits a contemporary religious dispute, in this case, the controversy over infant baptism (Fig. 19.2). What in the narrative seems merely an illustration of female willfulness and susceptibility to fits of passion is revealed on the title page to be an example of the frightening results of misplaced faith. Much less developed and sympathetic than *A Pittilesse*

Mother, Bloody Newes from Dover relates the crime in less than half a page: John Champion, an honest tradesman, seeks to have his newborn baby christened. His wife (unnamed in the text, but named Mary and labeled an "Anabaptist" on the title page) refuses, greatly perplexing her husband (and the reader because the text itself says nothing about her religious beliefs and presents her actions as totally lacking in motivation). Six or seven weeks pass, until one day while the husband is away, "this wicked minded woman" takes "a great knife and cuts off the child's head." When the husband returns home, the wife calls him into the parlor, points to the bloody infant, and utters, "Behold husband, thy sweet babe without a head, now go and baptize it, if you will, you must christen the head without a body: for here they lye separated."[13] Lacking the ambivalence of other texts, this pamphlet preys on cultural anxieties about various non-conforming religious sects that denied infant baptism, a fundamental tenet of the Church of England.[14] The entire story is told on the sensational title page, where the mother gruesomely offers the severed head to her shocked husband. Nonetheless, despite its stereotyping of the mother as a fiendish "Anabaptist" (a term used indiscriminately during the period for any radical sect),[15] the woodcut's emphasis on the literal head of the child at least points toward the metaphoric battle for the position of household head.

Religion is the locus of maternal anxiety in these narratives because it offers women the potential for power, even if this power was not often realized. Many sects recognized the necessity for educating women so that they might read and understand scripture and pass this knowledge on to their children. Further, although Protestantism may have actually increased paternal authority, virtually all churches sanctioned wifely disobedience in the name of true faith.[16] Some sects ostensibly allowed women equal participation in religious matters, occasionally even legitimizing political action.

Beyond spiritual sustenance, the mother was also responsible for the physical nurturance of her children, and other pamphlets relate the sad stories of mothers who kill their children because they cannot afford to feed them. In a single page broadsheet entitled, "The Distressed Mother, or a Sorrowful Wife in Tears," the mother murders her two young children because they are starving. As the title suggests, the writer is completely sympathetic to the mother and places total blame for the tragedy on the profligate husband who has squandered the family's estate through riotous living, extravagance and drink. In an especially pitiful passage, the author describes the murder after the child begs his mother for food: "Mother saith one, a little food, or I die." The mother sighs, "Where shall I get it? Your father hath lost his Patience, and his Wealth, and we all our Hopes, with his Mishaps. Alas! Alas! what shall become of me, or who shall succour you, my children? Better it is to Die with one Stroke, than so languish in a continual Famine." And with that explanation, the mother slits the children's throats and prepares to kill herself as well. Before she can commit suicide, however, the husband returns, "laden with wine" and she resolves to kill him instead: "Thou shalt Die, thou negligent Man, since thy ill Government hath been the Ruine of me and my Children." In a masterstroke of understatement, the pamphlet writer offers this moral: "Wives should beware of too much Fury, and Husbands [should] be more circumspect in their Families."[17] Instead of confirming female agency and will, this narrative serves to reinforce patriarchal power. The father is held completely responsible for the death of his family; his presence and careful supervision could easily have averted the tragedy. Without his good government over the household, the family is completely destroyed.

Still other accounts represent the mother's mental weakness and susceptibility to melancholy. Although their intent is to challenge motherly authority, they seem instead to indict the institution of marriage as oppressive and detrimental to the mother. The various narratives of Mary Cook, a suicidal mother who kills her favorite child, a two year old daughter, offer a good example of a mother driven to murder because she places no value on her own life. There are three versions of this story: *Blood for Blood*, *The Cruel Mother*, and *Inquest After Blood*. That this story attracted so much attention suggests the extent to which seventeenth-century England was grappling with its construction of motherhood.

Blood for Blood opens like *A Pittilesse Mother* with a description of the mother's good character. A 37-year-old wife and mother of eight children,[18] Mary Cook "was of a very civil and sober life and conversation, living in the neighborhoud very inoffensively," but the writer also cautions that she was "of a very melancholy temper, which is the Anvil that the Devil delights to forge upon."[19] As discussions of hysteria, appropriately called "the mother" in the Renaissance, explain, women were considered prone to various fits of temperament and melancholia. The womb, the source of women's salvation and power but also of her shame and frailty, was thought to wander, either from lack of sex or from retention of menstrual fluid. This wandering womb could cause all sorts of strange behaviors, from sorrow and depression to convulsions and disorientation.[20] The "remedy – a husband and regular sexual intercourse – declares the necessity for male control of this volatile female element," as Coppélia Kahn notes.[21] *The Cruel Mother* offers an additional reason for Cook's crime – but an equally female one – when it reports that she miscarried while she was in prison. Since the early modern period often viewed pregnancy as a disease that could bring about irrational longings and fits of temperament, the murder can be explained as the result of periodic, natural female processes. In defining pregnancy negatively as a disease that subjects the woman to frightful bodily changes over which she has no control, medical literature from the period pathologized and diminished reproductive power. Like other writings from the period, these narratives are deeply suspicious of female reproductive ability.[22]

Like other pamphlets that we have looked at, *Blood for Blood* holds the husband partially responsible for the tragedy that follows. As the narrative represents her, Mary Cook is frustrated because her husband is frequently absent and neglects his business at home. In a desperate cry of self-assertion, she tries to commit suicide numerous times over the course of a year and a half. Paradoxically, she endeavors to assert herself by erasing herself. Although her husband finally realizes that she is suicidal and knocks down all the hooks and nails in the cellar to prevent her from hanging herself, he never really hears her cries for help. After several aborted attempts at suicide, Cook finally kills her youngest child, not out of malice, but at least in this account, because she fears what will happen to the child after she is dead. Later, when asked why she had perpetrated so atrocious an act, she replies, because "she is weary of her own life."

The killing of the child because she is "weary of her own life" suggests that in a strange way she associates the child's life with her own. In fact, *The Cruel Mother* makes the connection between the mother's life and the child's explicit, explaining that she killed the child so that "she by that means [should] come to her own end."[23] The murder in this instance derives largely from the mother's own lack of self-worth, and she projects that worthlessness onto her only daughter. In fact, she verbalizes her disgust with herself in terms of womanhood: "God had convinced her that her own righteousness was but unrighteousness, even as a filthy menstruous clothe, and therefore desired out of the sense of her own nothingness, and utter emptiness to go out of herself."[24] That Cook defines her self-disgust in terms of menstruation, the signal of potential motherhood, suggests a complex intermingling of selfhood and motherhood. As Marilyn Francus contends, "the roles of wife and mother frequently – perhaps usually – required the erasure of the self; and one suspects that her frustrations were profoundly typical (and perhaps all the more horrifying for that reason) as Mary Cook the person was eclipsed by Mary Cook the wife and mother."[25] Further, perhaps she surmises that her only female child will suffer the same sense of worthlessness that she herself does and seeks to save the child from the pain the mother suffers.[26] Apparently, this obsessive identification with the child was not unusual.[27] Indeed, Cook seems so completely defined by her role as mother that she fails to distinguish herself from her child. She views the child as merely an extension of herself, so much so that after she confesses to murder she worries that the child may suffer damnation because of the state of *her* soul. As such, the narrative posits the need to circumscribe domestic nurturance; as Frances Dolan explains, "maternal subjectivity is threatening when its boundaries expand to include – even consume – the offspring."[28]

In Mary Cook's case, the pamphlet writers are forced to confront an example of female agency and subjectivity in a way that those who write about unmarried infanticidal mothers are not. And taken together, these three accounts of Mary Cook's crime are remarkable for the various motivations they attribute to the mother, almost all of which seek to rob her of that agency. Both *Blood for Blood* and *The Cruel Mother* depict the mother's depression as a kind of satanic possession, and *Blood for Blood* even reports a rumor that Satan actually appeared to her. The narrators clearly want the reader to view her as a victim, describing her as "more like a Lamb going to the slaughter than a Murderer going to the Gallows." In one account religion is blamed ("she was under trouble of mind about Religion," *Blood for Blood*), as it is in *A Pittilesse Mother* and *Bloody Newes from Dover*, but Cook denies this assertion: "There was nothing of any Religious Concernment in it" (34). *Inquest After Blood* constructs her as insane and reports that her husband brought forth several witnesses to attest to her madness. This defense fails because Cook provides lucid responses in her deposition.[29] In particular, she proves her competency by answering questions about the maintenance of the household. Ironically, as Francus point out, "Cook succeeded at the technical aspects of homemaking even as she subverted the ideological criteria."[30] Nonetheless, the various strategies to deflect maternal agency only serve to make it more ambivalent.

Although the account of Cook's fragile psychological state suggests that she was not really in control of her actions, the text remains ambivalent on this point. Cook's actions express at least a limited challenge to patriarchal prerogative. In one tragic assertion of selfhood, she threatens to kill her youngest child if her husband goes out, but his compliance prevents this. Further, the murder occurs completely within the context of maternal and wifely duty, the husband in the background demanding his Sunday clothes and the baby in the cradle crying for its breakfast. Suddenly, in one shocking moment, the picture of domestic bliss goes haywire: "But she laying aside all motherly Bowels, took the Babe out of the cradle, set her on her lap, took the knife out of her skirt, laid her left hand upon its face and chin, and with the other hand cut her throat at one stroke" (15). Then, curiously, she stamps her foot to call for her husband! (Interestingly, the forwardness represented by the stamping of the foot is transformed into acquiescence on the scaffold, where she stamps her foot to indicate that she is willing and ready to die.) Before she is conveyed to Newgate, she takes off her rings, cuts the silver chaps from her scarf and gives her husband all the keys of the trunks, chests and boxes in a symbolic ceding of her domestic place. And in one final jab at her husband's neglect, she chides, "O, if you had been more careful to look after me, you might have hindered me from doing this" (20). Although these actions hint that the murder is a contest for power in the household, the greater weight given to the husband's neglect and to the wife's mental state actually serves to reinforce paternal authority by denying maternal power.

And yet maternal power remains conflicted in these texts. In one final attempt at recognition, Mary Cook asks that her story be recorded and published. If we agree with Mary Beth Rose that "the ideal society is based upon the sacrifice of the mother's desire,"[31] Cook remains dangerous despite the pamphlet writers' attempts to explain away her agency because she continues to assert herself even after death by seeking to have her story heard. Given the various retellings of her story, she is at least partially successful. The woman whose voice was ignored in life will finally be heard, if only because of her notoriety.

The mother's desire to have her voice heard is the most striking feature of the last pamphlet that I will discuss, *A Fairwarning to Murderers of Infants: Being an Account of the Tryal, Condemnation and Execution of Mary Goodenough*. Although Goodenough is not a married woman but a widow, her story belongs in this study because the text examines her authority, first as a criminal and then as a mother. Unlike the other women we have examined, however, her "good mothering" comes after the death of her baby. The narrative begins with the death of Goodenough's child, but the bulk of the pamphlet is devoted to a lengthy letter that the mother ostensibly dictates for her surviving children. As in other criminal accounts, the "ideology of chastity" that "made silence an equivalent of bodily purity" is suspended in this text.[32] Yet the voice here is louder because Goodenough speaks not just from her position as criminal but from her authorized position as mother. And she speaks not in confession but in a long treatise of advice to her children. Mary Beth Rose convincingly argues that within literary and domestic texts of the period "maternal desire and agency ... can be represented visibly (corporeally) only as dangerous, subordinate, or peripheral in relation to public, adult life" unless the mother is absent or dead. The "best mother is ... a dead mother."[33] Although Rose is explaining the phenomena of the mother's advice book, a genre that at once transgresses and replicates patriarchal dictates, her argument seems equally valid for this text. Goodenough's letter, entitled "Advice of your Dying Mother," exhibits the same characteristics of the mothers' advice books, and whether actually dictated by the mother or not, suggests that Dorothy Leigh and other writing mothers were influential enough for the pamphleteer to use them as models for his repentant mother.

Like Leigh's *The Mother's Blessing*, Goodenough's letter of advice enjoys a liminal status poised between life and death and is offered as the mother's legacy to her children. And exactly like Elizabeth Jocelin's *The Mothers Legacie to her Unborn Child*, Goodenough seeks to provide the spiritual and moral guidance she will be unable to supply her children because she is dead. She speaks with a voice of maternal love and authority, thus becoming an exemplar of maternal solicitude, an irony apparently lost on the pamphleteer.

Goodenough's letter to her children extends the compulsory public confession of the typical crime pamphlet and transforms it into a pseudo-mother's manual. The mother's manual is a genre that is itself contradictory – both public and private.[34] Likewise, the female criminal on the scaffold – and in the pamphlets – disrupts the normative opposition of public/male space and private/female space. The letter in *Fairwarning* further problematizes the two categories.[35] In addition, the fact that the advice in this instance comes from a mother who killed one of her children makes the form doubly fractured. What at first seems the grand irony of a murdering mother writing in support of family values is not so strange after all when we consider the ambivalent position of both the female criminal and the mother in the early modern period. She has already been made public through her crime and is no longer bound by the dictates of silence and modesty. Oddly enough, because she is already transgressive, her writing reincorporates her into society and refocuses the readers' attention on her role as good mother.

Yet one of the strange things about this case is that Goodenough fails to provide the requisite confession. Her boldness in leaving a written legacy to her children is partially negated by her inability to speak publicly in confession. The refusal here is not depicted as a conscious act of will and self-assertion, but rather as a sign of her physical and mental impairment. The author apologizes for this breach of custom, explaining, "it could not be expected she should say much more; for she must needs be in great Confusion and Surprize, who in less than Two month's time, was Committed, Try'd, Condemn'd and Executed for her Crime. Besides, she seem'd never to have had any great Faculty or Freedom of Speech …"[36] Her letter to her children, then, serves to replace the missing confession, and while this omission emphasizes her weakness, the letter foregrounds her power as mother.[37]

The street literature of seventeenth-century England preys on cultural anxiety about motherhood by carrying the mother's legitimate power to its most extreme manifestation and intermingling maternal power with other anxieties. The writers depict criminal mothers as "good mothers," but they pervert the ideal of the good mother by exaggerating and distorting maternal nurturance. By depicting violence as deriving from maternal duty, the popular press makes all mothers suspect. Although these texts are often sympathetic to their subjects, their sympathy brands these women as weak and provides further justification of the need to circumscribe maternal authority.

As these pamphlets suggest, the woman's role as wife *and* mother in early modern English society was highly conflicted. Although the crime pamphlets describe events that were extreme and extraordinary, they provide vivid examples of the period's interrogation of the proper scope of maternal authority. The texts discussed here illustrate how the murdering mother embodies both her society's expectations and its anxieties about motherhood by showing motherhood to be at once empowering and destructive. That the popular press's obsession with murdering mothers occurs at the same time that women were gaining greater recognition and authority within the domestic sphere is crucial. Paradoxically enough, while these accounts criminalize female subjectivity, they often also attempt to qualify maternal authority by casting the mother's actions as reactions to her own weakness or to patriarchal neglect and irresponsibility. Maternal power is thus partially undermined and made less threatening.

Notes

1. Christopher Newstead, *An Apology for Women: or Women's Defence* in *Renaissance Women: Constuctions of Femininity in England*, ed. Kate Aughterson (New York: Routledge, 1995), 116.
2. Betty Travitsky, "Child Murder in English Renaissance Life and Drama," *Medieval and Renaissance Drama in England: An Annual Gathering of Research, Criticism and Reviews* 6 (1993): 64. See also, Travitsky, "The New Mother of the English Renaissance: Her Writings on Motherhood" in *The Lost Tradition: Mothers and Daughters in Literature,* eds. Cathy N. Davidson and E.M. Broner (New York: Frederick Ungar Publishing, 1980), 33–43 and Patricia Crawford, "The Construction and Experience of Maternity in Seventeenth-Century England" in *Women as Mothers in Pre-Inductrial England*, ed. Valerie Fildes (New York: Routledge, 1990), 3–38.
3. Deborah Willis, *Malevolent Nurture: Witch-Hunting and Maternal Power in Early Modern England* (Ithaca: Cornell University Press, 1995), 17–19.
4. Mary Beth Rose, "Where Are the Mothers in Shakespeare? Options for Gender Representation in the English Renaissance," *Shakespeare Quarterly* 42.3 (1991): 308.
5. Anxiety about maternal nurture was everywhere present in England at this time, and the mother's role from conception through childhood was a contested site of female empowerment. Midwives, for example, came under increased scrutiny and regulation. For an example of the popular press's participation in the demonizing of midwives, see *The Murderous Midwife, with her Roasted Punishment* (London, 1673). The practice of wet-nursing was also heatedly critiqued because mother's milk was thought to hold an almost mystical power over the development of the child. See, for example, the case of Abigail Hill, a wet nurse who brutally murdered four infants in *A True Relation of the Most Horrid and Barbarous Murthers Committed by Abigail Hill of St. Olaves Southwark* (London, 1658) and *Conceal'd Murther Reveil'd* (London, 1699), a broadside that relates the drowning murder of an infant by her nurse. The mother's womb carried an equally important function, subjecting the unborn child to all its mother's whims and fancies. For a popular example of the birth of a monstrous baby caused by the mother's thoughts before giving birth, see *The True Description of a Childe with Ruffes* (London, 1566). Even the witch-hunts have been read as a fear of maternal power. The search for the witch's teat – itself a perversion of the mother's nurturing breast –

suggests a parallel construction of motherhood as malevolent and dangerous. For a more detailed account of the connection between motherhood and witches, see Deborah Willis, *Malevolent Nurture.*

6. The first widespread prosecutions of women occurred during this period. Unmarried women were increasingly prosecuted for infanticide, an action newly criminalized during the period; widows were prosecuted as witches. On the criminalization of female agency, see Christina Larner, "Crimen Exceptum? The Crime of Witchcraft in Europe," in *Crime and the Law: The Social History of Crime in Western Europe since 1500,* eds. V.A.C. Gatrell, Bruce Lexman, and Geoffrey Parker (London: Europa, 1980), 49–75 and Frances Dolan, *Dangerous Familiars: Representations of Domestic Crime in England, 1550–1700* (Ithaca: Cornell University Press, 1994).

7. R. W. Malcolmson, "Infanticide in the Eighteenth Century," in *Crime in England, 1550–1800,* ed. J. S. Cockburn (Princeton: Princeton University Press, 1977), 192.

8. The pamphlet *Deedes Against Nature and Monsters by Kind* (London, 1614), for example, constructs the crime as a result of the woman's unrestrained sexuality – her "lusty body, strong nature, and feare of shame." Repeatedly, the mother is called a "strumpet" or a "harlot," and her crime is depicted as monstrous and unnatural. She is a "Caterpillar of nature, a creature more savage than a shee woolf, more unnatural than either bird or beast." For further discussion of unmarried infanticidal mothers, see Laura Gowing, "Secret Births and Infanticide in Seventeenth-century England," *Past and Present* 156 (1997): 87–115 and Mark Jackson, *New-Born Child Murder: Women, Illegitimacy and the Courts in Eighteenth-Century England* (New York: St. Martin's, 1996).

9. Elizabeth Jocelin, *The Mother's Legacie to Her Unborn Child* (London, 1624), Sig. B 34v.

10. Betty Travitsky, "'A Pittilesse Mother': Reports of a Seventeenth-Century Filicide," *Mosaic* 27.4 (1994): 60.

11. *A Pittilesse Mother* (London, 1616), A2v.

12. Travitsky, "Reports of a Seventeenth-Century Filicide," 60.

13. *Bloody Newes from Dover* (London, 1647), n.pag.

14. For a discussion of the various controversies surrounding baptism during the period, see David Cressy, *Birth, Marriage and Death: Ritual, Religion, and the Life-Cycle in Tudor and Stuart England* (New York: Oxford University Press, 1997), 97–194.

15. Cressy, *Birth, Marriage, and Death,* 101.

16. See Patricia Crawford, *Women and Religion in England 1500–1720* (London: Routledge, 1993).

17. "The Distressed Mother," (London, no date), British Library 515.l.2 (12).

18. There is some discrepancy in the accounts about the number of children Cook had. *The Cruel Mother* reports that she has three, two boys and one girl.

19. N. Partridge and F. Sharp, *Blood for Blood* (London, 1670), 9–10.

20. See Audrey Eccles, *Obstetrics and Gynaecology in Tudor and Stuart England* (Kent: Kent State University Press, 1982), 76–7.

21. Coppélia Kahn, "The Absent Mother in *King Lear*" in *Rewriting the Renaissance,* eds. Margaret W. Ferguson, Maureen Quilligan, and Nancy J. Vickers (Chicago: University of Chicago Press, 1986), 34.

22. For a discussion of pregnancy as disease, see Eccles, *Obstetrics and Gynaecology* and Lori Schroeder Haslem, "'Troubled with the Mother': Longings, Purgings, and the Maternal Body in *Bartholomew Fair* and *Duchess of Malfi*," *Modern Philology* 92.4 (1995): 438–59.

23. *The Cruel Mother* (London, 1670), 5.
24. *Blood for Blood*, 38.
25. Marilyn Francus, "Monstrous Mothers, Monstrous Societies: Infanticide and the Rule of Law in Restoration and Eighteenth-Century England," *Eighteenth-Century Life* 21.2 (1997): 139.
26. Francus, "Monstrous Mothers," 139.
27. Michael MacDonald, *Mystical Bedlam: Madness, Anxiety, and Healing in Seventeenth-Century England* (Cambridge: Cambridge University Press, 1981), 84.
28. Dolan, *Dangerous Familiars*, 148.
29. Although MacDonald points out that married women were likely to be pardoned as insane for the murder of their children, such is not the case here. See *Mystical Bedlam*, 13ff.
30. Francus, "Monstrous Mothers," 141.
31. Rose, "Where Are the Mothers?" 307.
32. Margaret Ferguson, "A Room Not Their Own: Renaissance Women as Readers and Writers," in *The Comparative Perspective on Literature: Approaches to Theory and Practice* (Ithaca: Cornell University Press, 1988), 97.
33. Rose, "Where Are the Mothers? 307.
34. Kristen Poole, "'The fittest closet for all goodness': Authorial Strategies of Jacobean Mothers' Manuals," *Studies in English Literature* 35 (1995): 172.
35. On the collapsing of public/private space in mothers' advice books, see Elaine V. Beilin, *Redeeming Eve: Women Writers of the English Renaissance* (Princeton: Princeton University Press, 1987), 247–85.
36. *Fairwarning to Murderers of Infants* (London, 1692), 3.
37. Dolan discusses the necessity for public confession and notes the omission here in "'Gentlemen, I have one more thing to say': Women on Scaffolds in England, 1563–1680," *Modern Philology* 92.2 (1994): 169.

CHAPTER TWENTY

"I fear there will a worse come in his place": Surrogate Parents and Shakespeare's *Richard III*

Heather Dubrow

Although revisionist studies of *A Midsummer Night's Dream* have posited the suppression and violation of its female characters, a related but significantly different form of resentment splinters the surface of the play in its opening lines. "She lingers my desires," Theseus observes of the moon, "like to a stepdame or a dowager, / Long withering out a young man's revenue" (I.i.5–7).[1] A dowager by definition assumed the rights and privileges of her dead husband, so the linkage between such women and stepmothers crystallizes the issue of surrogacy; it is no accident that this play, one of only two dramas in which Shakespeare refers repeatedly to dowagers, also mentions that other substitute, the stepparent. Because this allusion to stepdames and dowagers appears in a simile, the line rhetorically enacts their roles as substitutes, as people who are both like and unlike, who both fill and draw attention to an absence.

The preoccupation with stepparents in this passage recurs throughout the texts of early modern England. Sidney, too, mentions a stepmother, that deflected version of maternal origins, in the originary, opening sonnet of *Astrophil and Stella*. The plot of *The Faerie Queene*, like that of many romances, often pivots on substitute parents. Other, non-literary cultural texts are equally concerned with stepparents and their implications; thus in his influential marriage manual *Of Domesticall Duties* (1622) William Gouge alerts his readers to the "fearefull tragedies" and "lamentable mischiefes" that can issue from the machinations of these conniving guardians.[2]

Surrogate parents of many types also recur throughout Shakespeare's own canon, where, as in *A Midsummer Night's Dream*, literally realized stepmothers and -fathers often figure other types of proxy. *All's Well That Ends Well*, a play in which both the king and the Countess of Rossillion replace dead parents, achieves its comedic closure through other forms of substitution. Claudius is stepfather as well as uncle, a role of which contemporaries would have been more aware than most recent critics have been. Claudius's position as a substitute tropes the broader preoccupation with replacement, replacement, and the connections between them that structures the play: the villain who has taken the place of a king insists that the king's son resume his own place at court, Hamlet survives because one letter is substituted for another, Laertes dies because swords are exchanged, and so on. The substitute parents in Shakespearean romance flag the ways that genre rescripts tragic closure by emphasizing the viability of surrogates, whether a new husband for Paulina or a new couple in lieu of the daughter who has married in far distant Tunisia. Indeed, a more detailed comparison of how Shakespeare's genres variously deploy the closural and anti-closural force of substitution would crystallize many central distinctions among them.

Why and how, then, do his plays, like so many early modern texts, represent the phenomenon of stepparenting and other types of surrogacy, and why do they engage with the problems adumbrated by Theseus? These questions are as broad as they are significant, encompassing as they do not only the material issues that interest so many critics today but also the workings of gender, of representation, and of literary tropes.

* * *

Generalizations about the prevalence of surrogate parents must be bracketed with cautions, thus providing an exemplary instance of the potentialities and dangers of practicing cultural history. Mortality statistics vary from one region to another, yet again demonstrating the perils of basing generalizations on London and the court. Social and economic historians disagree among themselves about rates of death and remarriage and therefore about the precise likelihood of what would today be called blended families.[3] Nonetheless, the early death of parents was indisputably frequent: scholars have estimated that about one-third to one-half of the population had witnessed the death of at least one parent by the time they themselves married.[4] Because of the mortality crisis of 1557–1559, a period when death rates rose sharply in a number of regions, many members of Shakespeare's audience were especially likely to have endured the loss of a mother or father early in their own lives. And remarriages occurred often enough for bereaved children to experience the anxiety expressed by the third plebian in *Julius Caesar*: "I fear there will a worse come in his place" (III.ii.111).

Many texts of Tudor and Stuart England emphasize the threats created by such surrogates. A Renaissance translation of Petrarch, the *Phisicke against Fortune*, conflates such dangers with the devastation of fire: "Who so having children by his first marriage, bringeth a Stepmother among them, he setteth his house afire with is [*sic*] owne handes."[5] More immediate to the early modern period are Gouge's warnings in *Of Domesticall Duties*. He insistently emphasizes the responsibilities of stepparents, flagging the danger that they might instead prove irresponsible and exploitative. Tales of such exploitation also appear in the account of the eponymous hero's problems with his stepfamily in Lucy Hutchinson's *Memoirs of the Life of Colonel Hutchinson*.[6] Ilana Krausman Ben-Amos's *Adolescence and Youth in Early Modern England* issues a shrewd warning about the accuracy of biographical narratives written long after the event even as it acknowledges the pervasive traumas occasioned by parental loss.[7] But however one evaluates the reliability of a given record like the Hutchinson memoir, it is clear that in the early modern period as today, stepmothers and -fathers were widely regarded as very threatening.

A culture whose history had included Lord Protectors like Richard, Duke of Gloucester, men rightly perceived as primarily protecting their own interests, is likely to have been particularly conscious of analogous perversions of guardianship in the domestic sphere. And antagonism originally and guiltily directed towards the dead parent might readily be deflected onto stepparents and other guardians, especially if they provided some rationale for doing so. But the anxieties expressed by writers like Gouge and Hutchinson also stem more immediately from the institution of stepparenthood itself. To begin with, Gouge's linguistic usage when he stresses that stepparents serve in the stead of mothers and fathers draws attention to semiotic and epistemological threats. Stepparenthood signals the complexities of representation in general and substitution in particular and in so doing carries with it implications for arenas ranging from the workings of rhetorical tropes to the problematics of gender. Surrogate parents both are and are not the parents they represent; if the dead are absent presences, so too in this sense are the living stepparents. Thus on one level they draw attention to the vulnerability of the individual family members they replace while on the other hand testifying to the longevity of family roles. The mother is dead, long live the mother – an emotionally charged statement whether maternity is perceived as beneficient, as suffocating, or as both at once. And such assertions are further destabilized in that the death of one mother reminds one of the vulnerability of her substitutes as well. These types of instability may help to explain the tendency, noted above and traced acutely by Marianne Novy, of splitting parents into good and evil versions.[8] Similarly, self-serving stepparents and guardians at once signified protection and ironically redefined that concept in ways that suggested that protection and signification itself were as vulnerable as the life of a parent.

From yet another perspective the introduction of a stepparent could complicate mourning in several ways. Clearly the processes of substitution might help a child redefine a relationship with the dead parent, thus achieving the decathectization of which Freud writes.[9] On the other hand, it is not hard to imagine scenarios in which new parents too quickly or too insensitively attempt to impose themselves as substitutes, thus interrupting the trajectories of mourning.

Whereas parental substitutes could complicate the workings of grief, arguably the changes in religious and social modes of mourning that resulted from the Reformation in turn complicated familial surrogacy. These shifts in customs and rituals threatened patterns of grieving and recovering in that certain highly significant ways of expressing grief and in so doing maintaining a reassuring relationship with the dead, notably practices connected with Purgatory, were curtailed in the course of the sixteenth century. Anthony Low finds in *Hamlet*'s repression of references to Purgatory an enactment of that radical change.[10] "The emotional and psychological consequences of the abolition of the doctrine of purgatory and curtailment of prayers for the dead," the social historian Ralph Houlbrooke observed, "constituted one of the great unchartable revolutions of English history."[11]

Houlbrooke goes on to speculate, persuasively enough, that this rejection of Catholic mourning rituals might decrease fear of suffering in the next world; but Joshua Scodel's suggestion that the same change emphasized the barrier between the dead and living is equally persuasive and more significant to an analysis of early parental loss.[12] In particular, at the beginning of the sixteenth century the culture that built the ritual of parental blessing into quotidian domestic practices offered a continuation of that ritual in the belief that a dead parent could intercede for the living.[13] In denying the possibility of that sort of intercession, Protestantism again displaced the dead parent. Not the least reason *A Midsummer Night's Dream* and other texts are so concerned with substitution, then, is that truncating the relationship with the dead parent put more pressure on its alternative, the several forms of surrogacy we have explored.

Bereaved children were liable not only to, as it were, wicked stepmothers and stepfathers but also to many other apparently well-meaning guardians. The records of the Court of Orphans testify to the machinations of unscrupulous stepfathers as well as other male relatives.[14] Uncles clearly had many opportunities for such exploitation, and it is telling that the villain in the popular ballad "The Children in the Wood" is one – as are his analogues in *Hamlet* and *Richard III*. Given the emphasis on threatening male relatives in these and other renditions of parental loss, the focus on stepmothers rather than stepfathers in so many literary texts, notably *Pericles* and *Cymbeline*, provides a particularly telling instance of the gendering of anxieties.

In addition, many abuses resulted from the workings of wardship, an institution that deserves more attention than it has yet garnered from students of early modern literature.[15] Developed by the Tudors as a source of revenue, the system exemplifies the pragmatic efficiency of those monarchs. Wardship, which was based on medieval conceptions of financial obligation and of marriage practices, again demonstrates the need to nuance generalizations about proto-capitalism with the recognition that feudal practices survived – and were skillfully deployed – in the laws regulating wardship no less than in land law. And most germane to this study is its profound effect on the material as well as the affective consequences of parental loss. Fathers sometimes attempted to avert those sorry effects through such devices as passing on property while they were still alive, but nonetheless the potentially abusive system continued to flourish.[16]

Whereas the monarch might benefit financially by retaining a wardship, it was through their sales that most benefit accrued to the crown. And it was through such sales that a number of abuses indisputably arose. Ascertaining just how corrupt the national administrators of the system were remains problematical. Lord Burghley, Master of Wards between 1561 and 1598, took gifts, but so too did many other Tudor officials; weighing the evidence against him, the historian Joel Hurstfield does not wholly exonerate him but persuasively asserts that he was generally fair and judicious.[17] Whether or not one seconds that verdict, however, it could not be pronounced on many of the guardians created by the wardship system. Anticipating the antics of twentieth-century ambulance chasers, they were known to file petitions in anticipation of the death that would turn a child into a ward. Many of these so-called guardians were more concerned with the financial profit they could gain from their ward than the child's education or spiritual well-being; witness among a host of other examples the marriages into which wards were often forced.

Moreover, both the policies of the wardship system and the practices of individual guardians intensified the displacement associated with parental death. The surviving mother received little if any preference in the assignment of wardships, but the temptation merely to read this as yet another instance of the disempowerment of women needs to be qualified by the recognition that when male relatives sought to become guardians, their relationship to the child did not necessarily ensure that they would succeed. In the reign of Edward VI, only one-fifth of wardships were sold to the mother, a relative, trustees chosen by the father, or the own use of the ward his- or herself; during Mary's reign the figure came close to one in three, but in the opening years of Elizabeth's reign, it declined again to one in four. In 1587–90 one-third of all grants went to such parties, an improvement but hardly a reversal of a disturbing pattern.[18] Because of it, a child who had suffered the loss of a parent might well be forced to move far from home and in effect lose the other parent as well, thus suffering another loss of control. The unscrupulous guardians provided by the wardship system not only displaced parents but in another sense often effected the geographical displacement of their charges, and their manipulations could turn the mourning child from the subject who pitches the reel in *fort-da* to that object itself.

Yet one needs to remember that although the primary effects of wardship or other types of guardianship were more likely to be traumatic than liberating, bereaved families, like unhappy ones, are not all alike. It is not hard to imagine comedic scenarios culminating in relief, emancipation, and the formulation of a new society, as it were, around a beneficient stepparent. In his autobiography the Renaissance minister Richard Baxter explains that shortly after his mother's death his father married a woman "whose Holiness, Mortification, Contempt of the World, and fervent Prayer" were "Exemplary"; this paragon was, he announces a "Special Blessing to our Family."[19] Though, as we have seen, autobiographies famously distort what they claim to report, the passage reminds us that stepparents might be perceived or represented or both very positively. As Quintilian observes in VIII.vi, the term a trope substitutes for the original one may be better than that original.

Nor were the social institutions of early modern England inevitably exploitative of bereaved children. The dog that does not bite the man stands less chance of headlines; the social institutions that oppose exploitation and the individuals who disdain it are likely to be neglected in an academic culture that prizes conflictual paradigms for social interactions. In fact, preventing the abuse of children was one agenda of another cultural institution, the Court of Orphans. Nonetheless, the fact remains that on the whole the material and emotional consequences of parental surrogacy were indeed threatening. Moreover, though the contrast between cultural myths about unscrupulous surrogate parents and the more positive behavior of some of them was no doubt sometimes a source of relief, it could again erode categories, spinning judgments and perceptions until they whirled as dizzyingly as a Van Gogh cypress.

Stepparents, other relatives, and the guardians appointed by the wardship system had a profound impact on not only the affective but also the material consequences of the early loss of a parent.[20] Those who live in a society of life insurance, pension plans, and so on may too easily forget the financial devastation that the death of a breadwinner could bring. In the discussion in *Of Domesticall Duties* cited above, Gouge devotes considerable attention to the economic results of parental death. Warning of the disasters that can result from the machinations of unscrupulous stepparents or other guardians, he sedulously urges parents to prepare a will and ensure that reliable surrogates will be responsible for their children (esp. 569–74, 580–83, 585–6). He proceeds to assert that the majority of guardians, rather than protecting the child, are all too likely to pursue their own financial interests.

Studying early parental death invites us to rewrite one of the most common new historicist generalizations about early modern England. It has become common, indeed commonplace, in studies of that period to trace crises of representation to the theater. Though much of the criticism in question is incisive, yet again we need to acknowledge that the domestic realm anticipates, glosses, and nuances events often associated largely or entirely with the court and theater of London. Critics have noted the theatricality of deathbed scenes, but the remarriages that succeeded them were in certain senses no less theatrical.[21] A generation that had grown up seeing mothers and sons assuming the roles of a deceased paterfamilias and stepparents representing and misrepresenting the progenitors they replaced learned a great deal about theatricality, performance, and cross-dressing without going to the Globe.

* * *

Loss and his "imperial jointress" (*Hamlet*, I.ii.9) recovery are the reigning monarchs in Shakespeare's conception of history; they quarrel, struggle with each other for supremacy, flirt with other partners, yet repeatedly seize each other in the embrace that generates the narrative of these plays. The history plays enact the relationship between deprivation and recuperation generically through the interplay between tragedy and history, though merely to associate the former with loss and the latter with recovery is to oversimplify their dynamic since each genre typically traces the interaction of both states. As the prologue to *Henry V* insists, the monarchs in question also stage the relationship of loss and recovery metatheatrically. And much as *Henry VI* opens with the body of a monarch on the stage, so throughout the history plays the death of a parent, whether he be the father of a small child or a nation, is both harbinger and figure of other types of loss, many of them related to surrogacy.

In none of Shakespeare's history plays, however, is the interplay between loss and recovery more central or intriguing than it is in *Richard III*. That dynamic subsumes and unites many other issues that have interested readers of the drama, such as the viability of providential interpretations and the extent to which characters other than Richard himself, notably Richmond, are untrustworthy or even evil.[22] The extraordinary encounter between the grieving Anne and Richard, though usually analysed in characterological terms, is in fact as well a paradigm of how the relationship between loss and recuperation works throughout this drama. For in a sense this play, like *Macbeth*, is all about whether one can securely bury one's dead – that is, whether one can negotiate the consequences of loss in ways that discourage the repetition of it, notably in the form of ghostly visitations, and that protect the living from those who attempt to take the place of the dead. Thus when Richard interrupts the funeral procession, he demonstrates his predilection for interruption of all types; the man whose untimely birth obstructed the normal gestation period breaks into Margaret's curse in I.iii.233, breaks into patterns of succession, and, similarly, his late arrival cuts short plans to crown his nephew. Hence by obstructing linearity as realized in the spatial movement of the funeral procession, he stages the ways he will obstruct narrative movements from loss to recuperation.

The interaction of loss and recuperation that structures the whole play is at its most intriguing, and its most relevant to this study, in relation to the loss of parents and the resulting patterns of surrogacy that result. In a text that stages the demise of not one but two kings and famously pivots on that of innocent children, several incidents also draw attention to the immediate fears and long-term consequences of the death of parents, implicitly but insistently relating the public and private spheres. To begin with, then, Act II, scene ii, the episode in which Clarence's children learn of his death, does not serve any significant narratological or characterological functions; instead, it not only anticipates the fate of their cousins, who have also lost a father, but also gestures towards the larger issues intertwined with the death of parents in the play. The dialogue here insists on the danger that event creates for the young: "Why do you look on us, and shake your head, / And call us orphans, wretches, castaways" (II.ii.5–6). The answer to that question, the play suggests, is not that such children are all alone but rather that they may be surrounded by too many unscrupulous relatives, notably uncles, a point with obvious relevance not only to members of the royal family but also, as we have seen, to the many members of Shakespeare's audience who had lost a parent early in their lives. Similarly, the wailing of the royal women in this scene hints at their recognition that they are powerless to protect these children, a situation that echoes the plight of many widows whose offspring entered the wardship system.

Yet most suggestive, and most predictive of the ways the play will subsequently analyse the loss of parents, is Clarence's son's description in this scene of how his "good uncle Gloucester" (20) behaved: "Bade me rely on him as on my father, / And he would love me dearly as a child" (25–6). For these lines, in which the connective "as" echoes the syntax of a simile, represent the first of many times this play acknowledges the link between the substitutions effected by parental death and those created by metaphoric language. Familial substitution as it were tropes troping: in both cases the replacements are unlike and like, a dual role signalled by the connective "as," and in both cases the process of linkage destabilizes and complicates. And in both "as" at once exposes an absence and promises, however reliably, to fill it. In particular, on one level Richard's assertions are just heavily ironic, while in another their uncle hopes that Clarence's offspring will indeed be like children to him – those who turn to him for guidance, those whom he hopes to manipulate even more easily than adults. The lines also remind us yet again that if Richard, like other Vices, creates unnatural separations and divisions, he also delights in generating unnatural familial bonds.[23]

Many issues raised by Clarence's children recur when their cousins the princes arrive in London in Act III, scene i. In drawing attention to the surprising absences of his other uncles, his mother and brother, and Hastings, Prince Edward reminds the audience that literal, material absences represent as well the absence of a stable political and personal family and of protection he can trust. These gaps in who appears on stage also gesture towards the role of ghostly presences throughout the play: the dead and dying kings who represent lost hopes for reconciliation and stable leadership, the dead personages enumerated in the hypnotic wailing of the women. It is not surprising that a coffin figures early in the play and ghosts make their cameo appearances towards its end, for the drama, like *A Midsummer Night's Dream*, *Pericles*, and *Cymbeline*, concerns the presence of those who are not present and the absence of those who should be.

As the scene progresses, it engenders another type of gap. Its emphasis on seizing the Duke of York from sanctuary signals the literal permeability of the religious house in which he resides, a material manifestation of the corruptibility of religious leaders in this scene and elsewhere in the play, men whose principles can readily be permeated with specious arguments, men whose perceptions are as soft and easily spoiled as a strawberry. And the decision to take away the young duke also variously represents the unreliability and the frailty of metaphoric sanctuaries, whether they be the Tower in its ambivalent role as such, the tellingly named Lord Protector, or the armor of wit this ill-fated young man attempts to wear.

Above all, however, the episode demonstrates the limitations on the maternal body in its role as sanctuary for a child denied a father and other more powerful guardians. Notice the wording of Buckingham's command: "And from her jealous arms *pluck* him perforce" (36; italics inserted). Later, in a line that does not refer specifically to the mother's arms, the reference to "seizing" (47) suggests the necessity of a more violent act. But the fact that the Duke of York can be plucked, a verb that might be used for, say, those strawberries (or the godly gardener who arranges for their delivery), suggests that maternal arms offer little protection indeed. Many studies of the play have emphasized the limited agency of its women, and others have reactively drawn attention to the power of their curses, but this passage, again like the experience of many widows and their young children, provides a new and chilling perspective on one crucial type of impotence.

In the most telling power play of the scene, and the most intense reminder of the dangers facing those who have a Lord Protector – or a guardian from the wardship system – rather than a reliable father, Richard arranges his charges' accommodation. As acute about the significance of space as any contemporary Marxist critic, this uncle, who earlier directed the body of one of his victims away from Chertsey and to White-Friars, here pretends to give his nephew the choice of where to stay:

> *Glou.* Where it seems best unto your royal self.
>   If I may counsel you, some day or two
>   Your Highness shall repose you at the Tower;
>   Then where you please, and shall be thought most fit
>   For your best health and recreation. (63–7)

On one level the speech simply endows the prince with the major decision about long-term accommodations while offering a firm recommendation about temporary plans. But observe too how the deference of the first line and the tentativeness of the conditional segue into the "shall" (65), whose insistence is immediately blurred by the emphasis on choice in the final lines. And then the Machiavel who delights in manipulating others to do his bidding revealingly qualifies the ascription of choice to the prince in a line that could refer to himself but elides subject and agency: "shall be thought most fit" (66). In the Olivier film, this speech reduces the prince to a quavering child, an impression intensified by the high angle shot. The Tower, an ostensible guardian that is instead the site of betrayal, is the inanimate analogue to the Lord Protector Richard.

Tyrrel's description of the princes' murder intensifies several issues raised by this scene. Their prayer book reminds us of the church and churchmen who failed to offer them sanctuary; their sleeping in each other's arms recalls the maternal arms from which the younger prince was plucked. They are embracing each other in a world that has failed to embrace and protect them, a failure facilitated by their loss of a father and realized in the figures of false or weak would-be protectors. In particular, if we accept the argument that the embrace recalls the popular ballad to which I referred earlier, "Children in the Wood," one of the most telling links between the two plots is that both cast an uncle as the principal villain, reflecting the cultural suspicions about that role I have posited.[24] Thus Tyrrel's description demonstrates the broader implications of parental loss in *Richard III*: the child deprived of a parent loses one form of protection and acquires what may variously be reliable substitutes and simulacra.

Indeed, as this passage reminds us, *Richard III* engages throughout with both familial and national resonances of protection and protectors. The drama draws on remembrances of England's recent history under a Lord Protector, playing them against the role of such figures when Henry VI and Prince Edward were in their minority. Perhaps too such debates also reflect remembered anxieties of what would ensue if Elizabeth produced a child late in life, hence opening the possibility of a protectorship, maybe even one with a foreign husband in that role. In any event, it is revealing that in a play with as many choric interludes as a Bach passion, the citizens comment chorically on only one issue other than their immediate decision about the kingship of the cunningly devout, devoutly cunning Richard. In Act II, scene iii they discuss in some detail the situation of a country with a child ruler, debating whether his uncles would be a source of wise counsel or dangerous "emulation" (25), thus signalling the significance of such problems to Shakespeare and his audience.

In a text that so repeatedly relates the familial to the national, the ambiguous status of a Lord Protector mimes the instabilities of familial roles; the civil war engulfing England is staged through uncivil behavior, and worse, among the family members in the play. Those familial roles are repeatedly travestied, as when Richard insistently declares that Queen Elizabeth is his mother. In particular, family members who might be expected to guard and nurture do the opposite; to signal the importance of that issue, of all the incidents on which he might have opened his story, Shakespeare begins it when the king, far from caring for Clarence, imperils him, and when Richard, ostensibly caring for Clarence, betrays him. It is telling, too, that Clarence's dream suggests that he harms himself when hoping to protect Richard: "Strook me (that thought to stay him) overboard" (I.iv.19); this is but one of many times in the text when a family member who thinks to stay a fall in fact cannot or will not do so. In short, if the lust for power distorts sexual encounters in the play, so too does it twist the *caritas* that should characterize familial relationships; the situation of a child who, after losing a parent, is surrounded by dubious surrogate caretakers is a synecdoche for the situation of families as a whole and for that family the state.

All these connections between the surrogate parents of a child and the Lord Protector of a state draw attention to the complex workings of patriarchal paradigms. On one level, of course, Richard's behavior towards his unfortunate nephews merely mimes and glosses his relationship to England. Yet the princes are in no sense responsible for their fate, whereas in the national arena a series of fools and knaves colludes, variously wittingly and unwittingly, with Richard's machinations, a contrast that gestures towards contemporaneous debates about the responsibilities of the subjects of a tyrant. Here, as is so often the case, patriarchalism functions not by simply equating king, father, and husband but rather by establishing a dynamic of both comparisons and contrasts.

The bereft children who must rely on surrogates crystallize not only analogous political issues but also the relationship between surrogacy and representation. We have already observed how Richard's pious claim that he will love the late Clarence's son "as a child" (II.ii.26) gestures towards the instabilities of figurative language and their connections to a range of different forms of substitution.[25] As Marjorie B. Garber points out, in Clarence's dream metaphor masks the lineaments of his subconscious, and, similarly, one might add, other dreams and prophecies rely on the surrogacy of figuration.[26] That form of substitution has mixed results in the play, but they are generally negative or at least dubious. If, as Garber elsewhere suggests, Richard's deformity is catachresis,[27] the play invites us to speculate on whether metaphor itself can in fact be distinguished from catachresis. How often is it too deformed? In any event, metaphor indubitably conceals truths from those who cannot read it properly, as in Clarence's and Hastings's misinterpretation of dreams. And so *Richard III* demonstrates the necessity – and the difficulty – of reading both substitute words and substitute guardians accurately.

Other types of surrogacy in *Richard III* extend and further complicate the play's valuation of it. The text's preoccupation with substitution is manifest in its repeated appearance even in more neutral contexts, such as Stanley's statement, "I, by attorney, bless thee from thy mother" (V.iii.83). But more often surrogacy involves danger and, like the other ghosts in the play, recalls what is missing, what has been displaced and replaced. When Queen Margaret uses the verb "usurp" (IV.iv.109) in reference to Queen Elizabeth's putative stealing of her place as queen, she reminds us of the political ramifications behind certain types of substitution, and in fact that verb is repeatedly used for Richard's behavior (see, for example, V.iii.112). Richard, as we have already seen, famously promises to replace the husband and father he has murdered. And throughout the play we witness characters suborning others to do evil in their stead; Tyrrel is like his employer in this and many other ways.[28] And yet the play qualifies its emphasis on surrogacy's potentiality to deform. It is no accident, I think, that the dying King Edward not just once but twice uses terminology that draws attention to Christ's role as substitute for sinful man, in the first instance even deploying polyptoton to reinforce the point and in the second referring to a cognate form of replacement, representation: "I every day expect an embassage / From my *Redeemer* to *redeem* me hence" (II.i.3–4; italics inserted), and "The precious *image* of our dear *Redeemer*" (II.i.124; italics inserted).

* * *

My study of stepparenthood and surrogacy within *Richard III* also gestures towards a range of broader questions, including challenges posed by our own institutional and critical practices. The fraught role of external reviewers in personnel cases, for example, might profitably be reexamined in terms of the issues about surrogacy this essay has raised. The threats associated with substitution might even help us to gloss our responses to that realm where the surrogate is monarch and tyrant, cyberspace; particularly thought-provoking is the increasing role in the academy of email, the simulacrum of traditional correspondence. More immediately, this essay represents an attempt to reconcile a number of critical approaches and in so doing to emphasize the continuing symbiosis of social and cultural history and of literary and cultural studies. It is as common as it is unfortunate to regard newer critical methods as surrogates that displace their predecessors rather than as supplements that might interact with them. To what extent will the current move to study the rhetorical rather than the literary facilitate and to what extent frustrate a renewed and revitalized interest in the workings of language and the recognition that issues of form unite both literary and non-literary texts?

Notes

1. I cite *The Riverside Shakespeare*, ed. G. Blakemore Evans (Boston: Houghton Mifflin, 1974).
2. William Gouge, *Of Domesticall Duties* (London, 1622), 581. Subsequent citations of this book will appear in parentheses within my text.
3. The most comprehensive study of death rates and the problems of studying them is E.A. Wrigley and R.S. Schofield, *The Population History of England 1541–1871: A Reconstruction* (Cambridge: Cambridge University Press, 1981). On differing rates of remarriage, see esp. Vivien Brodsky, "Widows in Late Elizabethan London: Remarriage, Economic Opportunity and Family Orientation," in Lloyd Bonfield, Richard M. Smith, Keith Wrightson, eds., *The World We Have Gained: Histories of Population and Social Structure* (Oxford: Basil Blackwell, 1986), esp. 123–4. Also cf. my essay "The Message from Marcade: Parental Death in Tudor and Stuart England," in Betty S. Travitsky and Adele F. Seeff, eds., *Attending to Women in Early Modern England* (Newark and London: University of Delaware Press and Associated University Presses, 1994), which includes a preliminary exploration of a few of the ideas in the current essay.
4. On the odds of losing a parent, see esp. Ralph Houlbrooke, *The English Family 1450–1700* (London: Longman, 1984), chap. 4.
5. Francesco Petrarch, *Phisicke against Fortune*, trans. Thomas Twyne (London, 1579), sig. Nviii^V.
6. Lucy Hutchinson, *Memoirs of the Life of Colonel Hutchinson*, ed. James Sutherland (London: Oxford University Press, 1973), 24–5.
7. Ilana Krausman Ben-Amos, *Adolescence and Youth in Early Modern England* (New Haven: Yale University Press, 1994), 49–50.
8. See Marianne Novy's study, "Reading Adoption and Shakespeare." I am grateful to the author for making her work available to me before publication, though I regret that I did not see it until this chapter was virtually complete.
9. Freud's oeuvre includes many analyses of death and mourning, but his principal statement on the subject is "Mourning and Melancholia," in vol. 14 of *The Standard Edition of the Complete Psychological Works of Sigmund Freud*, trans. James Strachey, 24 vols. (London: Hogarth Press, 1953–1974). Also see "Anxiety, Pain and Mourning," in vol. 20 of *The Standard Edition* and letter #239 in *Letters of Sigmund Freud 1873–1939*, ed. Ernst L. Freud, trans. Tania and James Stern (London: Hogarth Press, 1970).
10. Anthony Low, "*Hamlet* and the Ghost of Purgatory: Intimations of Killing the Father," in press. I thank the author for making his manuscript available to me prior to publication.
11. Ralph Houlbrooke, "Death, Church,and Family in England Between the Late Fifteenth and the Early Eighteenth Centuries," in Houlbrooke, ed., *Death, Ritual,*

and Bereavement (London: Routledge in association with the Social History Society of the United Kingdom, 1989), 36.

12. Joshua Scodel, *The English Poetic Epitaph: Commemoration and Conflict from Jonson to Wordsworth* (Ithaca: Cornell University Press, 1991), 21.

13. On parental blessings as a form of intercession, see Bruce W. Young, "Ritual as an Instrument of Grace: Parental Blessings in *Richard III, All's Well That Ends Well*, and *The Winter's Tale*," in Linda Woodbridge and Ralph Berry, eds., *True Rites and Maimed Rites: Ritual and Anti-Ritual in Shakespeare and His Age* (Urbana: University of Illinois Press, 1992), 170–73.

14. See Charles Carlton, *The Court of Orphans* (Leicester: Leicester University Press, 1974), 44.

15. For a useful overview of wardship, see H. E. Bell, *An Introduction to the History and Records of the Court of Wards and Liveries* (Cambridge: Cambridge University Press, 1953); Joel Hurstfield, *The Queen's Wards: Wardship and Marriage Under Elizabeth I*, 2nd ed. (London: Frank Cass, 1973). Exceptions to the neglect of this system by students of early modern literature include the brief but useful commentaries on wardship and inheritance in Lisa Jardine, *Still Harping on Daughters: Women and Drama in the Age of Shakespeare* (Harvester Press and Barnes and Noble: Brighton, Eng. and Totowa, NJ, 1983), 80–84; Marilyn L. Williamson, *The Patriarchy of Shakespeare's Comedies* (Detroit: Wayne State University Press, 1986), 61–4.

16. The ante mortem passing on of property is the central thesis of Lloyd Bonfield, "Normative Rules and Property Transmission: Reflections on the Link between Marriage and Inheritance in Early Modern England," in Bonfield et al., eds., *The World We Have Gained*.

17. Hurstfield, *Queen's Wards*, chaps. 10, 12, 13.

18. Bell, *Court of Wards*, 115–6.

19. Baxter, *Reliquiae Baxterianae* (London, 1696), 12.

20. For a revisionist analysis of aristocratic inheritance practices, see Eileen Spring, *Law, Land, and Family: Aristocratic Inheritance in England, 1300 to 1800* (Chapel Hill: University of North Carolina Press, 1993).

21. On the theatricality of death, see, e.g., Michael Cameron Andrews, *This Action of Our Death: The Performance of Death in English Renaissance Drama* (Newark and London: University of Delaware Press and Associated University Presses, 1989), 14–16.

22. One of the best analyses of the connections between Richmond and Richard III is Barbara Hodgdon, *The End Crowns All: Closure and Contradiction in Shakespeare's History* (Princeton: Princeton University Press, 1991), 113–5.

23. On his propensity for creating those divisions see William B. Toole, "The Motif of Psychic Division in 'Richard III,'" *Shakespeare Survey* 27 (1974): 21–32.

24. An early argument for the connection with the ballad appears in Sharon Turner, *The History of England During the Middle Ages*, vol. 3 (London: Longman, Hurst, Rees, Orme, Brown and Green, 1825), 487. Also cf. David R. Carlson, "The Princes' Embrace in *Richard III*," *SQ* 41 (1990): 344 n.2.

25. For a different but compatible view of rhetorical substitution, also see Russ McDonald, "*Richard III* and the Tropes of Treachery," *PQ* 68 (1989): 470–71.

26. Marjorie B. Garber, *Dream in Shakespeare: From Metaphor to Metamorphosis* (New Haven: Yale University Press, 1974), 23.

27. Marjorie Garber, *Shakespeare's Ghost Writers: Literature as Uncanny Causality* (New York: Methuen, 1987), 36.

28. On Richard's propensity for delegating his evil deeds see Robert Ornstein, *A*

Kingdom for a Stage: The Achievement of Shakespeare's History Plays (Cambridge: Harvard University Press, 1972), 66; R. Thomas Simone, *Shakespeare and 'Lucrece': A Study of the Poem and Its Relation to the Plays* (Salzburg: Institut für Englische Sprache und Literatur, 1974), 113.

Index